I. David L. Bogle, Tomasz R. Sosnowski (Eds.)

Chemical Engineering Principles Applied to Medicine

Also of interest

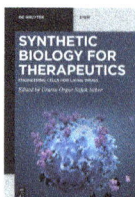

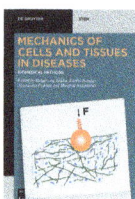

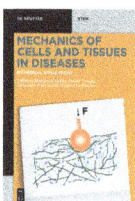

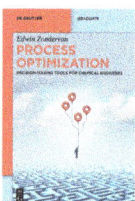

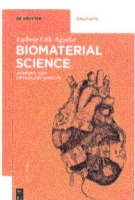

Chemical Engineering Principles Applied to Medicine

—

Modeling Physiology, Disease and Drug Delivery

Edited by
I. David L. Bogle and Tomasz R. Sosnowski

DE GRUYTER

Editors

Ian David Lockhart Bogle
University College London
Department of Chemical Engineering
Torrington Place
WC1E 7JE
London
Great Britian

Tomasz R. Sosnowski
Warsaw University of Technology
Faculty of Chemical and Process Engineering
ul. Waryńskiego 1
00-645 Warsaw
Poland

ISBN 978-3-11-139454-1
e-ISBN (PDF) 978-3-11-139455-8
e-ISBN (EPUB) 978-3-11-139489-3

Library of Congress Control Number: 2025940575

Bibliographic information published by the Deutsche Nationalbibliothek
The Deutsche Nationalbibliothek lists this publication in the Deutsche Nationalbibliografie; detailed biblio-graphic data are available on the Internet at http://dnb.dnb.de.

Cover image: Ilya Lukichev / iStock / Getty Images Plus
Typesetting: TNQ Tech Private Limited, Chennai, India

https://www.degruyterbrill.com
Questions about General Product Safety Regulation:
productsafety@degruyterbrill.com

Preface

Chemical Engineering and Chemical Engineers analyze, design, operate and manage complex processes that involve chemical and physical change: manufacturing systems, environmental systems, water systems and many others. The premise of this book is that the Chemical Engineering skillset can also apply to another system that involves chemical and physical change: human physiology and medicine.

Medicine has become increasingly complex because of the huge development in understanding of genetics, metabolism, anatomy and physiology and the influence of diet and an increasingly wide array of sophisticated medicines often used in combination. The medical profession has become increasingly fragmented with all its specialisms. We believe that the time is ripe to develop the engineering systems approach to assist in analysis and design of medical systems to assist the medical profession with decision support in the same way that computational systems are now used in complex chemical manufacturing. In this way the body can again be seen as a system of systems with computational tools based on our understanding of physiology (and possibly aided by Artificial Intelligence where appropriate) to help to explore the complex systems and the use of combinatorial and synergistic effects of multiple actions in a way that is impossible for an individual clinical specialist. Of course the human body is a much more complex system than manufacturing systems but there is now a more comprehensive set of mathematical models to describe many aspects of physiology making it possible to bring to bear quantitative engineering methodologies to human physiology and medicine. The area is still early in development but we hope this book will help provide a stimulus for more Chemical Engineers to work on such problems.

The book genesis has come alongside the formation of a new Section of the European Federation of Chemical Engineers called 'Chemical Engineering as Applied to Medicine'. Through this group we aim to create a stronger community of researchers, and eventually practitioners, working in applying Chemical Engineering approaches, tools and methodologies to aspects of physiology and medicine (particularly in Europe but also beyond).

Engineers and clinicians are both problem solvers. The analogy even works in our distinctive language: 'analysis' of the problem is often referred to as diagnosis, 'simulation' could be used for prognosis, 'design' for determining the best therapeutic actions, and 'control' for managing symptoms. The new EFCE Section had its inaugural meeting in Paris in 2022, the second meeting in Salerno in 2024 and has contributed to the ECCE conferences, the EFCE Spotlight talk series and a Special issue of Chemical

https://doi.org/10.1515/9783111394558-201

Engineering Science. We look forward to a growing activity and future meetings and publications.

The book has four parts. The first (Bogle and Martin) is a perspective article developing the idea of Systems Medicine and the role of Chemical Engineering and Chemical Engineers in this new world of quantitative systems medicine. The second part, Modeling and Physiology, looks at developing models in specific parts of physiology: the liver (Liao et al.), the lungs (Sosnowski and Kuczaj), the skin (Sebastia-Saez et al.) and the kidneys (Zarghamidehaghani et al.). The third part, Disease and Treatment, has contributions on specific diseases such as hyperthyroidism (Manca), those such as diabetes which rely on glucose measurement (Guati et al.), transport models for oncology drugs in cancer tissues (González-Garcinuño et al.), haemodialysis for liver disease (Cancilla et al.), atherosclerosis (Jędrzejczak et al.) and von Willebrand disease (Galvanin et al.). The fourth part, Pharmacokinetics and Drug Delivery, begins with an introduction to Quantitative Systems Pharmacology for Chemical Engineers from two industrial practitioners (Abbiati and Pichardo) and contributions on drug delivery for brain cancer (Dluska et al.), gene therapy for haemophilia B (Jamili et al.) and delivery of nucleic acids (Baldino). There is of course some overlap between parts since they all focus on aspects of physiology, disease and drug delivery but this organization helps signal the key focus of each contribution and helps the reader navigate. It is certainly not meant to be comprehensive but to reflect the activity that is underway at the beginning of what we hope will be a fast growing community.

We hope you find these contributions stimulating in introducing you to aspects of physiology and medicine from the view of the Chemical Engineering community and that it stimulates you to become more involved in this exciting and fast developing field.

David Bogle (University College London) and Tomasz Sosnowski (Warsaw University of Technology)

Contents

Tomasz R. Sosnowski and Arkadiusz K. Kuczaj

Daniel Sebastia-Saez, Tao Chen, Benjamin Deacon and Guoping Lian

Maryam Zarghami Dehaghani, Thomas Fabiani and Maria Grazia De Angelis

Part III: **Disease and treatment**

Davide Manca

Carlota Guati, Lucía Gomez-Coma, Marcos Fallanza and Inmaculada Ortiz

Álvaro González-Garcinuño, Antonio Tabernero and Eva Martín del Valle

Nunzio Cancilla, Luigi Gurreri, Michele Ciofalo, Andrea Cipollina, Alessandro Tamburini and Giorgio Micale

Krystian Jędrzejczak, Arkadiusz Antonowicz, Krzysztof Wojtas, Wojciech Orciuch, Malenka
Bissell and Łukasz Makowski

Federico Galvanin, Chun Fung Lee and Yuxuan Yang

List of contributing authors

Roberto A. Abbiati
Roche Pharma Research and Early Development
Predictive Modeling and Data Analytics
F. Hoffmann-La Roche Ltd
Grenzacherstrasse 124
4070 Basel
Switzerland
E-mail: roberto.abbiati@roche.com
https://orcid.org/0000-0002-6052-5736

Maria Grazia De Angelis
School of Engineering
Institute for Materials and Processes
University of Edinburgh
King's Buildings
Robert Stevenson Road
EH9 3FB, Edinburgh, SCO
UK
E-mail: grazia.deangelis@ed.ac.uk
https://orcid.org/0000-0002-1435-4251

Arkadiusz Antonowicz
Faculty of Chemical and Process Engineering
Warsaw University of Technology
Waryńskiego 1
00-645 Warsaw
Poland
and
Eurotek International Sp.z o.o.
Skrzetuskiego 6
02-726
Warsaw
Poland

Lucia Baldino
Department of Industrial Engineering
University of Salerno
Via Giovanni Paolo II, 132
84084 Fisciano, SA
Italy
E-mail: lbaldino@unisa.it
https://orcid.org/0000-0001-7015-0803

Malenka Bissell
Leeds Institute of Cardiovascular and Metabolic
Medicine
University of Leeds
Leeds
UK

I. David L. Bogle
Sargent Centre for Process Systems Engineering and
COMPLEX
(Centre for Computation, Mathematics and Physics in
the Life Sciences and Experimental Biology)
Department of Chemical Engineering
University College London
London
UK
E-mail: d.bogle@ucl.ac.uk

Nunzio Cancilla
Dipartimento di Ingegneria
Università Degli Studi di Palermo
Viale Delle Scienze Ed. 6
90128 Palermo
Italy
E-mail: nunzio.cancilla@unipa.it
https://orcid.org/0000-0003-3065-3291

Manuel Cardamone
Department of Industrial Engineering
University of Salerno
Via Giovanni Paolo II, 132
84084 Fisciano, SA
Italy

Tao Chen
School of Chemistry & Chemical Engineering
University of Surrey
Guildford, GU2 7XH
UK
E-mail: t.chen@surrey.ac.uk

https://doi.org/10.1515/9783111394558-202

Michele Ciofalo
Dipartimento di Ingegneria,
Università Degli Studi di Palermo
Viale Delle Scienze Ed. 6
90128 Palermo
Italy
E-mail: michele.ciofalo@unipa.it

Andrea Cipollina
Dipartimento di Ingegneria,
Università Degli Studi di Palermo
Viale Delle Scienze Ed. 6
90128 Palermo
Italy
E-mail: andrea.cipollina@unipa.it

Nathan A. Davies
Institute for Liver and Digestive Health
UCL Division of Medicine
Royal Free Campus
Rowland Hill Street
University College London
London
UK

Benjamin Deacon
School of Chemistry & Chemical Engineering
University of Surrey
Guildford, GU2 7XH
UK

Maryam Zarghami Dehaghani
School of Engineering
Institute for Materials and Processes
University of Edinburgh
King's Buildings
Robert Stevenson Road
EH9 3FB, Edinburgh, SCO
UK
E-mail: mzargham@ed.ac.uk

Ewa Dluska
Faculty of Chemical and Process Engineering
Warsaw University of Technology
Warsaw 00-645
Poland
ewa.dluska@pw.edu.pl
https://orcid.org/0000-0001-8833-2744

Vivek Dua
Department of Chemical Engineering
The Sargent Centre for Process Systems Engineering
University College London
Torrington Place
London WC1E 7JE
UK
E-mail: v.dua@ucl.ac.uk
https://orcid.org/0000-0002-0165-7421

Thomas Fabiani
School of Engineering
Institute for Materials and Processes
University of Edinburgh
King's Buildings
Robert Stevenson Road
EH9 3FB, Edinburgh, SCO
UK
E-mail: T.Fabiani@sms.ed.ac.uk

Marcos Fallanza
Chemical and Biomolecular Engineering Department
University of Cantabria
39005 Santander
Spain

Federico Galvanin
Department of Chemical Engineering
University College London
London
UK
E-mail: f.galvanin@ucl.ac.uk

Álvaro González Garcinuño
Department of Chemical Engineering
University of Salamanca
Salamanca, Spain
E-mail: alvaro_gonzalez@usal.es
and IBSAL
Institute for Biomedical Research of Salamanca
Salamanca
Spain

Lucía Gomez-Coma
Chemical and Biomolecular Engineering Department
University of Cantabria
39005 Santander
Spain

Carlota Guati
Chemical and Biomolecular Engineering Department
University of Cantabria
39005 Santander
Spain
E-mail: carlota.guati@unican.es (C. Guati)

Luigi Gurreri
Dipartimento di Ingegneria Elettrica
Elettronica e Informatica
Università di Catania
Viale Andrea Doria 6 Ed. 3
95125 Catania
Italy
E-mail: luigi.gurreri@unict.it

Krystian Jędrzejczak
Faculty of Chemical and Process Engineering
Warsaw University of Technology
Waryńskiego 1
00-645 Warsaw
Poland
and
Leeds Institute of Cardiovascular and Metabolic
Medicine
University of Leeds
Leeds
UK

Elnaz Jamili
Department of Chemical Engineering
Centre for Process Systems Engineering
University College London
Torrington Place
London, WC1E 7JE
UK

Arkadiusz K. Kuczaj
Department of Applied Mathematics
Faculty EEMCS
University of Twente
Enschede
The Netherlands
and
PMI R&D
Philip Morris Products S.A.
Quai Jeanrenaud 5
Neuchâtel
Switzerland

Chun Fung Lee
Department of Chemical Engineering
University College London
London
UK

Guoping Lian
School of Chemistry & Chemical Engineering
University of Surrey
Guildford, GU2 7XH
UK
and
Unilever R&D Colworth
Bedfordshire, MK44 1LQ
UK

Yunjie Liao
Sargent Centre for Process Systems Engineering
Department of Chemical Engineering
Torrington Place
University College London
London
UK
and
Institute for Liver and Digestive Health
UCL Division of Medicine
Royal Free Campus
Rowland Hill Street
University College London
London
UK
E-mail: y.liao@alumni.ucl.ac.uk

Łukasz Makowski
Faculty of Chemical and Process Engineering
Warsaw University of Technology
Waryńskiego 1
00-645 Warsaw
Poland
E-mail: Lukasz.Makowski.ichip@pw.edu.pl

Davide Manca
PSE-Lab
Process Systems Engineering Laboratory
Dipartimento di Chimica, Materiali e Ingegneria
Chimica "Giulio Natta"
Politecnico di Milano
Piazza Leonardo da Vinci 32
20133 Milano
Italy
E-mail: davide.manca@polimi.it
https://orcid.org/0000-0003-2055-9752

Agnieszka Markowska-Radomska
Faculty of Chemical and Process Engineering
Warsaw University of Technology
Warsaw 00-645
Poland
E-mail: agnieszka.markowska@pw.edu.pl

John Martin
Centre for Cardiovascular Science
Division of Medicine
University College London
WC1E 7JE
London
UK

Giorgio Micale
Dipartimento di Ingegneria,
Università Degli Studi di Palermo
Viale Delle Scienze Ed. 6
90128 Palermo
Italy
E-mail: giorgiod.maria.micale@unipa.it

Amit C. Nathwani
Department of Haematology
UCL Cancer Institute
University College London
London
UK

Wojciech Orciuch
Faculty of Chemical and Process Engineering
Warsaw University of Technology
Waryńskiego 1
00-645 Warsaw
Poland

Inmaculada Ortiz
Chemical and Biomolecular Engineering Department
University of Cantabria
39005 Santander
Spain
E-mail: ortizi@unican.es

Cesar Pichardo
AstraZeneca R&D
Systems Medicine
Clinical Pharmacology & Quantitative Pharmacology
The Discovery Centre
1 Francis Crick Avenue
Cambridge CB2 0AA
UK

Ernesto Reverchon
Department of Industrial Engineering
University of Salerno
Via Giovanni Paolo II, 132
84084 Fisciano, SA
Italy

Sonia Sarnelli
Department of Industrial Engineering
University of Salerno
Via Giovanni Paolo II, 132
84084 Fisciano, SA
Italy

Daniel Sebastia-Saez
School of Chemistry & Chemical Engineering
University of Surrey
Guildford, GU2 7XH
UK

Tomasz R. Sosnowski
Faculty of Chemical and Process Engineering
Warsaw University of Technology
Warynskiego 1
00-645 Warsaw
Poland
E-mail: tomasz.sosnowski@pw.edu.pl
https://orcid.org/0000-0002-6775-3766

Antonio Tabernero
Department of Chemical Engineering
University of Salamanca
Salamanca
Spain
and
IBSAL
Institute for Biomedical Research of Salamanca
Salamanca
Spain

Alessandro Tamburini
Dipartimento di Ingegneria,
Università Degli Studi di Palermo
Viale Delle Scienze Ed. 6
90128 Palermo
Italy
E-mail: alessandro.tamburini@unipa.it

Eva Martín del Valle
Department of Chemical Engineering
University of Salamanca
Salamanca, Spain
and IBSAL
Institute for Biomedical Research of Salamanca
Salamanca
Spain
E-mail: emvalle@usal.es
https://orcid.org/0000-0003-3506-2546

Krzysztof Wojtas
Faculty of Chemical and Process Engineering
Warsaw University of Technology
Waryńskiego 1
00-645 Warsaw
Poland

Yuxuan Yang
Department of Chemical Engineering
University College London
London
UK

Part I: **Chemical engineering and medicine**

I. David L. Bogle* and John Martin

1 A systems engineering approach to medicine

Abstract: Human physiology is a complex system of systems such that it is impossible for clinicians to be able to consider all elements in a diagnosis. Medicine is becoming more quantitative and predictive mathematical models are becoming much more common and are being used to help in diagnosis and treatment. Chemical engineers have much experience of developing and using methodologies to tackle systems analysis for example with chemical manufacturing systems consisting of complex chemistry, fluid flow and collections of connected units. The paper seeks to show parallels with the complex metabolism, blood flow and interconnected systems of organs and how engineering methodologies are needed to make the use of these systems of models to help clinicians make most use of all information available and to manage risks associated with complexity. Examples are drawn from cardiology, cancer and liver disease where some progress has been made.

Keywords: complex systems; systems engineering; quantitative medicine; cardiology; liver disease

1.1 Introduction

We know the causes of a heart attack right? However, it seems that it is not so straightforward - it results from a set of complex interacting physiological and metabolic systems influenced by many factors. The blockage of the coronary artery can be caused by several mechanisms arising from physical, chemical and metabolic changes in the body. Monaco, Mathiur and Martin [1] have discussed the causes of acute coronary syndrome and divided them into those arising from the role of the vessel wall and those from the role of the blood. Both arise from complex physical and chemical changes and can be treated chemically using medicines provided the correct diagnosis leads to the right therapy. However the cause in a specific case is rarely clear because this is a very complex system.

Engineers solve problems of analysis, simulation, optimisation and control of complex systems. These have very close parallels in medicine: analysis seeks to understand in order to make a diagnosis, simulation predicts short or long term behaviour enabling a

*Corresponding author: I. David L. Bogle, Sargent Centre for Process Systems Engineering and COMPLEX (Centre for Computation, Mathematics and Physics in the Life Sciences and Experimental Biology), Department of Chemical Engineering, University College London, London, UK, E-mail: d.bogle@ucl.ac.uk
John Martin, Centre for Cardiovascular Science, Division of Medicine, University College London, WC1E 7JE London, UK, E-mail: j.martin@ucl.ac.uk

As per De Gruyter's policy this article has previously been published in the journal Physical Sciences Reviews. Please cite as: I. D. L. Bogle and J. Martin "A systems engineering approach to medicine" *Physical Sciences Reviews* [Online] 2024. DOI: 10.1515/psr-2024-0050 | https://doi.org/10.1515/9783111394558-001

prognosis, optimisation aims to find a set of actions – therapy – which can result in an optimal outcome, and control systems implement a set of real time actions that keep a process stable - healthy or at least clinically stable – through feedback and the addition of agents (medicines) that can bring a system back to its stable state to manage the condition [2].

This paper arose from discussions between a chemical engineer and a clinical cardiologist about the depth of complexity facing medical practitioners. We aim to show how engineering methodologies (with a particular bias towards chemical engineering because of the chemical nature) can help to find solutions to complex medical and physiological problems and that this is a fascinating area where chemical engineers working together with clinical colleagues can contribute much.

Taking the cardiology case further, in a heart attack artherosclerotic lesions in the arteries can restrict the blood flow but this is not usually blood-limiting. It seems the causes arise from the two sources mentioned above: the cell wall and the blood interacting. Those arising from the role of the cell wall can come from plaque rupture, endothelial disfunction (expression of certain molecules causing a loss of anti-coagulant properties), or plaque thrombogenicity where exposed tissue factor initiates a blood coagulation cascade arising from metabolic processes. The blood has several components that can activate clotting: increased platelet (blood clot cells) reactivity and volume, alteration of the physiological balance between coagulation and fibrinolytic (breaking down of clots) cascades resulting from expression of coagulant factors, the well-known effect of cholesterol and other lipo-proteins, and inflammation which can cause changes in lipoprotein balance, susceptibility to infection agents or antigens disturbing the auto-immune process. All of these are the result of changes in physiology and metabolism arising from a host of short and long term effects. Monaco et al. [1] concluded that when intracoronary thrombosis occurs the exact chain of events that might cause the final event is not fully understood. Indeed many diseases (so called) are not diseases but syndromes i.e. a collection of signs and symptoms. The prevention of heart attacks will not be achieved until the specific diseases causing the syndrome are identified as specific cellular of metabolic changes contributing to a system's failure.

The heart is at the centre of the cardiovascular system. But even within this there are systems such as the one that regulates the platelet cells (the megakaryocyte-platelet system [3]). The complexity of medical problems such as heart attack (myocardial infarction) confronting clinicians is huge and increasing as understanding of biology increases. How can clinicians keep on top of all of this information let alone navigate a path to appropriate diagnosis and treatment without decision-support systems? With the advent of molecular biology biological scientists have lost the ability to think in systems.

Physiology and clinical medicine have become splintered into specialists in very specific areas. Knowledge has become much deeper on all physiological processes making it impossible to be able to view the whole body and to understand system level interactions which may be affected by phenomena or defects at genetic, metabolic, vascular or organ level. The knowledge is being codified by researchers through data models and predictive models which can be brought together to assist in understanding whole body physiology and of the effects of health, diet and disease but there is still much to do to have models of sufficient accuracy and to bring these models together to make systems that might be of use to clinicians.

1.2 Physiological systems and complexity

Physics is inherently simple in so far as its complexity is predictable. Biology is inherently complex; even though it ultimately obeys the rules of physics in its parts, it is not predictable in its totality. This property of biology affects our ability to understand how biology works and how it can malfunction. This is a formidable challenge for the scientist whose job is to unravel the function of biological systems and brings difficulties for the clinician who needs to understand how mammalian biology malfunctions. The problem is amplified by the therapeutic pharmacologist who wants to make molecules that interfere in biological malfunction. In experiments to probe malfunction single molecules are used to observe change in function. The constraint is that the biological system probed by pharmacology is complex even if it is a single cell. Cells make tissues then tissues make organs and then organs make systems within an individual animal. The information gained from such experiments is greater the less complex the system: more information from a cell, less information from an organ. However, often the information gained from a cell is less useful than the information gained from a whole organ. The agents used to probe biological systems may become therapeutic drugs. However the complexity of the systems being probed means that the process of discovering new therapeutics is inherently hit and miss. It is inefficient, costly and time consuming. The pharmaceutical company Pfizer invested $3.5 billion per year for three years into pharmacological discovery and discovered nothing useful. So, the complexity of biological systems is a fundamental problem for the understanding of biology and creating new drugs to change it when it goes wrong.

This is true in many systems, however there are differences. If the endocrine system malfunctions it is relatively easy to intervene therapeutically. For example in hypothyroidism the diagnosis is made by measuring the level of the hormone thyroxine in the blood. If the level is low it needs replacing. This is a replacement therapy which is the simplest form of therapeutics. However in more complex diseases the problem of treating the totality of the disease, as in hypothyroidism, is almost impossible. Cancer and cardiovascular disease are the two most common diseases which cause death in developed society. The former is caused by a change at the level of the cell. The latter is caused by the interaction of changes in many different cells, different tissues and different organs. The development of drugs to change cardiovascular disease has taken place over the last 50 years. However cardiovascular disease still kills more people prematurely in developed society than any other disease. The mismatch between the effort of research and achievement is probably a reflection of the inherent complexity involved. Tools to understand that biological complexity are lacking.

Models and their use in systems analysis could be useful for both clinicians and biological scientists: "A biological scientist … must question whether the various mechanisms form part of a single process … or whether each proposed mechanisms is capable of giving rise to the syndrome by itself. Similarly, a clinical scientist should question whether we should tackle therapeutically all components together … or each component individually." [1].

Although there is still so much yet to be understood there are some predictive models of physiological systems. As these are put together into computational systems of systems (through project such as the virtual physiological human http://www.vph-institute.org, the Physiome Project http://physiomeproject.org/ and HumMod http://hummod.org/) there is a need for engineering tools to make best use of the systems of connected models.

There is a similar mindset between clinicians and engineers: both are problem solvers. "Engineers make things, they make things work and they make things work better" (http://www.raeng.org.uk/education/what-is-engineering#sthash.q8O7jQXK.dpuf.). Complex physiological systems can be approached in the way that chemical engineers tackle manufacturing problems through analysis, modelling and design of complex "flowsheets". In the 1930s Kahn presented the idea of "Man as Industrial Palace" with a set of cartoons illustrating five cycles within the human factory: respiration, blood circulation, digestive circuit, control centre (brain), and metabolism (see http://www.industriepalast.com/ for an animation). In the 1950s Guyton [4, 5] pioneered the use of systems analysis in the cardiovascular system integrating many factors affecting peripheral circulation, the heart, the endocrine system, the autonomous nervous system, the kidneys and body fluids. Noble developed the first computational model of the heart including electrical, mechanical and chemical elements which has been used by the Food and Drug Administration for drug testing [6]. Recently Christ et al. [7] demonstrate how computational modelling and systems medicine can be used in surgery of the liver.

When considered in this light we can see that Engineers have a role to play in helping to make the most of the knowledge of physiology that is becoming increasingly quantified, modelled and computational. Engineers have much experience with modelling, optimising and controlling complex systems involving chemical and physical change. Some chemical engineers in particular have been involved in modelling and experimental investigations in medical fields. For example Yin [8] consider challenges in virology and Netti et al. [9] in fluid transport in tumours. Peppas and Langer [10] reviewed the contributions of chemical engineers to biomedical engineering over the years concentrating on biomaterials, drug delivery and tissue engineering. Engineers have been engaged in looking at the systems engineering of medicine (see [11–13] for recent reviews and [14] for an example for inflammation response to infection or trauma). The report Convergence–The Future of Health" [15] sets out the range of challenges for bringing together disciplines, including Chemical Engineering, to solve healthcare problems highlighting imaging, nanotechnology, regenerative engineering and medicine, and big data.

Our aim in this paper is to look in particular at the challenges where modelling and Systems Engineering techniques can explore and manage the complexity to find effective solutions and help manage the risk associated with making decisions about very complex interacting systems.

The paper is presented in four parts: "how complicated can this really be?" exploring in more detail the interconnected complexity, "The power of purpose" which influences the modelling approach, "Do we really understand?" very briefly discusses the state of the art of quantitative modelling, and "What can we do?" looks at how we might be able to deploy our skills and toolboxes. The references in this paper are not meant to be comprehensive and the examples are drawn mostly from the authors' own experience and discussions with other medical colleagues.

1.3 How complicated can this really be?

The human system functions through the operation of a number of interacting systems [16]: cardiovascular (includes heart, veins, lymphatics and arteries carrying the blood), digestive, endocrine (chemical communications using hormones), integumentary (skin, hair, nails, seat and other glands), lymphatic (immune system), muscular, skeletal, nervous, renal, reproductive, respiratory and sensory systems. These all involve networks of chemical reactions and transport of fluids within and between cells and organs. Primary transport of fluids is via the blood and lymph both of which are chemically very complex, and air in the respiratory system from which oxygen is absorbed into the blood stream. These fluids transport nutrients and waste around the body between organs, or what Engineers call "unit operations" such as reactors or separators in manufacturing operations, including the heart, liver, lungs, pancreas stomach and so on as shown in Figure 1.1.

Standard Chemical Engineering assumptions consider any system as a collection of unit operations connected by fluid transport and by information networks through a control system. In chemical manufacturing processes this is an approximation with operations by no means confined to the units themselves. The flow of information in human physiology is even more complex through the nervous system, genetics, and through a range of complex chemical signalling entities.

Manufacturing control aims to achieve stable operation through fixed "set points" for certain variables to achieve safe and efficient operation and is achieved by valves, controllers and an information system. The objectives for human operation are not simple. The control of the body, homeostasis, requires smooth and steady operation but this does not necessarily mean that key variables need to track a set point such as a fixed temperature. The system needs to keep these variables within bounds. Homeostasis ensures the following entities are "kept, by carefully regulated mechanisms, within the narrow limits compatible with life": nutrients, O_2, CO_2, waste, pH, water, salts and other electrolytes, blood pressure and volume, and temperature [16]. For example glucose in the bloodstream needs to be kept within bounds to ensure no hyperglycaemic or

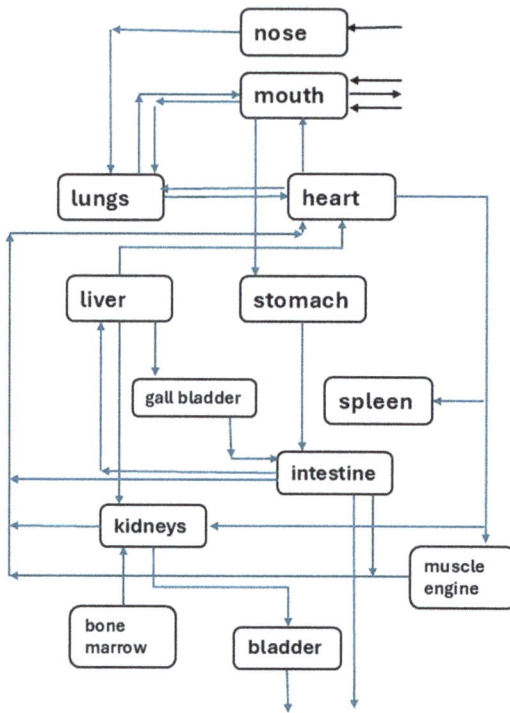

Figure 1.1: An idealised "unit operations" perspective of the human body.

hypoglycaemic attacks. Many controls that are given to the system are periodic and provide a stimulus that keeps the operation within bounds–such as feeding and drug dosages.

The chemistry and biochemistry in these systems is hugely complex. The chemistry of life is a dynamic process governed by very complex reaction networks, is affected by personal genetics, and is spatially distributed by being localised in some parts of organs and of cells. Reactions are of course not confined to the "unit operations". There has been huge progress in unravelling the chemistry of life with vast databases of pathways, genetics, transcription factors and so on which can be exploited in analysis and operation. We would need to be able to quantify fluid and transport properties (through cells, across membrane boundaries, and within fluid streams) where there has been considerable theoretical work but there is considerable need for more modelling across scales and data [17]. This makes the need for a systems approach all the more necessary, not only to help link and solve the complexity but also to identify what really crucial information is missing.

Time varying treatment is common in hospital to keep key functions within safe operating limits. But time varying dosage may be in for more radical reappraisal with the aim of exploiting and regulating changes in the cell cycle. Lee et al. [18] recently demonstrated with very comprehensive experimental and clinical programmes that using a deferred dosage of a second chemotherapy drug 8 h after the first drug had beneficial effects to cancer patients by exploiting changes in the cell behaviour during its natural cycle. This opens up a new set of opportunities for treatment that will require engineering analysis of dynamic systems once models are available.

This complex system of interacting networks, with chemical and genetic signals, has time and space dependent responses which are mostly not measurable (for now anyway). However it is one where decisions are currently made on very partial information and yet where there is much more relevant information that could influence actions if brought together for the whole system.

1.4 An example: the cardiovascular system

The commonest cause of cardiovascular disease is an occlusion of an artery by a thrombus. This leads to lack of blood flow to the organ supplied by that artery. If the artery supplies the brain then a stroke is caused, if a limb then leg ischaemia is caused, if a coronary artery is involved then myocardial infarction (heart attack) is caused. This latter is an example of the effects of complexity at many levels: chemical signalling, cell-cell interaction, tissue interaction, whole organ interaction and physical forces such as flow.

The final event in the cause of myocardial infarction is a single catastrophic failure. However this event only occurs on a background of pathological change over decades. The single happening has its own complexity which is at a different level from the complexity of the very slow change which precedes it. Autopsies performed on soldiers killed in Vietnam and Korea showed that the start of the slow change, atherosclerosis, probably starts in some people in their late twenties. This change progresses mostly imperceptibly until the final infracting event which occurs at a mean age of around 65.

1.4.1 The arterial wall

In engineering terms the artery is simple: it is a conduit for blood. However the flow of blood has to be regulated through rapid change in diameter along the length of the artery. To achieve this both local and systemic signalling molecules interact with the contractile muscle cells that comprise the bulk of the artery. These signals vary from very low molecular weight molecules like NO to very large proteins like VEGF, many thousand times larger than NO. The lining of the artery, the endothelium, is essential in this signalling process. It also produces agents which act on the blood. Both the smooth muscle and the endothelium is composed of cells which are not all of one type; there are variations in structure and function. The outer layer of the artery, the adventitia has been neglected by researchers. However it has a complex structure. In particular there are small blood vessels within it that penetrate the muscle layer of the artery. These vasa vasorum supply oxygen to the outer layers of the muscular zone. They themselves can undergo the changes that conduit vessels do. A micro thrombus forming in these vessels can cause change in function of the main artery. Thus the structure and function of the normal artery is complex in itself and in its relationship to signalling systems in the whole body.

Vascular disease is a consequence of malfunction of any component of the vessel wall or its signalling system. A single event, like thrombus formation in the artery, only occurs on a background of years of change in structure and function. The endothelial lining is damaged slowly by high blood pressure, by smoking and by high cholesterol levels in the blood. The latter effect is partly via an effect of the cholesterol on a blood cell, the macrophage, which is stimulated to enter the vessel wall from the blood and cause damage in the wall. Such damage can progress over decades with several blood cells being involved until a plaque of atheroma is formed. Eventually this may become hardened with calcium within it. This process is not simple but involves slow change in components of the wall and blood. Some caused by external influences some by internal ones such as ageing. Most of these changes are, in part, due to a disturbance of a dynamic equilibrium between cells and signalling systems.

1.4.2 The blood

The blood is composed of cells flowing in a medium of soluble elements, mostly proteins. The red cells carry oxygen from lungs to tissues. The white cells have a myriad of types each with a specialised function, mostly being involved in different elements of defence. Platelets are structurally unique as they have no nucleus: an essential element of all other cells. Why this is remains a mystery. Platelets are very small cells with a relatively large surface area. They are essential in stopping bleeding but if they are inappropriately active they can form into a mass which stops the flow of blood in arteries. This function of aggregating into a mass is controlled by more than a dozen signalling systems. Probably the most important being NO and a large prostaglandin called prostacyclin. These two act synergistically to damp down platelet aggregation through modulation of proteins in the platelet which in turn cause changes in the signalling of calcium within the platelet. This small element of the normal function of the artery is itself very complex. It is a system that is held in tension for years then might be activated in a millisecond. The complexity of the platelet system is enhanced as the platelet is produced from a cell which matures in the bone marrow and travels to the lungs where one of these megakaryocytes fragments into 3,000 small functional units, platelets. Every step in this complex process of platelet production can affect the function of the circulating platelet.

1.4.3 The catastrophic event

In an adult human being the gross function of the artery in delivering blood to the heart muscle can remained unchanged for decades while slow deterioration occurs in its component parts. These slow changes produce no symptoms. However myocardial infarction produces sudden massive pain in the chest. Autopsy studies demonstrate that this pain is caused by the formation of a blood clot in the artery taking blood to the heart. This clot is initiated by platelet aggregation. The source of the agents that cause the aggregation is a sudden rupture of a plaque of atheroma in the arterial wall. This has been likened to the catastrophic breaking of an aircraft wing after years of metal fatigue. The contents of the plaque pore out into the blood delivering a high concentration of agents which stimulate platelets to aggregate. This produces a chain reaction among platelets so they react as though the body was suffering a life-threatening bleed. This causes the production of more procoagulant platelets from the bone marrow. This in turn caused protein ropes to form over the platelet aggregate to stabilize it, making it resistant to forces which can break up clot. A consequence of this catastrophic biological event is sudden death or long-term damage to heart muscle causing chronic heart failure.

1.4.4 Therapeutics

Therapeutic intervention to prevent or treat these pathological processes is based on the study of normal tissues in the laboratory. For example small pieces of rat artery can be suspended on a wire and agents applied to them which cause then to contract or relax. Once such a deterministic system has mapped the normal function of an artery, agents which modify the function can be tested. These tests may be considered as binary, giving rise to one agent which may become a drug which modifies one element in a very complex system. The same applies to platelets which can be suspended in plasma in the laboratory and caused to aggregate in a quantifiable way. Although the experimental output is elegant dynamic dose response curves again the experiments can be considered as binary: the results for one agent produce one blocker of a process which can give rise to one drug. Even though aspirin was developed for the prevention of platelet aggregation and statins were developed to prevent the slow effect of cholesterol over many years on the artery wall, people taking both aspirin and statins still suffer fatal myocardial infarction. The binary study of individual events has not solved the problem of treating or preventing myocardial infarction.

1.4.5 The system

It is understandable that a complex system has been understood only in part through deterministic steps since only deterministic experimental methods were used. However the failure of 50 years of therapeutic science to produce a definitive therapeutic approach to the prevention or treatment of myocardial infarction must question the use of deterministic experimentation as the only approach to therapeutics. The biological system which delivers blood to the heart in a controlled way is the product of 120 million years of mammalian evolution which has produced a complex system. (The simplicity of physics did not evolve). Both the evolution of the system and the present function of the system need to be examined as a whole. Modern laboratory science has in fact gone in a different direction. Molecular biology has the power to examine the products of thousands of genes in samples taken from cells. This science can in fact be considered a regression from physiology to anatomy: the study of structure; the structure involved in smaller and smaller events. What may be lacking is progress from physiology and pathophysiology to study of the complex system as a whole. In this way patterns of function which are crucial to function might be identified. Further crucial choke points in dynamic systems might be identified as places where effective intervention might produce effective therapeutics. In particular the slow change in the arterial wall leading to atherosclerosis could be modelled and compared to the instantaneous catastrophic change which causes myocardial infarction. The study of dynamic systems has not been undertaken in therapeutics since it requires a different language to be applied. The change from thinking in deterministic quanta to a systems approach requires a cross disciplinary connection which has been lacking.

1.5 The power of purpose

Diagnosis and disease management will need different models and data. Clinicians use their experience for diagnosis requesting specific diagnostics based on their analysis of the symptoms. The choice of measurements depends on experience and they can be vague and conflicting. Systems models could aid this process but as engineers know the requirements of a model depend very much on purpose to which it is being put [19]. Here are a few examples where the purpose dictates model requirements.

Much chemical engineering is based on models which assume homogeneity ("lumped" models) as are some organ models. If we are interested in glucose regulation in the bloodstream for diabetes for example, lumped models of liver and pancreas give good prediction of behaviour and allow discovery of system behaviour characteristics [20]. Metabolic dysfunction-associated steatotic liver disease (MASLD) is a condition of accumulation of lipids and fats in the liver and liver cells (hepatocytes) arising from malfunction in the hepatocyte metabolic processes. Conditions such as MASLD (and also paracetamol poisoning) do affect the liver cells across the liver in a differential way resulting in the need for the "distributed" model [21] shown in Figure 1.2. This figure is explored in more detail in one of the companion articles [22].

Many patients have long standing chronic liver disease resulting in complex management, hospitalisation, and eventually death. Patients' condition can be stable for extended periods and then experience a sudden degradation in their condition without warning. There are many causes and indicators for this to occur but in this case an early warning system would need many data points where some causative models may be

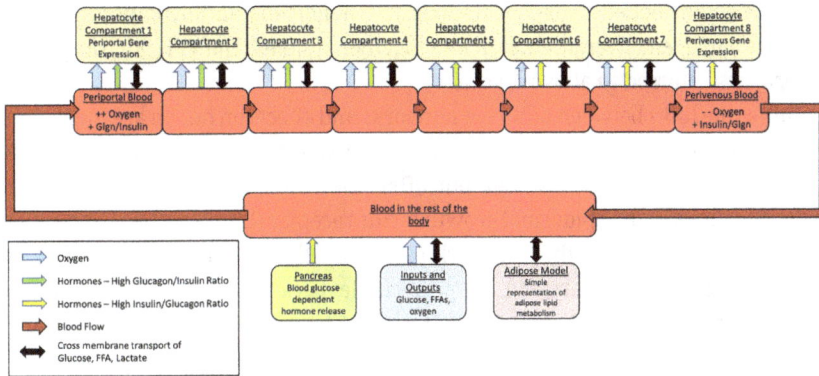

Figure 1.2: An engineering representation of zonated behaviour of hepatocyte cells processing nutrients from the blood across the liver (from [21]).

more useful than detailed predictive models [23]. The architecture of fault detection systems used in manufacturing could be used [24].

To control the production of insulin to manage type 1 diabetes Percival et al. [25] developed and implemented a real time control system using feedback of the glucose signal to adjust insulin flow in real time. Control algorithms require a precise and quantifiable objective to enable calculation of control actions. Their controller is a traditional engineering controller (an Internal Model Control tuned Proportional-Integral action controller) and has been used successfully on patients.

If we are interested in well-being of non-diseased populations or individuals a model could be used to investigate the impact of different foods, as defined by their key chemical ingredients, on metabolism and potential fat accumulation. The model could be used to explore efficient energy utilisation of nutrients for example.

The optimization and control of physiological processes to treat disease are very ambitious goals currently with significant limitations. Their effectiveness will depend on the quality of model predictions. To solve any design or optimisation problem we need to articulate clearly the design objectives and be able to determine the precise quantifiable objective function of the optimisation problem. Modellers need to ensure that the key phenomena related to the required purpose are included. At the moment this is still a matter of judgement.

1.6 Do we really understand?

Modelling of physiological processes is widespread. There is a huge range of models from the very simple to the very complex, from the entirely data driven to the fully deterministic and all points in between (see for example collections of papers in [26, 27]). Many models have been developed to explore individual phenomena and hypotheses. Fewer look at systems and even fewer attempt to link together systems. The VPH, Physiome and HumMod projects referred to above do this.

The multi-scale links between different networks and effects on health are important and not well integrated yet. Cancer is the result of metabolic defects causing cell proliferation. Causes are varied and unclear but often the result of genetic changes. For example malfunctions in the epidermal growth factor receptor (EGFR) network is a cause of some cancers. It is a well-studied network [28] and yet the behaviour and effects of treatments are not fully understood or predictable because of the huge data requirements for properly characterising its behaviour. The network is very complex and pathway bypasses can give the cell more robustness resulting in greater proliferation. Multiple drug targets are necessary which would need to be identified by network optimisation techniques.

The models to treat MASLD of the liver require both the equations for the metabolism describing the processing of nutrients to fats and lipids together with the ability to predict differentiated amounts across the plate of liver cells. Figure 1.2 shows an engineering representation which uses the approach used for industrial chemical reactors. This requires information on a range of metabolic processes, but particularly accurate information on the insulin sensitivity which causes the disease. This is not directly measurable but can be inferred from experiments allowing the effectiveness of the system to different treatments to be explored [21]. The behaviours are not fully understood but the engineering approaches to modelling help to direct experimental investigations towards key data and information required to predict behaviour.

There is still much that is not well understood about human physiology which limits the contribution modelling can make. But that was also said at the start of the modelling and simulation revolution in the process industries in the 1950s. Progress can be made by developing systems, solving partial problems (but considerably more complete than single individuals can do now), linking these models of systems within systems, and helping to identify important information that is lacking. This sort of systems biology work is going on already (see [29] for a recent review) but mostly to aid understanding. As well as models this requires fitting models together, bringing in data often available in significant amounts but with mixed quality, and then directing further experiments resulting in an iterative process between model and experiment.

1.7 What can we do? An expanded role for engineers

Healthcare is a matter of such concern and interest to society that engineering would like to play a greater role in it. Chemical processes are central to the way our physiology functions. Physiological processes are much more complex than those we are used to tackling in manufacturing but engineers have the skill set to help make progress.

Engineers are adept at using models for solving problems so there is much scope for using the tools of control and optimization with models and interlinked groups of models in medicine. A model can be used to optimise an objective such as minimise energy or minimise a particular metabolic product. Solutions are almost always on constraints which are often poorly characterised. In the first instance solutions would be most useful in indicating actions and highlighting their consequences in the systems involved in the model to highlight physiological effects which might not otherwise be expected because of the complexity of the system. By bringing together patient databases, with a wide range of data on patients' condition, models can become richer and used to understand potential wider effects of treatments. Precision medicine [30] cites the use of large datasets for guiding therapy but it needs a framework of models to help integrate the data and incorporate known predictable quantitative behaviour in an efficient way, particularly for predicting beyond the range of the individual's known data.

Engineering became a very quantitative discipline many years ago by developing predictive models and using them to design, control and troubleshoot complex chemical manufacturing processes. The life and medical sciences is becoming more quantitative. Engineers are adept at using complex models for decision making, sometimes instructing decisions in real time or in an advisory capacity. Working together with medical colleagues engineers are in a position to help deploy these techniques of design, control and optimisation in medicine.

By bringing together all information relevant into a model or system of models engineering methods could help answer questions such as: what is the optimal drug dosage, timings and location for effective treatment? amongst all the competing phenomena what according to the system models what is the most likely cause of a condition? amongst all the information available which affect the outcomes most and need therefore to be most accurate? These are ambitious goals that elude us at the moment but the explosion of data and models and the deployment of engineering problem-solving tools will give sufficient information in the future.

The chapters in this book demonstrate some of the progress that chemical engineers have made in modelling and systems analysis of certain physiological systems.

Engineering methodologies can have a very significant role to play in the future as the world works towards model-based personalised medicine. It needs joint teams of engineers, biologists and clinical scientists working together to tackle complex systems using all information available.

Acknowledgments: The authors would like to thank several medical colleagues for discussions and collaboration over many years in particular Prof Daniel Hochhauser (UCL Cancer Institute), Prof Rajiv Jalan (UCL Institute for Liver and Digestive Health) and Prof Nathan Davies (UCL Institute for Liver and Digestive Health). The authors also thank William Ashworth for Figure 1.2.

References

1. Monaco C, Mathiur A, Martin JF. What causes coronary syndromes – applying Koch's postulates. Athersclerosis 2005;179:1.
2. Bogle IDL, Allen R, Sumner T. The role of computer aided process engineering in physiology and clinical medicine. Comp Chem Eng 2010;34:763–9.
3. Martin JF, Kristansen SD, Mathur A, Grove EL, Choudry FA. The causal role of megakaryocyte-platelet hyperactivity in acute coronary syndromes. Nat Rev Cardiol 2012;9:658–70.
4. Guyton AC, Lindsey AW, Kaufmann BN. Effect of mean circulatory filling pressure and other peripheral circulatory factors on cardiac output. Am J Physiol 1955;180:463–8.
5. Hall JE. The pioneering use of systems analysis to study cardiac output regulation. Am J Physiol Regul Integr Comp Physiol 2004;287. https://doi.org/10.1152/classicessays.00007.2004.
6. Noble D. Modeling the heart – from genes to cells to the whole organ. Science 2002; 295, 1678-82, 2002
7. Christ B, Dahment U, Herrmann K, Konig M, Reichenbach JR, Ricken T, et al. Computational modeling in liver surgery. Front Physiol 2017;8:906.
8. Yin J. Chemical engineering and virology: challenges and opportunities at the interface. AIChE J 2007;53: 2202–9.
9. Netti TA, Baxter LT, Boucher Y, Skalak R, Jain RK. Macro- and microscopic fluid transport in living tissues: application to solid tumors. AIChE J 1997;43:818–34.
10. Peppas NA, Langer R. Origins and development of biomedical engineering within Chemical Engineering. Aiche J 2004;50/3:536–46.
11. Bogle IDL. Recent developments in process systems engineering as applied to medicine. Curr Opin Chem Eng 2012;1:453–8.
12. Vodovotz Y, An G, Androulakis IP. A systems engineering perspective on homeostasis and disease. Front Bioeng Biotechnol 2013;1:6.
13. Androulakis IP. A chemical engineer's perspective on health and disease. Comput Chem Eng 2014;71: 665–71.
14. Parker RS, Clermont G. Systems engineering medicine: engineering the inflammation response to infectious and traumatic challenges. J R Soc Interface 2010;7:989–1013.
15. Sharp P, Jacks T, Hockfield S. Convergence: the future of health. Cambridge: MIT; 2016.
16. Sherwood L Human physiology: from cells to systems, 7th ed. Baltimore: Brook/Cole; 2010.
17. Kapellos GE, Alexiou TS, and Payatakes AC. Theoretical modeling of fluid flow in cellular biological media: an overview. Math Biosci 2010;225/2:83–93
18. Lee MJ, Ye AS, Gardino AK, Heijink AM, Sorger PK, MacBeath G, et al. Sequential application of anticancer drugs enhances cell death by rewiring apoptotic signalling networks. Cell 2012;149:780–94.
19. Hangos KM, Cameron IT. Process modeling and model analysis. Cambridge: Academic Press; 2001.
20. Sumner T, Hetherington J, Seymour RM, Li L, Varela RM, Margoninski O, et al. A composite computational model of liver glucose homeostasis. Part 2: exploring system behaviour. J R Soc Interface 2012;9/69:701–6.
21. Ashworth W, Davies N, Bogle IDL (2016) A computational model of hepatic energy metabolism: understanding zonated damage and steatosis in NAFLD. PLoS Comput Biol. 2016;12:e1005105.
22. Liao Y, Davies N, Bogle IDL. Computational modelling of the liver system and liver disease. Phys Sci Rev 2025;10:51–78.
23. Schuppan D, Afdhal NH. Liver cirrhosis. Lancet 2008;371:838–5.
24. Reis MS, Gins G. Industrial process monitoring in the big data/industry 4.0 era: from detection, to diagnosis, to prognosis. Processes 2017;5:35.
25. Percival MW, Dassau E, Zisser H, Jovanovic L, Doyle FJ. Practical approach to design and implementation of a control algorithm in an artificial pancreatic beta cell. Ind Eng Chem Res 2009;48:6059–67.

26. Batzel JJ, Bachar M, Karemaker JM, Kappel F. Merging mathematical and physiological knowledge: dimensions and challenges. In: Batzel JJ, editors. Mathematical modeling and validation in physiology. Lecture notes in Mathematics 2064. Berlin: Springer; 2013.
27. Coveney PV, Diaz V, Hunter P, Viceconti M. Computational biomedicine: modelling the human body. Oxford, UK: Oxford University Press; 2014.
28. Avraham R, Yarden Y. Feedback regulation of EGFR signalling: decision making by early and delayed loops. Nat Rev Mol Cell Biol 2011;12:104–17.
29. Allen R, Ridley A, Bogle IDL. A model of localised Rac1 activation in endothelial cells due to fluid flow. J Theor Biol 2011;280/1:34–42.
30. Bahcall O. Precision medicine. Nature 2015;526:335.

Part II: **Modelling physiology**

Yunjie Liao*, Nathan A. Davies and I. David L. Bogle

2 Computational modelling in liver system and liver disease

Abstract: The liver, our body's chemical factory, is central to metabolism, homeostasis, and detoxification. The advent of systems biology and computational modelling has revolutionised our understanding of the liver system and its diseases. This chapter focuses on the application of computational modelling, specifically a kinetic model of fructose metabolism, to explore the relationship between fructose and liver disease progression. We begin by reviewing the fundamental aspects of liver anatomy and physiology, setting the stage for an in-depth discussion on the alarming crisis of metabolic dysfunction-associated steatotic liver disease (MASLD). Through a specific case study, we provide insights into the metabolic events triggered by fructose intake and illustrate how computational models can predict disease progression and identify potential therapeutic targets, paving the way for personalised treatment plans. The chapter concludes by discussing the challenges and future directions in the field, emphasising the transformative potential of engineering principles in medicine.

Keywords: systems biology; computational modelling; MASLD; fructose metabolism

2.1 The liver – the Body's chemical factory

For chemical engineers the liver can be thought of as 'the body's chemical factory'. It performs a broad range of biochemical functions for the maintenance of metabolic and energetic homeostasis, including the synthesis and catabolism of proteins, the regulation of carbohydrates, the moderation of lipids, the storage and metabolism of micro-nutrients, and the excretion of toxic xenobiotics [1]. The liver operates as part of a wider system for several of its functions. A key function is glucose homeostasis – the regulation of glucose in the blood stream to provide energy for human activity – which is done together with the pancreas, fatty tissue and the blood stream.

*Corresponding author: Yunjie Liao, Sargent Centre for Process Systems Engineering, Department of Chemical Engineering, Torrington Place, University College London, London, UK; and Institute for Liver and Digestive Health, UCL Division of Medicine, Royal Free Campus, Rowland Hill Street, University College London, London, UK, E-mail: y.liao@alumni.ucl.ac.uk
Nathan A. Davies, Institute for Liver and Digestive Health, UCL Division of Medicine, Royal Free Campus, Rowland Hill Street, University College London, London, UK
I. David L. Bogle, Sargent Centre for Process Systems Engineering, Department of Chemical Engineering, Torrington Place, University College London, London, UK

As per De Gruyter's policy this article has previously been published in the journal Physical Sciences Reviews. Please cite as: Y. Liao, N. A. Davies and I. D. L. Bogle "Computational modelling in liver system and liver disease" *Physical Sciences Reviews* [Online] 2024. DOI: 10.1515/psr-2024-0051 | https://doi.org/10.1515/9783111394558-002

There are several ways of exploring physiology modelling: by organ, but the organs work together as systems so this has limitations; by exploring specific diseases such as diabetes or cirrhosis, which again involves multiple organs and communication channels; or by physiological function such as glucose homeostasis, where it can be difficult to draw suitable boundaries to make study possible. In this chapter we will focus on glucose and fructose homeostasis, where the liver is central but other organs are involved. Altered homeostasis has a particular role in diseases like metabolic dysfunction-associated steatotic liver disease (MASLD), which has been becoming increasingly common in the developed world, and type 2 diabetes.

The chapter will first outline specific features of the liver to help chemical engineering readers understand some of its functions, discuss some of the key diseases that affect the liver and associated systems, and then present work on modelling the chemical functions of the liver in regulating glucose and fructose derived from our diet which affect normal function and are impaired in the case of certain diseases, with results exploring the effects of diet and medicines.

2.2 Liver physiology – fundamentals of hepatic function

2.2.1 Anatomy and structure

As the largest solid organ, a healthy human liver accounts for approximately 2–3% of the total body weight in an adult. It normally resides in the right upper quadrant of the abdomen, below the diaphragm. As depicted in Figure 2.1, the liver is divided into a large right lobe and a small left lobe from an anatomical perspective. In terms of functional anatomy, the liver can be further divided into eight functional segments.

The liver is comprised of four types of vasculature: the portal vein, hepatic artery, hepatic vein, and liver sinusoid [2]. These hepatic vascular networks play a crucial role in exchanging a substantial amount of nutrients, hormones, and oxygen within the liver, as well as between the liver and the rest of the body [3]. Approximately four-fifths of the blood flow in the liver is derived from the portal vein, while the remaining one-fifth is supplied by the hepatic artery [4]. The portal vein serves as the primary blood supply to the liver, collecting the majority of absorbed nutrients from the digestive system and serving as the site for the release of pancreatic hormones and gastrointestinal peptides. Blood then exits the liver through hepatic veins into the systemic circulation [5].

In terms of histological structure, the liver comprises approximately one million hepatic lobules (Figure 2.2). Each lobule is a multilateral (diamond-shaped) structure of functional tissue (parenchyma) surrounding the central vein [6, 7]. There are two types of cell typically found in the liver: parenchymal cells, principally hepatocytes which play the major role in accomplishing the liver's functions particularly those related to the

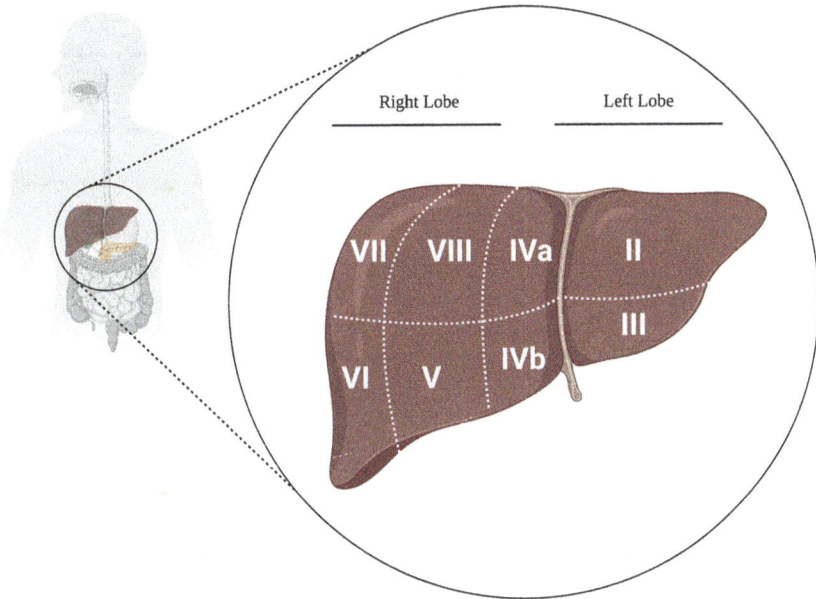

Figure 2.1: Anatomical structure and functional anatomy of the liver (created with BioRender.com).

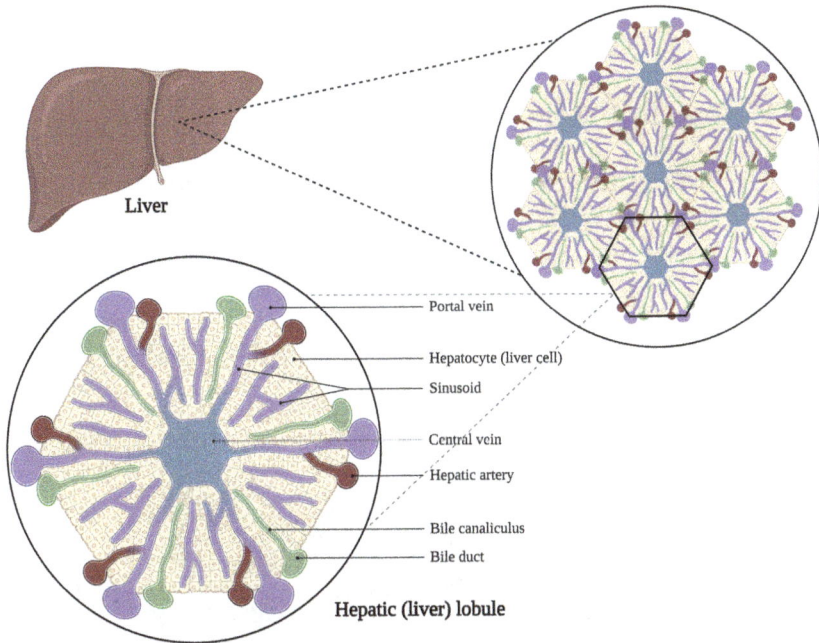

Figure 2.2: The structure of liver lobules (created with BioRender.com).

Table 2.1: Cell types and essential functions in the liver.

Cell type	% of the hepatic volume	Essential function
Parenchymal cell		
Hepatocytes	80	Metabolism of protein, carbohydrate, lipid, micronutrients and xenobiotics, also bile secretion
Non-parenchymal cells		
Liver sinusoidal endothelial cells (LSECs)	2.8	Filtration and transport of nutrients from the blood; blood clearance and endocytosis; secretion of inflammasome molecules
Kupffer cells	2.1	Phagocytosis of bacteria, cytokine production responsible for inflammatory response and liver regeneration; iron metabolism
Stellate cells	1.2	Fat-storing cells; vitamin a storage; secretion of growth factors
Pit cells	Minor	Liver-specific natural killer cells; antitumor function
Biliary epithelial cells	3.5 % of cell mass	Cytokine secretion, regulation role in inflammation, regulation of hepatic glutathione

metabolic function, contributing about 80 %–90 % of the hepatic volume and around 60 % of liver cell numbers; and non-parenchymal cells, including liver sinusoidal endothelial cells (LSECs), Kupffer cells, stellate cells, pit cells and biliary epithelial cells [2]. The types of hepatic cells and their functions are summarised in Table 2.1.

2.2.2 Liver Sinusoid and Hepatic Zonation

The hepatic lobule is regarded as the fundamental unit of the liver. Each individual lobule receives a mixed blood supply from the liver bile ducts, portal veins and hepatic arteries, and drains it into central veins and eventually to the hepatic vein which feeds into the vena cava [3].

The blood flow across the liver sinusoid is displayed in Figure 2.3. Along the direction of the hepatic bloodstream, hepatocytes are exposed to different concentrations of

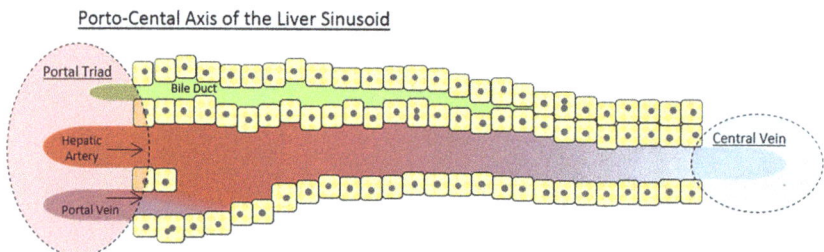

Figure 2.3: The structure of liver sinusoid (adopted from Ashworth [8]).

nutrients, hormones and oxygen according to their position. Liver cells react to changes in the constituents and rates of substrate delivery vary depending on their distance from the entry of the blood from the portal vein [5].

The distributed nature of nutrient exchange between the blood flow and hepatocytes is known as 'zonation' – a type of 'distributed system'. The 'acinus' model, widely accepted to describe this phenomenon, delineates three zones across the liver sinusoid: the periportal, intermediate, and perivenous zones [3, 7, 9]. Hepatocytes in each zone exhibit different metabolic capacities [10].

Abnormal metabolic changes within liver cells would be expected to lead to hepatic lipid deposition, which can subsequently result in advanced liver diseases. Remarkably, the liver can maintain all its normal functions with as little as one fifth of its original mass. It stands as the only internal organ capable of regenerating back to full size in approximately three months (on average), even if 80 % of its tissue mass has been removed [11]. Consequently, there are only a few warning signals or symptoms prior to severe hepatic impairment. Asymptomatic liver damage can continue for as long as 20 years [12].

2.3 Liver disease – the leading cause of death in UK

According to the British Liver Trust [12], liver disease has become the third leading cause of mortality in those aged under 75 years old in the United Kingdom (UK), only after cardiovascular disease and cancer. Surprisingly, liver disease is now the commonest cause of death in the 35–49 age group, accounting for approximately 10 % of deaths.

2.3.1 Classifications of liver disease

Liver disease can be broadly classified into two categories: chronic liver disease lasting over six months, and acute liver failure, which occurs within three months of the first signs of liver injury [13, 14].

Acute liver failure (ALF) denotes a sudden and severe hepatic dysfunction that progresses rapidly, typically within hours or weeks, without preceding liver damage [15]. This rare clinical condition often leads to jaundice, blood clotting disorders, neurological impairment (hepatic encephalopathy, HE), and multisystem failure [16]. Viral infections (such as hepatitis A, B, and E viruses) and drug poisoning are identified as the predominant triggers of ALF in developing and developed countries, respectively [17]. Apart from spontaneous recovery and cause-oriented interventions, emergency liver transplant is considered the most effective treatment for ALF [16, 17].

In contrast, chronic liver disease (CLD) refers to hepatic impairment characterised by progressive changes over a period of six months or more. While the incidence of ALF is approximately one to six individuals per million population worldwide per year [15], the incidence of CLD is estimated to be around 20 per million population [18]. A dynamic process called liver cirrhosis should be noted. Caused by various mechanisms of liver damage, cirrhosis is often considered the end-stage liver disease, characterised by necroinflammation and fibrogenesis, leading to hepatic functional abnormalities. Histologically, cirrhosis is distinguished by the presence of scar tissue and collapse of liver structures, resulting in alterations in hepatic vascular architecture [19].

2.3.2 MASLD – the alarming crisis

Although more than 86 % of mortality from liver diseases result from alcohol over-consumption, it is important not to overlook the rising prevalence of other lifestyle-induced liver-related deaths [12]. Among these, metabolic dysfunction-associated steatotic liver disease (MASLD) stands out as the most common chronic liver condition, affecting approximately 38 % of the global population, and is often associated with obesity, type 2 diabetes mellitus (T2DM), and metabolic syndrome [20–22].

MASLD, the latest nomenclature and definition for steatotic liver disorders (previously called non-alcoholic fatty liver disease or NAFLD), encompasses a spectrum of conditions resulting from excess lipid accumulation in the liver without excessive alcohol consumption. Additionally, the new term MetALD now includes patients with MASLD whose alcohol consumption exceeds 140–350 g per week for females and 210–420 g per week for males [23].

MASLD can progress from simple steatosis (intrahepatic lipid deposition, also referred to as metabolic dysfunction-associated fatty liver, MAFL) to metabolic dysfunction-associated steatohepatitis (MASH), a more severe stage characterised by the combination of steatosis and inflammation. Subsequently, MASH has the potential to progress to fibrosis (excessive fibrous connective tissue) and cirrhosis (an advanced stage of liver scarring), and in some cases, may lead to hepatocellular carcinoma [21, 24]. Notably, while steatosis and MASH are reversible, high levels of fibrosis and cirrhosis are typically considered irreversible [25]. The pathologic manifestations of MASLD are shown in Figure 2.4. Data was adopted from Lekakis and Papatheodoridis [23].

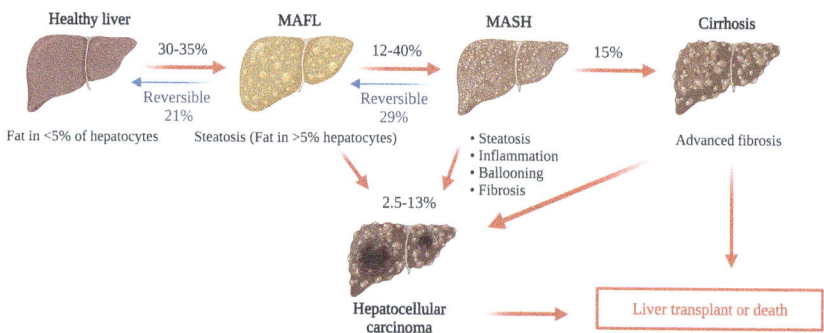

Figure 2.4: The spectrum of MASLD progress (created with BioRender.com). (MAFL: Metabolic dysfunction-associated fatty liver; MASH: Metabolic dysfunction-associated steatohepatitis).

In the U.K., it is speculated that one in three people have pro-steatosis conditions (the early phrase in MASLD development) and around 3.3 million individuals have MASH. In the last decade, the number of liver transplantation procedures resulting from MASLD has increased tenfold [12].

Among obese subjects, an estimated 30–37 % have MASLD [26], while among the non-obese population (including normal weight and overweight) the prevalence of MASLD is still as high as 12 % [27]. The classification of obese and non-obese can be found in Table 2.2. In addition, MASLD has been reported to be highly associated with T2DM. Among T2DM patients, there are around 56 % and 37 % individuals that are also living with MASLD and MASH, respectively [28].

Diagnosis of MASLD is based on the detection of hepatic steatosis (>5 % fat are observed in the hepatocytes [29]) in adults, along with one of the following three criteria: overweight/obesity, T2DM, or evidence of metabolic dysregulation determined by the presence of ≥2 metabolic risk abnormalities [23]. Additionally, even though liver enzymes such as alanine aminotransferase (ALT) and aspartate transaminase (AST) serve as hepatic biomarkers in regular liver function blood tests, they cannot be used as the indicators for MASLD diagnosis. Approximately up to 80 % MASLD patients are tested as having normal levels of ALT. Also, there is no difference in histological observation between normal and abnormal liver enzyme level within MASLD population [29, 30]. Therefore, the actual number of people with MASLD might be highly underestimated and a novel, accurate, non-invasive diagnostic methodology is urgently needed.

The pathogenesis of MASLD is widely accepted as multifactorial, involving genetic, environmental, dietary, and metabolic factors. However, the ambiguity in the underlying mechanism of MASLD has led to a lack of effective therapeutic interventions. Currently, lifestyle intervention is commonly recommended for MASLD and MASH patients, focusing on weight loss through improved dietary choices and increased physical activity [31].

In addition, a few other medical treatments can be introduced to alleviate MASLD-associated symptoms and dysfunctions, such as glucagon-like peptide-1 (GLP-1) receptor agonists [32] and Orlistat for obesity [33], angiotensin-converting enzyme inhibitors for hypertension [34], and metformin for T2DM [35]. Despite the fact that there are almost 30 potential medicines that have been experimentally explored and

Table 2.2: Calculation and classification of BMI.

Body Mass Index $(BMI) = \frac{Weight(kg)}{Height^2(m)}$	Classification
BMI < 18.5	Underweight
18.5 ≤ **BMI** ≤ 24.9	Normal weight
25 ≤ **BMI** ≤ 29.9	Overweight
30 ≤ **BMI** ≤ 39.9	Obese

tested [36, 37], to date, only one pharmaceutical drug (resmetirom) has been approved specifically targeting MASH [38].

2.4 Glucose & fructose – a "sweet" burden

Given the significant impact of liver disease on human health, understanding the intricate metabolic processes within the liver becomes paramount. Most carbohydrates and sugars are broken down into glucose in the digestive system before entering the blood stream through the intestine. The metabolic pathways of glucose and fructose play a pivotal role in liver physiology, orchestrating a delicate balance between energy production and storage.

Glucose, fructose, and galactose are the three primary dietary monosaccharides. Among them, glucose is the body's predominant energy source. Metabolic transformations of glucose and fructose predominantly occur within the liver. Despite sharing the same chemical formula ($C_6H_{12}O_6$), fructose and glucose exhibit distinct structural compositions. Unlike glucose and galactose, which are aldohexoses, fructose is the only ketohexose that exists in the body in a notable quantity.

Historically, fructose was championed as a beneficial sweetener, particularly advocated for individuals with obesity or diabetes. Its unique ability to avoid triggering insulin secretion and its potential for reducing postprandial hyperglycaemia were among the reasons for this recommendation. The dramatic increase (from ~20 g/day to ~70 g/day) in fructose consumption over the past century has transformed dietary habits, with fructose now constituting a significant portion of daily energy intake (from 5 % to 15–25 %) [39, 40]. This rise is largely driven by the widespread availability of refined and processed fructose, utilised as a cost-effective sweetener in ultra-processed food and beverage products. In the U.K. it has been reported that the average intake of sugar sweetened beverages is 106 g per day for adults during the period 2016–2019 [41]. However, the consumption of high levels of fructose has been linked to a spectrum of health concerns, including metabolic syndrome, obesity, type 2 diabetes, and MASLD [42]. And it is suggested that the strong association of fructose with these chronic health conditions is attributed to its distinct metabolic pathways.

The primary difference between the fructose metabolism and glucose metabolism lies in their phosphorylation processes (as shown in Figure 2.5). In the glucose metabolism, glucose is first metabolised into glucose-6-phosphate (G6P) by the enzyme glucokinase. G6P is then transformed into glucose-1-phosphate (G1P) by phosphoglucomutase, which aids in glycogen synthesis. Subsequently, G6P is converted into fructose-6-phosphate (F6P) by phosphofructokinase. F6P is further converted into fructose-1,6-bisphosphate, which is subsequently broken down into glyceraldehyde-3-phosphate (GA3P) and dihydroxyacetone phosphate (DHAP). These intermediates are ultimately converted into pyruvate, which enters the tricarboxylic acid (TCA) cycle within the mitochondria [43].

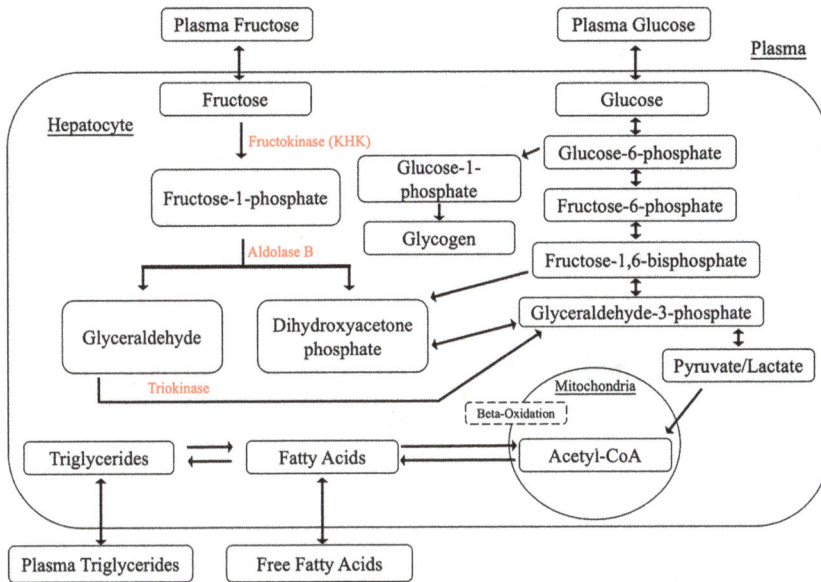

Figure 2.5: Hepatic fructose VS glucose metabolism.

As displayed in Figure 2.5, upon entering the liver, fructose is rapidly phosphory-lated by fructokinase (ketohexokinase, KHK) to produce fructose-1-phosphate. This pathway bypasses the key regulatory enzyme of glycolysis, phosphofructokinase, observed in the glucose metabolism. Fructose-1-phosphate is subsequently converted to DHAP and glyceraldehyde (GA) by aldolase B, providing intermediates for further glycolysis. Triokinase, serving as the third essential enzyme, phosphorylates glyceral-dehyde to form GA3P, generating additional intermediates for subsequent reactions. Beyond this point, both the glucose and fructose metabolisms converge at the pro-duction of GA3P and proceed identically [24, 44–46].

While glucose serves as the primary energy source for the body, fructose's unique metabolism in the liver, bypassing key regulatory steps in glycolysis, highlights its complex relationship with metabolic health.

2.5 Systems biology approach–the rising star

The concept of systems biology was first introduced 20 years ago. The core of this modern cross-disciplinary field is to apply mathematics, statistics, bioinformatics and computer science to support complex biological research at a systematic scale, from genomics, proteomics, pathways, to cells, tissues, organs, organisms, populations and ecologies [47]. The conventional framework of the systems biology approach is an iterative cycle: the "make-test-validate-refine" process normally combines mathematical and computational modelling with quantitative experiments.

Despite the fact that abundant studies have highlighted the important role fructose plays in liver-related metabolic diseases, the lack of a model that only focuses on the fructose metabolism motivated this work. A few models [25, 48, 49] have placed emphasis on the hepatic fructose metabolism but without reflecting the underlying dynamic mechanism of the fructose metabolism and MASLD development. A brief comparison of these models is listed in Table 2.3.

2.6 Computational modelling of fructose-induced lipid deposition and MASLD

MASLD is a complex disease influenced by multiple factors, including genetics, dietary habits, and physical activity. While overnutrition and a sedentary lifestyle have long been implicated, compelling evidence from clinical and experimental studies suggests that the

Table 2.3: What has and has not been done in the existing fructose models.

The existing fructose models	What has been done	What has not been done
Allen and Musante [48]	1) Two fructose-specialised enzymes were included in the model (fructokinase and aldolase B); 2) The relationship between fructokinase deficiency and essential fructosuria was explored; 3) Urine fructose concentration was included in the model.	1) Downstream fructose pathways after aldolase B were excluded; 2) The relationships between fructose and other metabolic conditions were not explored.
Allen and Musante [49]	1) The relationship between fructose and *de novo* lipogenesis was discussed; 2) Simplification method has been applied in metabolic pathway of the fructose-pyruvate-fatty acids-triglyceride axis.	1) The relationship between fructose and MASLD has not been explored; 2) The model does not have other inputs such as glucose.
Maldonado, Fisher, Mazzatti et al. [25]	1) The relationship between fructose and MASLD has been investigated; 2) A fructose model was constructed that integrated the transport and signalling network with a hepatocyte-specific human genome-scale metabolic network (HepatoNet1). 3) Glucose input was included in the model.	1) The human genome-scale metabolic network produces static predictions but did not represent the dynamic flows of metabolic reactions; 2) The fructose metabolism in the disease state has not been considered.

increasing consumption of fructose may also play a critical role [24, 50–53]. This growing body of research highlights the significant link between fructose intake and MASLD development.

The surge in research interest in this area is evident in the dramatic increase in publications over the past two decades (Figure 2.6). In 2005, only two publications addressed the relationship between fructose and NAFLD/MASLD, whereas over 150 papers were published in 2023.

Biomedical studies and clinical trials often focus on discovering one specific molecule or component at a time, frequently lacking a holistic perspective to integrate the complex interactions within biological systems. Adopting a systems biology approach to explore the relationship between fructose consumption and the development of MASLD provides a comprehensive understanding and helps identify potential interventional targets.

This study follows an "experiment-model-experiment" process, reflecting the iterative nature of systems biology approach. In this study, a kinetic and dynamic computational model of the fructose metabolism has been developed to explore potential pathophysiological mechanisms. The model can generate predictions of the regulatory and metabolic consequences of fructose under both healthy and disease conditions. Additionally, it can assess potential interventional targets for reversing and treating fructose-induced fatty liver during the early stages of disease progression.

2.6.1 Experimental Attempt and Exploration

Before constructing a computational model of fructose metabolism, two preliminary studies were performed to investigate the effects of a high-fructose diet on liver health. These experiments aimed to determine if a fructose-enriched diet could induce fatty liver and if the observed effects aligned with existing literature.

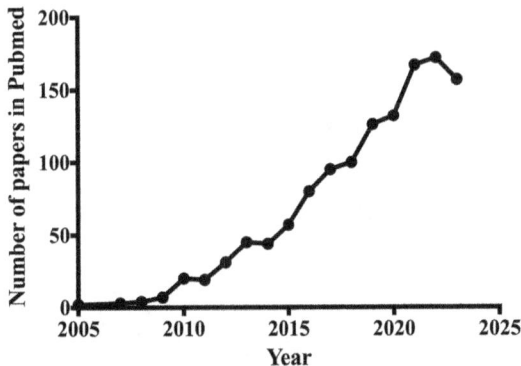

Figure 2.6: Searching results by year (2005–2023) in PubMed. (Keywords: Fructose & NAFLD; fructose and MASLD; fructose & MAFLD).

2.6.1.1 Experimental design of an *in vivo* study

Sprague Dawley rats were divided into two groups and fed different diets as described in Liao, Davies and Bogle [54]. One group received a control diet, while the other received a high-fructose diet containing 66.3 g of fructose per 100 g of chow, representing 69.6 % of total caloric intake. This animal model was established in collaboration with Aarhus University in Denmark.

2.6.1.2 Results and discussion

2.6.1.2.1 Animal sample characteristics

The data of body weight and liver weight in the animal experiment was recorded to summarise the sample characteristics. The comparison between two groups in body weight as well as in the ratio of liver/body weight are presented in Figure 2.7(A) and (B), respectively. Figure 2.7(C) exhibits the whole liver pieces (one representative from each group) for the visual comparison.

Our analysis of body weight and liver weight revealed interesting findings. There was no significant statistical difference in body weight between the two diet groups, with the control group even exhibiting a slightly higher average weight. However, the livers in the fructose group were significantly heavier compared to the control group, which can be observed directly from Figure 2.7(C). This led to a significantly higher liver-to-body

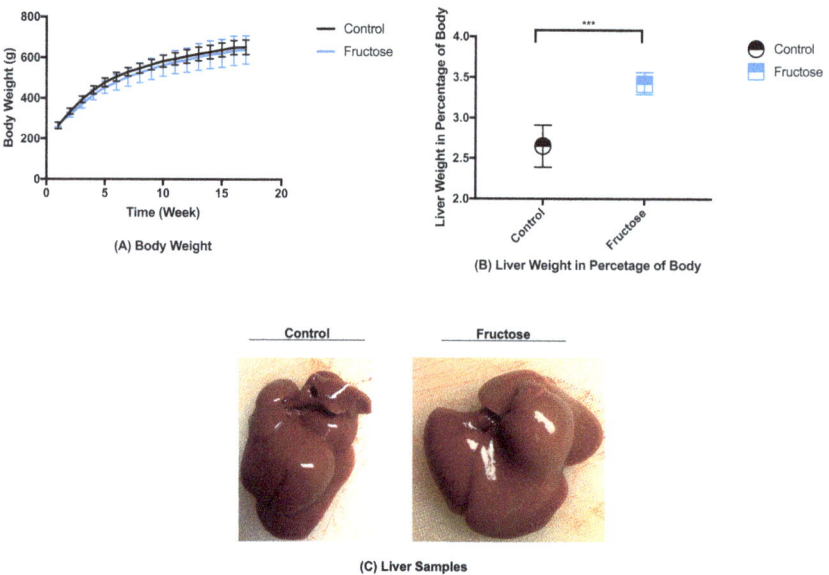

(A) Body Weight

(B) Liver Weight in Percetage of Body

(C) Liver Samples

Figure 2.7: Sample characteristics of body weight and liver/body weight ratio. (A and B: Mean ± SD, control: n = 10; fructose: n = 9). *$p < 0.05$, **$p < 0.01$, ***$p < 0.001$ vs. Control.

weight ratio in the fructose group (Figure 2.7(B)), supporting the notion of fructose-induced fatty liver. These findings suggest that high fructose consumption led to hepatic lipid accumulation (fatty liver) rather than systemic (whole body) fat storage. These initial observations are consistent with previous studies and provided a foundation for developing the computational model.

2.6.1.2.2 The effect of different carbohydrates on lipid accumulation

The rat liver pieces were used to quantify the impact of different diets on hepatic lipid accumulation. A total of 19 hepatic histological slides from both the control and fructose groups were analysed by ImageJ software to quantify the lipid area fraction. The results are presented in Figure 2.8.

In Figure 2.8(A), two histological images were displayed as the representatives: one from the control group and the other one from the fructose group. The image clearly shows a significant difference in lipid content, with a large amount of lipid droplets

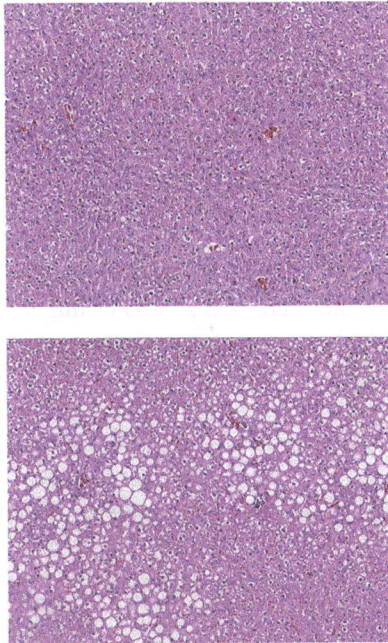

(A) Histology of liver tissues

(Upper: No.57 rat from the control group;

Lower: No.37 rat from the fructose group)

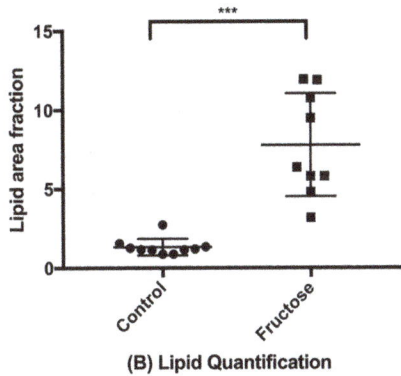

(B) Lipid Quantification

Figure 2.8: Lipid accumulation outcomes stimulated by different diets in the animal experiment. (B: Scatter plots with single value and means ± SD; control: $n = 10$; fructose: $n = 9$). *$p < 0.05$, **$p < 0.01$, ***$p < 0.001$ vs. Control.

(white spaces) observed in the liver of rat No. 37 from the fructose group, compared to minimal fat presence in rat No. 57 from the control group.

The quantified lipid area fraction for each sample (represented by black dots) and the group averages are shown in Figure 2.8(B). The control group exhibited an average hepatic lipid content of 1.33 ± 0.53 %, while the fructose-fed group had a significantly higher average of 7.78 ± 3.27 %. According to the biochemical criteria of hepatic steatosis, a liver is considered macroscopically steatotic when its lipid content exceeds 5 % [29]. Based on our findings and the visual observations in Figure 2.8, we can conclude that the fructose-enriched diet significantly contributes to the development of MASLD, which aligns with previous research.

2.6.2 Computational Model Development of Fructose Metabolism

This study constructs a kinetic and dynamic computational model to investigate the impact of fructose metabolism on MASLD development. The model development process involved a stepwise approach, progressively adding complexity to investigate different aspects of the system.

The initial stage focused on building a model for the fructose metabolism within the Section Hepatocytes (SH). This core model predicted the concentration of fatty acids and triglycerides produced by the liver. This stage served as a validation step to ensure the model functioned correctly and generated logical predictions.

The model was then expanded to include the glucose metabolism as an alternative dietary source. Additionally, compartments representing blood circulation (hepatic bloodstream (SHB) and bloodstream of the rest of the body (SBC)) were added to simulate the transport of metabolites throughout the body. This allowed for investigating the effects of different dietary compositions and individual variations in metabolic reaction rates.

In the third stage, the model was further refined to incorporate insulin resistance (IR), a hallmark characteristic of MASLD. This allowed us to explore how the model would respond under abnormal metabolic conditions, including predicting lipid deposition patterns under different dietary scenarios (isocaloric and hypercaloric diets) in the presence of IR.

Finally, the fourth stage focused on identifying potential therapeutic targets. The model was used to simulate the effects of modulating specific enzymes or pathways (pyruvate kinase (PK), fructokinase (KHK), and peroxisome proliferator-activated receptors alpha (PPARα)). By examining both individual and synergistic effects of these targets under various insulin resistance conditions, we aimed to assess the model's effectiveness in identifying potential treatment strategies.

The detail of the fructose computational model development was published in Liao, Davies and Bogle [55]. By starting with a core model and progressively adding complexity, we were able to validate each stage's functionality and gain deeper insights into the system's behaviours under different conditions. Simulations were conducted using MATLAB_R2019a (MATLAB, RRID:SCR_001622), employing the 'ode45' function to solve all ordinary differential equations concurrently. The simulations were designed to span a 12-h period, accounting for the inclusion of three meals.

2.6.2.1 Results and discussion

This section presents the key findings from the application of the computational model at each stage of development.

2.6.2.1.1 Stage one: basic model behaviour of hepatic fructose metabolism

The initial stage focused on evaluating the core model's functionality. Simulations predicted the concentration changes of key metabolites within the liver cells following fructose consumption. The simulations were conducted under the assumption that there is no further demand from utilisation or transportation of metabolites outside the liver.

Nine hepatic variables which were considered as distinctive components in the fructose pathways were included at this stage. Three meals with an equal quantity of pure fructose were simulated at time points 8:00, 12:00 and 16:00, respectively. An arbitrary number was assigned to fructose input since the range of fructose concentrations in clinical and experimental data can vary largely in magnitude depending on different detection methods: from 0.008 to 16 mM [39, 56]. Also, the effect of varying fructose intake on hepatic fatty acids and triglycerides was explored as a part of the model presentations. Three diets were simulated: a baseline diet, a high fructose diet (with a 25 % increase compared to baseline) and a very high fructose diet (with a 50 % increase compared to baseline). The initial values of all variables were set to zero.

The plots of the nine key variables are displayed in Figure 2.9, representing the basic model performance of hepatic fructose metabolism in response to fructose consumption. As shown in Figure 2.9, the black line shows that each input cycle takes 2 h to digest a fructose meal and to reach the peak value of hepatic fructose concentration. This behaviour is slightly different from the clinical data [57, 58], which achieves a summit in around 1 h and has a longer steadier decreasing tail after one meal. The discrepancy is caused by the simplification of dietary input, which was set as a high-power sine equation. However, this simplification is acceptable as it does not affect the subsequent model behaviour in lipid profiles.

Apart from acetyl-CoA, fatty acids and triglycerides, the concentrations of the other variables increased gradually after the meals and then dropped back to baseline along the time axis. For acetyl-CoA and fatty acids, their postprandial values were raised after breakfast and then fluctuated periodically within a certain range after lunch and dinner. These behaviours suggest that neither acetyl-CoA nor fatty acids were consumed completely by the liver after fructose feeding. However, they showed a tendency that they were able to reach an equilibrium state after three meals. Additionally, triglycerides

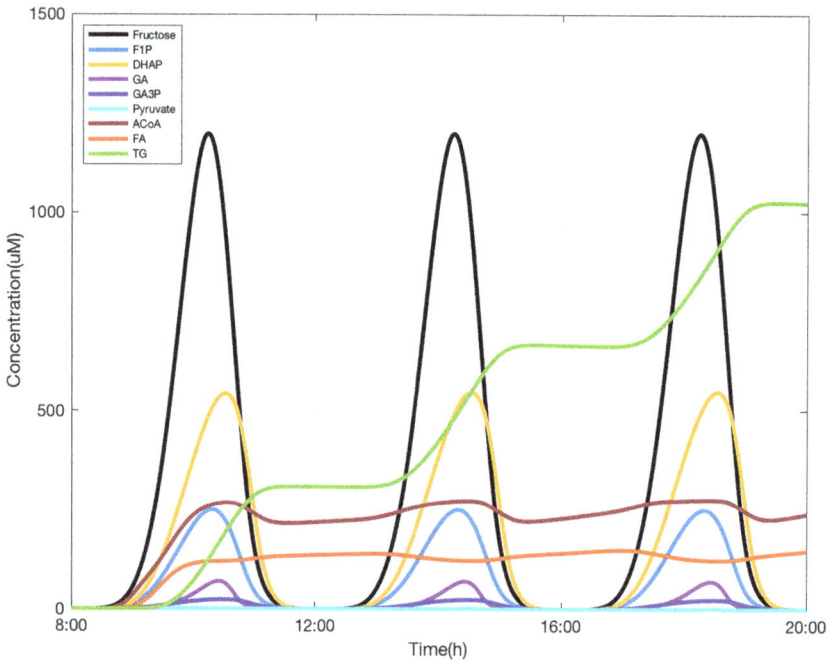

Figure 2.9: Baseline model behaviour of hepatic fructose metabolism. (F1P: Fructose-1-phosphate; DHAP: Dihydroxyacetone phosphate; GA: Glyceraldehyde; GA3P: Glyceraldehyde-3-phosphate; ACoA: Acetyl-CoA; FA: Fatty Acid; TG: Triglycerides).

presented a stable growth pattern with constant accumulation. This plot indicates that the fructose input has been converted into triglycerides over the three meals.

In addition, the results of hepatic lipid accumulation after high fructose diets are presented in Figure 2.10. As shown in Figure 2.10(A), when fructose exposure is increased by 25 % and 50 % per meal, the levels of hepatic fatty acids rise and fall more dramatically. Higher fructose intake results in more erratic fluctuations. In terms of hepatic triglycerides, in Figure 2.10(B) reveals that this product accumulates in a dose-dependent manner.

The model successfully captured the overall trends in these metabolite levels, including a gradual rise after meals and a subsequent decline. The model also demonstrated a dose-dependent effect of fructose intake on hepatic triglyceride accumulation, suggesting a logical response to varying dietary fructose levels. These observations confirmed the proper construction of kinetic equations and the model's ability to follow the law of mass conservation.

2.6.2.1.2 Stage Two: scenario construction and validation after model combination

Stage two involved expanding the model to include the glucose metabolism and blood circulation. This allowed us to investigate how dietary composition and individual

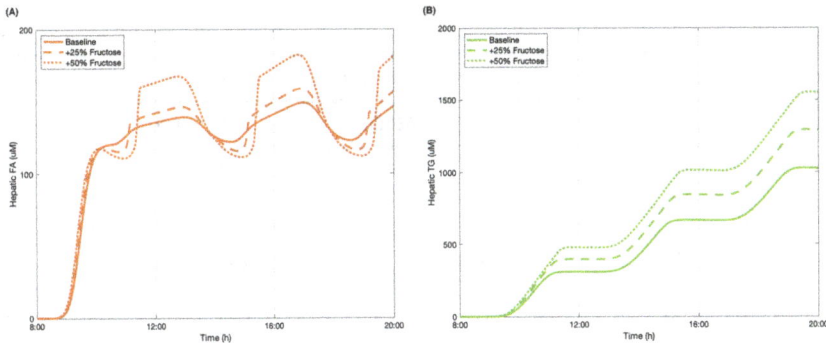

Figure 2.10: The change of hepatic lipid concentration after different fructose intakes. (A) Hepatic FA and (B) hepatic TG. (FA: Fatty Acid; TG: Triglycerides).

variations in metabolic rates affect the system. This stage included two scenarios: (1) The effect of varying carbohydrate intake on lipid accumulation, and (2) The effect of varying reaction rate constants on the hepatic metabolic process.

In Scenario One, the model's predictions were compared to clinical data under different dietary scenarios. This comparison demonstrated the model's ability to replicate the observed changes in metabolic activity. The details of these results can be found in Liao, Davies and Bogle [55].

In Scenario Two, a sensitivity analysis was performed to assess the model's robustness (see in [55]). Also, individual simulations (20 individuals) were conducted to examine the correlations between metabolic rate variations and the model's outputs (lipid production). Table 2.4 lists all the parameter values that were generated randomly within a set range. Figure 2.11 shows the variations in lipid production for each individual simulation, along with average values and standard deviations. Figure 2.12 compares the average lipid content across the simulations to the baseline condition.

As shown in Figure 2.11, the concentrations of various lipids (fatty acids and triglycerides in both the liver and bloodstream) fell within a specific range across the simulations. The distribution of fatty acid concentrations was more discrete compared to triglycerides. In Figure 2.12, the mean values of four kinds of lipids generated by the 20 simulated individuals are similar to the values produced using baseline parameter values. However, a slightly lower average on hepatic triglycerides could be spotted for the simulated subjects compared to the value emitted by standard parameters. Overall, the results showed minimal variation in predicted lipid profiles between the baseline and simulated individuals, indicating the model's stability and ability to generate consistent predictions under healthy conditions.

In conclusion, Stage Two successfully validated the model using clinical data and explored the impact of variations in metabolic rates. The results demonstrate the model's ability to replicate hepatic fructose metabolism and predict its effects on lipid production

Table 2.4: The random rate constants for the 20 simulated individuals.

Simulated Individuals	Rate Constants of Key Enzymes/Reactions										
	KHK	aldB	TPI	Tri	PK	PEPCK	PDC	FAS	boxi	TGS	Lply
1	4.45	1.69	2.63	7.12	94.21	36.23	16.43	4.28	3.54	9.46	0.080
2	4.73	1.68	2.94	6.74	91.92	37.83	13.61	3.80	3.43	9.72	0.087
3	4.59	1.72	2.44	6.96	83.44	37.86	14.48	4.07	3.45	9.41	0.078
4	4.75	1.80	2.88	6.31	80.94	36.73	16.42	4.35	3.40	8.83	0.085
5	4.15	1.77	2.77	6.76	93.05	33.32	14.60	3.64	3.31	9.79	0.091
6	4.93	1.83	2.72	6.97	91.96	36.33	14.43	3.64	3.19	8.56	0.092
7	4.81	1.55	2.78	7.31	83.01	32.42	13.86	3.62	3.41	9.06	0.085
8	4.10	1.60	2.82	6.63	82.26	32.36	16.25	4.15	3.05	9.82	0.081
9	4.47	1.69	2.48	6.14	83.89	32.84	13.91	4.08	3.07	8.58	0.088
10	4.34	1.86	2.90	6.11	92.73	32.52	14.50	3.69	2.98	8.55	0.092
11	4.62	1.80	2.44	6.87	92.61	35.60	16.19	4.24	3.61	9.77	0.085
12	4.26	1.68	2.59	7.10	88.23	32.01	15.00	4.09	3.61	8.22	0.093
13	4.57	1.64	2.53	6.96	88.25	37.26	15.35	3.66	3.05	8.64	0.080
14	4.59	1.55	2.93	6.49	83.28	36.56	15.25	3.66	3.28	9.16	0.078
15	4.59	1.78	2.47	7.30	90.46	37.98	15.59	3.71	3.40	8.47	0.082
16	4.45	1.70	2.74	6.73	92.15	34.95	13.59	4.23	3.16	9.24	0.083
17	4.08	1.60	2.77	7.31	85.98	36.08	15.08	3.67	3.47	9.54	0.084
18	4.51	1.68	2.78	6.13	86.06	37.73	13.60	3.79	3.34	9.00	0.082
19	4.42	1.59	2.90	6.31	86.40	35.27	15.98	3.79	3.25	9.27	0.088
20	4.15	1.79	2.46	7.07	83.16	33.48	14.52	3.68	3.15	9.53	0.078

(KHK, hepatic fructokinase; aldB, aldolase B; TPI, triose phosphate isomerase; TPI, triokinase; PK, pyruvate kinase; PEPCK, phosphoenolpyruvate carboxykinase; PDC, pyruvate dehydrogenase complex; FAS, fatty acid synthesis; boxi, beta-oxidation; TGS, triglyceride synthesis; Lply, lipolysis.

under healthy conditions. This paves the way for testing the model under abnormal conditions (like insulin resistance) to further investigate the link between fructose consumption and MASLD development.

2.6.2.1.3 Stage Three: model performance with insulin resistance simulation
Stage Three introduced insulin resistance, a hallmark of MASLD, into the model. The model's performance was evaluated under two scenarios: isocaloric carbohydrate intake and hypercaloric fructose intake, both with impaired insulin sensitivity. These scenarios were designed to test the model's ability to make robust predictions under pathological conditions. The detailed model settings and specific predictions can be found in the referenced publication [54].

2.6.2.1.4 Stage four: model based MASLD analysis and synergistic treatment exploration
The final stage focused on identifying potential therapeutic targets for early-stage MASLD. As shown in Figure 2.13, three key metabolic regulators – pyruvate kinase (PK),

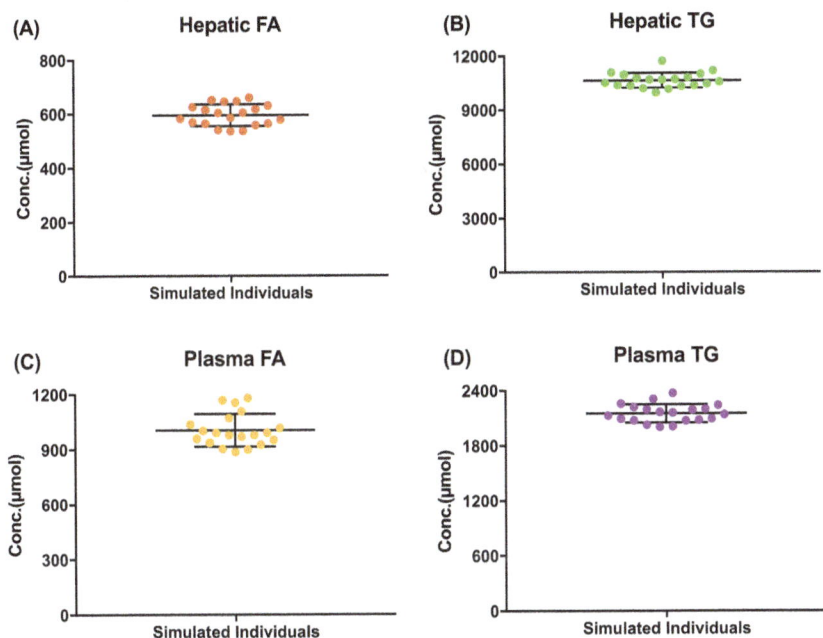

Figure 2.11: The concentrations of lipid compositions for the 20 simulated individuals. (Scatter plots with single value and means ± SD) (A) hepatic FA, (B) hepatic TG, (C) plasma FFA, and (D) plasma TG. (FA: Fatty Acid; TG: Triglycerides).

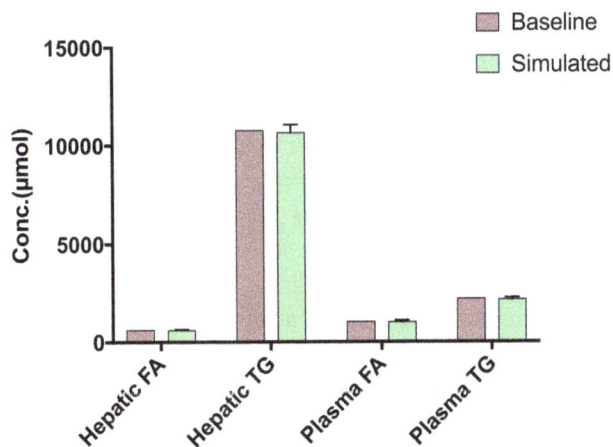

Figure 2.12: The comparisons of four lipid contents between baseline condition and simulated individual average. (FA: Fatty Acid; TG: Triglycerides).

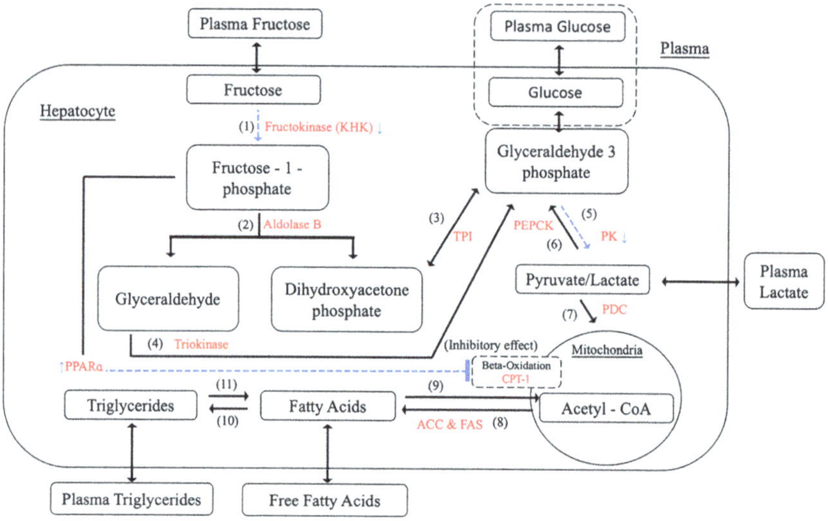

Figure 2.13: Hepatic fructose metabolism with interventional treatments. (The blue dash lines indicate reaction reduction).

fructokinase (KHK), and peroxisome proliferator-activated receptor alpha (PPARα) – were chosen for investigation. The model was used to simulate the effects of modulating these pathways. The rationale behind these targets is that they are three significant components in metabolic regulation.

To be specific, after glucose and fructose metabolisms merging at glyceraldehyde 3 phosphate (GA3P), PK is the rate limiting enzyme to break down GA3P to pyruvate, releasing essential substrates for lipid synthesis. Therefore, inhibiting PK at this point is considered to be a potential intervention which can productively reduce fatty acid synthesis.

As for KHK, this is not limited by adenosine triphosphate (ATP) or citrate availability (as is the case of glucokinase in the glycolytic pathway) as part of the fructose phosphorylation process. Since this reaction is the first step in the fructose metabolism within the liver and it is exclusively contributing to the fructose metabolic pathway, suppressing this process should effectively prevent fructose-induced lipid accumulation.

In terms of PPARα, recent research has shed a new light on its function, but its role in MASLD still remains unclear. It has been reported that the expression of PPARα might be inhibited by high production of fructose-1-phosphate, leading to the decrease of beta-oxidation activity. As a result, the clearance capacity of lipid contents would be impaired, contributing to the development of MASLD. Therefore, PPARα activation is considered as a promising intervention to protect the liver from developing MASLD after fructose over-consumption.

As described in Liao, Davies and Bogle [54], this stage employed a high fructose feeding scenario with each meal containing 62.5 g fructose and 50 g glucose. To represent varying degrees of pro-steatosis, simulations were run under both moderate and severe insulin resistance (IR) conditions. Three potential therapeutic interventions were introduced: suppression of PK, inhibition of KHK, and activation of PPARα. The combined effects of these interventions were also evaluated. This stage aimed to explore the model's effectiveness in predicting the efficacy of these interventions and its suitability for designing new therapeutic approaches.

Figure 2.14 depicts the effects of various interventions on hepatic triglyceride (TG) concentrations under conditions of moderate and severe insulin resistance. The simulations revealed that healthy individuals exhibited a baseline hepatic triglyceride concentration of approximately 11,000 µM after three meals. In contrast, the pro-steatosis condition, which represents a pre-disease state with increased susceptibility to fat accumulation, displayed significantly higher triglyceride levels under both moderate and severe insulin resistance conditions.

In the case of moderate insulin resistance (Figure 2.14(A)), individual interventions targeting PK inhibition, KHK inhibition, and PPARα activation all effectively reduced triglyceride levels back to the healthy baseline. Notably, PPARα activation exhibited the most significant reduction. Combining PK and KHK inhibition also resulted in a remarkable decrease in triglyceride concentration. Interestingly, the combination of KHK inhibition with PPARα activation showed an additive effect, achieving lower triglyceride concentrations compared to either intervention alone. Similarly, combining PPARα activation with PK inhibition yielded comparable results. The most significant reduction in triglyceride levels was achieved by the synergistic action of all three interventions.

However, under severe insulin resistance (Figure 2.14(B)), the model's predictions revealed a rather surprising outcome. Inhibiting PK resulted in a counterintuitive rise in triglyceride production, exceeding even the pro-steatosis levels. Even combining PK and KHK inhibition failed to bring triglyceride levels back to normal.

Conceptually, this unexpected finding might be explained by the Warburg effect, a metabolic phenomenon not explicitly incorporated into the model. The Warburg effect

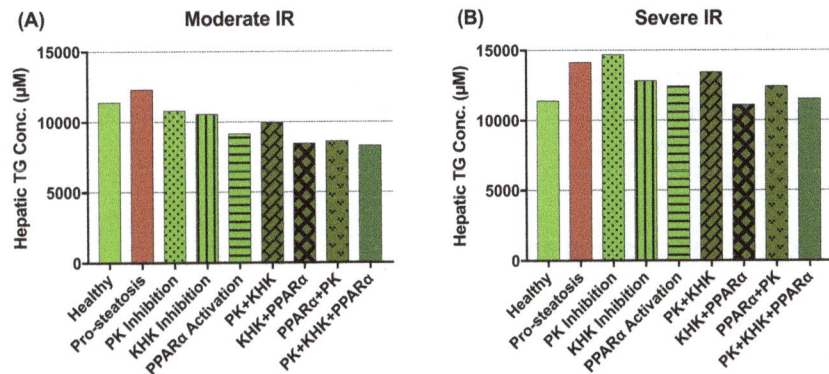

Figure 2.14: The effects of three interventions on hepatic triglycerides under insulin resistance conditions.

eludes catabolic oxidation deliberately to redirect the carbon substrate to generate lipid, protein or other biomass, resulting in the acceleration of cell growth and proliferation [59]. However, the model was built in a less complicated manner that it does not include the feedback mechanisms such as the Warburg effect. Within the model's framework, PK suppression leads to an accumulation of glyceraldehyde 3-phosphate (GA3P). While downstream metabolites following pyruvate are expected to decrease, excess GA3P appears to be diverted towards triglyceride synthesis, causing overproduction.

Despite the unexpected finding under severe insulin resistance, the simulations consistently highlighted the effectiveness of PPARα activation in reducing triglyceride levels, even under severe impaired insulin sensitivity. Additionally, combining interventions shows promise for achieving more substantial therapeutic effects in early-stage MASLD.

Overall, the results obtained throughout all four stages of development support the model's validity and effectiveness in simulating hepatic fructose metabolism and its impact on lipid production. The model demonstrates its potential to be a valuable tool for investigating the relationship between fructose consumption and the development of MASLD, as well as exploring potential therapeutic strategies. The simulations revealed that a synergistic intervention of PK, KHK and PPAR has been tested as the most effective in reducing the triglyceride production under both moderate and severe insulin resistance conditions. This finding highlights the potential of multi-targeted approaches for therapeutic development.

2.6.3 Experimental Assessment

Building on the model's findings, three potential interventional targets were identified: PK, KHK, and PPARα. Since the model focuses on protein levels, subsequent experimental assessment focused on protein analysis. Western blotting and enzymatic activity assays were performed on liver tissue samples from rats fed different diets to assess changes in expression levels and activity rates of these target proteins.

The results (presented in Liao, Davies and Bogle [54]) confirmed that high-fructose feeding in rats with fatty livers led to increased KHK secretion and activity, while PPARα expression was suppressed. These findings support the model's predictions regarding the three interventional targets.

2.6.4 Project Conclusions and Future work

2.6.4.1 Overview

This study employed a systems biology approach to investigate the metabolic mechanisms by which fructose consumption induces dyslipidaemia associated with MASLD, as well as to further explore the potential for reversing pathological conditions during the early stages of the disease.

A computational model of the hepatic fructose metabolism was developed. This kinetic model effectively captures the key features of MASLD and provides valuable qualitative insights for further research. In addition, the robust and detailed model successfully predicted the kinetic relationship between fructose and fatty liver under both healthy and insulin resistant conditions. By integrating model simulations with experimental results, we also identified and evaluated potential interventional targets for treating fructose-induced fatty liver.

The key findings include that the results support the hypothesis that excessive fructose consumption significantly influences MASLD development. Notably, the initial experimental design excluded confounding factors like excessive calorie intake and fat.

Another finding is that high-fructose intake combined with insulin resistance would greatly deteriorate hepatic lipid accumulation. This finding aligns with the proposed mechanism and strengthens the model's potential as a tool for identifying potential interventions.

Last but not least, with three regulatory points being assessed in the computational simulation, arousing KHK secretion and activity as well as suppress PPARα expression was confirmed in the high fructose feeding rats with the fatty livers, suggesting that they are suitable candidates for synergistic therapeutic treatment.

While confident in the model's potential, we acknowledge the need for further validation and expansion. The current limitations include: The model currently is incapable of generating precise quantitative predictions. Secondly, the model is designed for carbohydrate input only, neglecting the complexities of real-world dietary patterns. Thirdly, only acute effects of different carbohydrate diets could be represented by the current model. Simulation over a long period may result in cumulative errors. Last but not least, the structure of the liver is complex and the current simulations consider liver as an overly simplistic model that neglects zonation across the liver plate.

2.6.4.2 Future directions

The most pressing task is to improve the model's ability to generate quantitative predictions that closely match experimental/clinical data. Additional *in vitro* experiments will be conducted to further validate the model. These experiments will focus on inhibiting KHK, activating PPARα, and evaluating the combined effects.

Additionally, the model will be expanded to incorporate protein and fat as dietary inputs, reflecting a more realistic dietary pattern. This necessitates including the corresponding metabolic pathways for protein and fat. Subsequently, the effects of varying macronutrient distributions can be investigated. Also, the current model assumes identical meal sizes and rapid, simplified input. To simulate a more realistic scenario, the model will be refined to account for the passage of food through the digestive system, reflecting a more nuanced liver uptake rate.

In the medium term, the model will be further enhanced to include inflammatory and mitochondrial oxidative stress pathways to gain a deeper understanding of the mechanism of MASLD. This could involve setting a lipid content threshold to trigger cytokine release and integrating interactions between fructose metabolism, insulin resistance, and the innate immune system. Additionally, oxygen concentration will be considered as a factor in oxidative stress modelling.

In the long term, to simulate a more comprehensive biological system, the model could be expanded to integrate metabolism in adipose and muscle tissues, creating a multi-organ network. For a more nuanced understanding, the model could be further refined to incorporate zonated effects within the liver. Furthermore, to reflect the multifactorial and multisystemic nature of MASLD development, the model could be expanded to consider interactions with other diseases like diabetes, chronic kidney disease, and cardiovascular diseases, ultimately constructing a more sophisticated network representing these complex relationships.

By implementing these future directions, the model's accuracy and applicability in studying fructose-induced MASLD and designing therapeutic strategies will be significantly enhanced.

2.6.4.3 Potential impacts

A detailed kinetic model of fructose metabolism was constructed and as a result this computational model can directly serve as a tool to make predictions under both healthy and pathological conditions, providing a better understanding within the liver system. Furthermore, it can be used to identify and test potential interventional targets for MASLD and other related diseases. From a systematic perspective, this research can also be integrated into a more comprehensive and sophisticated biological network platform to explore the intrinsic complexity of human body.

In addition, this project can be beneficial to the subjects in a wider range of scope other than academia.

Firstly, this research enables to elevate the public awareness and facilitate public health policy development. Since asymptomatic liver damage can last for as long as 20 years [12], the majority of people tend to overlook this issue and often fail to realise the occurrence of liver diseases, especially MASLD. Additionally, the outcomes provide the evidence to support and encourage the current public health campaigns like sugar reduction programme to lessen daily fructose intake.

Secondly, the use of the constructed model would be of interest to pharmaceutical industry, as to date, only one pharmaceutical product is available for MASH. Therefore, biomarker identification by modelling can be transferable into diagnostic testing kit intervention and drug production. As reported by the British Liver Trust [12], around 25 %–64 % patients with MASLD would progress to MASH, but only approximately 7 % of which could currently be reversed. Therefore, if the combination therapy proposed by this project was to be successful, this population would be the main beneficiaries.

Last but not least, the ultimate and ideal goal of this project is to improve personalised medicine. This would result in enhancing survival rates and improving life quality for patients. With the aid of systems biology approach and engineering analysis, we can tailor each individual's therapeutic plans through adjusting rates, making the medical treatment more accurate, accessible and affordable.

2.7 Chapter conclusion

We believe that organ modelling *in silico* model systems will have numerous applications in developing future therapeutic strategies and represent a future growth area for disease modelling using the quantitative approaches applied by engineers to complex problems. These systems biology studies need to involve collaborations between engineers and clinical colleagues.

Acknowledgement: The authors would like to thank Professor Karen Louise Thomsen from Aarhus University for generously sharing the rat liver samples.

References

1. Baynes JW, Dominiczak MH. Medical biochemistry, 2nd ed. Philadelphia: Elsevier Mosby; 2005:555 p.
2. Enomoto K, Nishikawa Y, Omori Y, Tokairin T, Yoshida M, Ohi N, et al. Cell biology and pathology of liver sinusoidal endothelial cells. Med Electron Microsc 2004;37:208–15.
3. Hijmans BS, Grefhorst A, Oosterveer MH, Groen AK. Zonation of glucose and fatty acid metabolism in the liver: mechanism and metabolic consequences. Biochimie 2014;96:121–9.
4. Sibulesky, L, Normal liver anatomy. Clini Liver Dis 2013;2. https://doi.org/10.1002/cld.124.
5. Bizeau ME, Pagliassotti MJ. Hepatic adaptations to sucrose and fructose. Metabolism 2005;54:1189–201.
6. Chalhoub E, Hanson RW, Belovich JM. A computer model of gluconeogenesis and lipid metabolism in the perfused liver. Am J Physiol Endocrinol Metab 2007;293:E1676–86.
7. Jungermann K, Katz N. Functional specialization of different hepatocyte populations. Physiol Rev 1989;69: 708–64.
8. Ashworth W. A computational model of hepatic energy metabolism: Understanding the role of zonation in the development and treatment of non-alcoholic fatty liver disease (NAFLD). London: UCL; 2017.
9. Jungermann K, Keitzmann T. Zonation of parenchymal and nonparenchymal metabolism in liver. Annu Rev Nutr 1996;16:179–203.
10. Katz NR. Metabolic heterogeneity of hepatocytes across the liver acinus. J Nutr 1992;122:843–9.
11. Fausto N, Campbell JS, Riehle KJ. Liver regeneration. Hepatology 2006;43. https://doi.org/10.1002/hep.20969.
12. British Liver Trust, The alarming impact of liver disease in the UK 2019 [Online]. Available from: https://britishlivertrust.org.uk/wp-content/uploads/The-alarming-impact-of-liver-disease-FINAL-June-2019.pdf [Accessed 10 Feb 2021].
13. Pratt DS, Kaplan MM. Evaluation of abnormal liver-enzyme results in asymptomatic patients. N Engl J Med 2000;342:1266–71.

14. O'Grady J, Schalm S, Williams R. Acute liver failure: redefining the syndromes. Lancet 1993;342:273–5.
15. Amin AA, Agarwal B, Jalan R. Acute liver failure: updates in pathogenesis and management. Medicine 2019;
    47:838–42.
16. Dong V, Nanchal R, Karvellas CJ. Pathophysiology of acute liver failure. Nutr Clin Pract 2020;35:24–9.
17. Bernal W, Auzinger G, Dhawan A, Wendon J. Acute liver failure. Lancet 2010;376:190–201.
18. Moon AM, Singal AG, Tapper EB. Contemporary epidemiology of chronic liver disease and cirrhosis. Clin
    Gastroenterol Hepatol 2020;18:2650–66.
19. Tsochatzis EA, Bosch J, Burroughs AK. Liver cirrhosis. Lancet 2014;383:1749–61.
20. Williams R, Aspinall R, Bellis M, Camps-Walsh G, Cramp M, Dhawan A, et al. Addressing liver disease in the
    UK: a blueprint for attaining excellence in health care and reducing premature mortality from lifestyle
    issues of excess consumption of alcohol, obesity, and viral hepatitis. Lancet 2014;384:1953–97.
21. Cohen JC, Horton JD, Hobbs HH. Human fatty liver disease: old questions and new insights. Science 2011;
    332:1519–23.
22. Lim JS, Mietus-Snyder M, Valente A, Schwarz JM, Lustig RH. The role of fructose in the pathogenesis of
    NAFLD.and the metabolic syndrome. Nature Rev Gastroenterol Hepatol 2010;7:251–64.
23. Lekakis V, Papatheodoridis GV. Natural history of metabolic dysfunction-associated steatotic liver disease.
    Eur J Intern Med 2023. https://doi.org/10.1016/j.ejim.2023.11.005.
24. Ouyang X, Cirillo P, Sautin Y, McCall S, Bruchette JL, Diehl AM, et al. Fructose consumption as a risk factor for
    non-alcoholic fatty liver disease. J Hepatol 2008;48:993–9.
25. Maldonado EM, Fisher CP, Mazzatti DJ, Barber AL, Tindall MJ, Plant NJ, et al. Multi-scale, whole-system models of
    liver metabolic adaptation to fat and sugar in non-alcoholic fatty liver disease. NPJ Syst Biol Appl 2018;4:1–10.
26. Perumpail BJ, Khan MA, Yoo ER, Cholankeril G, Kim D, Ahmed A. Clinical epidemiology and disease burden
    of nonalcoholic fatty liver disease. World J Gastroenterol 2017;23:8263.
27. Ye Q, Zou B, Yeo YH, Li J, Huang DQ, Wu Y, et al. Global prevalence, incidence, and outcomes of non-obese or
    lean non-alcoholic fatty liver disease: a systematic review and meta-analysis. The Lancet Gastroenterol &
    Hepatol 2020;5:739–52.
28. Younossi ZM, Koenig AB, Abdelatif D, Fazel Y, Henry L, Wymer M. Global epidemiology of nonalcoholic fatty liver
    disease–meta-analytic assessment of prevalence, incidence, and outcomes. Hepatology 2016;64:73–84.
29. Petäjä EM, Yki-Järvinen H. Definitions of normal liver fat and the association of insulin sensitivity with
    acquired and genetic NAFLD. –a systematic review. Inter J Mol Sci 2016;17:633.
30. Fracanzani AL, Valenti L, Bugianesi E, Andreoletti M, Colli A, Vanni E, et al. Risk of severe liver disease in
    nonalcoholic fatty liver disease with normal aminotransferase levels: a role for insulin resistance and
    diabetes. Hepatology 2008;48:792–8.
31. Younossi ZM, Loomba R, Rinella ME, Bugianesi E, Marchesini G, Neuschwander-Tetri BA, et al. Current and
    future therapeutic regimens for nonalcoholic fatty liver disease and nonalcoholic steatohepatitis.
    Hepatology 2018;68:361–71.
32. Sarma S, Palcu P. Weight loss between glucagon-like peptide-1 receptor agonists and bariatric surgery in
    adults with obesity: a systematic review and meta-analysis. Obesity 2022;30:2111–21.
33. Zelber–Sagi S, Kessler A, Brazowsky E, Webb M, Lurie Y, Santo M, et al. A double-blind randomized placebo-
    controlled trial of orlistat for the treatment of nonalcoholic fatty liver disease. Clin Gastroenterol Hepatol
    2006;4:639–44.
34. Stokkeland K, Lageborn CT, Ekbom A, Höijer J, Bottai M, Stål P, et al. Statins and angiotensin-converting
    enzyme inhibitors are associated with reduced mortality and morbidity in chronic liver disease. Basic Clin
    Pharmacol Toxicol 2018;122:104–10.
35. Mazza A. The role of metformin in the management of NAFLD. Exp Diabet Res 2011:2012.
36. Dibba P, Li AA, Perumpail BJ, John N, Sallam S, Shah ND, et al. Emerging therapeutic targets and
    experimental drugs for the treatment of NAFLD. Diseases 2018;6:83.

37. Nguyen M, Asgharpour A, Dixon DL, Sanyal AJ, Mehta A. Emerging therapies for MASLD and their impact on plasma lipids. Am J Prevent Cardiol 2024;17. https://doi.org/10.1016/j.ajpc.2024.100638.

38. Kokkorakis M. Resmetirom, the first approved drug for the management of metabolic dysfunction-associated steatohepatitis: trials, opportunities, and challenges. Metab Clin Exp 2024;154.

39. Douard V, Ferraris RP. The role of fructose transporters in diseases linked to excessive fructose intake. J Physiol 2013;591:401–14.

40. Giussani M, Lieti G, Orlando A, Parati G, Genovesi S. Fructose intake, hypertension and cardiometabolic risk factors in children and adolescents: from pathophysiology to clinical aspects. A narrative review. Front Med 2022;9. https://doi.org/10.3389/fmed.2022.792949.

41. Public Health England and the Food Standards Agency, National diet and nutrition survey rolling programme years 9 to 11 (2016/2017 to 2018/2019) 2020. Available from: https://www.gov.uk/government/statistics/ndns-results-from-years-9-to-11-2016-to-2017-and-2018-to-2019 [Accessed 10 Feb 2021].

42. Basaranoglu M. Fructose as a key player in the development of fatty liver disease. World J Gastroenterol 2013;19:1166–72.

43. Berg J, Tymoczko J, Stryer L. Chapter 16, glycolysis and gluconeogenesis. Biochemistry. New York: W. H. Freeman; 2002.

44. Laughlin M. Normal roles for dietary fructose in carbohydrate metabolism. Nutrients 2014;6:3117–29.

45. Rutledge AC, Adeli K. Fructose and the metabolic syndrome: pathophysiology and molecular mechanisms. Nutr Rev 2007;65:13–23.

46. Havel PJ. Dietary fructose: implications for dysregulation of energy homeostasis and lipid/carbohydrate metabolism. Nutr Rev 2005;63:133–57.

47. Ideker T, Galitski T, Hood L. A new approach to decoding life: systems biology. Annu Rev Genom Hum Genet 2001;2:343–72.

48. Allen RJ, Musante CJ. Modeling fructose-load-induced hepatic de-novo lipogenesis by model simplification. Gene Regul Syst Biol 2017;11. https://doi.org/10.1177/1177625017690133.

49. Allen RJ, Musante CJ. A mathematical analysis of adaptations to the metabolic fate of fructose in essential fructosuria subjects. Am J Physiol Endocrinol Metab 2018;315:E394–03.

50. Jensen T, Abdelmalek MF, Sullivan S, Nadeau KJ, Green M, Roncal C, et al. Fructose and sugar: a major mediator of non-alcoholic fatty liver disease. J Hepatol 2018;68:1063–75.

51. Sellmann C, Priebs J, Landmann M, Degen C, Engstler AJ, Jin CJ, et al. Diets rich in fructose, fat or fructose and fat alter intestinal barrier function and lead to the development of nonalcoholic fatty liver disease over time. J Nutr Biochem 2015;26:1183–92.

52. Schultz A, Barbosa-da-Silva S, Aguila MB, Mandarim-de-Lacerda CA. Differences and similarities in hepatic lipogenesis, gluconeogenesis and oxidative imbalance in mice fed diets rich in fructose or sucrose. Food Funct 2015;6:1684–91.

53. Nomura K, Yamanouchi T. The role of fructose-enriched diets in mechanisms of nonalcoholic fatty liver disease. J Nutr Biochem 2012;23:203–8.

54. Liao Y, Davies NA, Bogle IDL. A process systems Engineering approach to analysis of fructose consumption in the liver system and consequences for Non-Alcoholic fatty liver disease. Chem Eng Sci 2022;263. https://doi.org/10.1016/j.ces.2022.118131.

55. Liao Y, Davies NA, Bogle IDL. Computational Modeling of fructose Metabolism and Development in NAFLD. Front Bioeng Biotechnol 2020;8. https://doi.org/10.3389/fbioe.2020.00762.

56. Patel C, Sugimoto K, Douard V, Shah A, Inui H, Yamanouchi T, et al. Effect of dietary fructose on portal and systemic serum fructose levels in rats and in KHK–/– and GLUT5–/– mice. Am J Physiol Gastrointest Liver Physiol 2015;309:G779–90.

57. Chong MF, Fielding BA, Frayn KN. Mechanisms for the acute effect of fructose on postprandial lipemia. Am J Clin Nutr 2007;85:1511–20.

58. Low WS, Cornfield T, Charlton CA, Tomlinson JW, Hodson L. Sex differences in hepatic de novo lipogenesis with acute fructose feeding. Nutrients 2018;10:1263.
59. Liberti MV, Locasale JW. The Warburg effect: how does it benefit cancer cells? Trends Biochem Sci 2016;41: 211–18.

Tomasz R. Sosnowski* and Arkadiusz K. Kuczaj

3 Inhaled aerosols as carriers of pulmonary medicines and the limitations of *in vitro– in vivo* correlation (IVIVC) methods

Abstract: Pulmonary drug delivery (PDD) involves flow and deposition of aerosol particles acting as carriers of drugs delivered onto the surface of the airways. As a direct consequence, optimal PDD requires controlling of drug aerosolization processes and deep understanding of multiphase flows in complex geometry of the airways including aerosol particle dynamics during the transient inhalation cycles. A chemical engineering-based approache can be effectively used to analyze these processes and help in designing optimized drug formulations and more effective drug delivery devices (inhalers). One of prerequisites of improved PDD is the knowledge of *in vivo–in vitro* correlation (IVIVC) for inhaled drugs that would allow establishment of the relationships between aerosol quality determined using *ex vivo* methods (such as determination of particle size, deposition in reconstructed anatomical structures, pharmacokinetics/pharmacodynamics using *in vitro* cellular systems, or *in silico* modeling of aerosol dynamics) in connection to the clinical effects. This manuscript discusses the challenges of the IVIVC analyses for aerosol delivery systems. The primary focus is given to the physical and physicochemical constraints in the PDD that can be effectively described and investigated using engineering approaches.

Keywords: aerosols; inhaled medicines; inhalers; testing methods; computational analysis; IVIVC

Abbreviations

ACI	Andersen cascade impactor
AINI	Alberta idealized nasal inlet
AIT	Alberta idealized throat
API	active pharmaceutical ingredient
CFD	computational fluid dynamics
COPD	chronic obstructive pulmonary disease
CT	computer tomography

*Corresponding author: Tomasz R. Sosnowski, Faculty of Chemical and Process Engineering, Warsaw University of Technology, Warynskiego 1, 00-645 Warsaw, Poland, E-mail: tomasz.sosnowski@pw.edu.pl. https://orcid.org/0000-0002-6775-3766

Arkadiusz K. Kuczaj, Department of Applied Mathematics, Faculty EEMCS, University of Twente, Enschede, The Netherlands; and PMI R&D, Philip Morris Products S.A., Quai Jeanrenaud 5, Neuchâtel, Switzerland

As per De Gruyter's policy this article has previously been published in the journal Physical Sciences Reviews. Please cite as: T. R. Sosnowski and A. K. Kuczaj "Inhaled aerosols as carriers of pulmonary medicines and the limitations of *in vitro–in vivo* correlation (IVIVC) methods" *Physical Sciences Reviews* [Online] 2024. DOI: 10.1515/psr-2024-0054 | https://doi.org/10.1515/9783111394558-003

DD	delivered dose, μg
DPI	dry powder inhaler
ED	emitted dose, μg
EMA	European Medicine Agency
FEV1	forced expiratory volume in 1 s, mL
FDA	Food and Drug Administration
FPD	fine particle dose, μg
FPF	fine particle fraction, %
HFA	hydrofluoroalkane
IoT	*Internet of Things*
IP	inertial parameter, μm^2 kg/min
IVIVC	in vivo-in vitro correlation
LRT	lower respiratory tract
MHRA	Medicines and Healthcare Products Regulatory Agency
MMAD	mass median aerodynamic diameter, μm
MPPD	multi-path particle dosimetry model
MRI	magnetic resonance imaging
NGI	next generation impactor
ND	nominal dose
OIP	orally inhaled products
PBPK	physiologically-based pharmacokinetics
PD	pharmacodynamics
PDD	pulmonary drug delivery
PEF	peak expiratory flow, mL/s
PIF	peak inspiratory flow, mL/s
PK	pharmacokinetics
PMDA	Pharmaceuticals and Medical Devices Agency
pMDI	pressurized metered dose inhaler
PSD	particle size distribution
QIVIVE	quantitative *in vitro* to *in vivo* extrapolation
RS	respiratory system
SMI	soft mist inhaler
URT	upper respiratory tract
USP	United States Pharmacopeia
VMN	vibrating mesh nebulizer

3.1 Introduction

Contemporary chemical engineering expands into new domains that extend beyond traditional industrial applications and technologies. Using the quantitative approach to multiphase flows and mass transfer phenomena [1], as fundamental pillars of the discipline, chemical engineering provides helpful methods in solving the challenges of physiology and medicine [2]. A straightforward example is the analysis of the flow and deposition of inhaled aerosol particles in the human respiratory system (RS) [3]. Airborne particles suspended in the atmospheric air, occupational environments or aerosolized medicines are inhaled and transported in the RS. Their behavior is governed by the physical principles that are identical as in many technological processes, such as pneumatic conveying or dust separation. Consequently, both experimental investigations and mathematical modeling of aerosol behavior in the RS should take advantage of methodologies commonly used in the chemical engineering, which is based on principles of chemistry, physics, mathematics, and biology.

On the other hand, specific features of aerosol inhalation have no direct analogy to the industrial systems. The respiratory flow is intrinsically unsteady and periodic (inspiration–expiration). In this case, adoption of the constant-flow approach, often present in the industrial processes, neglects the dynamic phenomena and leads to imprecise or incorrect results. The analysis is also complicated by other factors, especially regarding predictions of health effects from the mathematical modeling of particle deposition in the respiratory system and experiments that can be done *in vitro*. In general, this translation is called *in vivo-in vitro* correlation (IVIVC) [1, 4], and it is equally important both in pharmacotherapy and in assessing unfavorable effects of aerosol inhalation, where it is known as the quantitative *in vitro* to *in vivo* extrapolation (QIVIVE) [5]. Developed assessment methods are commonly used and established in assessing oral drugs dissolution, release and absorption [6]. In case of aerosol inhalation such evaluation requires detailed information on the physicochemical characteristics of tested substances including their physiological potential to be delivered and deposited in the human lungs. All alterations and losses of the initially released nominal dose (ND) present in the aerosol must be accounted in this process starting from the exposure and leading to biologically effective dose [7, 8].

This manuscript discusses the major challenges in IVIVC of inhaled aerosols, focusing mainly on inhalation therapy of the RS with aerosolized drugs. It starts in Section 3.2 with the general definition of IVIVC for inhaled aerosols, mainly pharmaceuticals although, in general, these concepts can be extended to all inhaled airborne particles regardless of their origin. In Section 3.3, the basics of aerosol dynamics in the respiratory system when delivered from different medical inhalers are presented. This part demonstrates the essential contribution that can be offered by chemical engineering to the analysis and mathematical modeling of aerosol flow and deposition mechanisms. In addition, chemical aerosol engineering also contributes to development of the reproducible generation methods for micrometer-size solid or liquid particles required for accurate drug dosing. In Section 3.4, drug devices for inhalation therapies are briefly summarized. Next, in Section 3.5, the basic limitations in IVIVC caused by the standard methods of aerosol characterization application are discussed, including particle size distribution (PSD) determination, inter-patient variability and related to adherence issues associated with human errors in using aerosol inhalers (presented in Section 3.6). These topics also may benefit from the chemical engineering-based approach to the understanding the critical factors of the correct inhaler design and operation with various aerosolization principles, taking an advantage of analogies to the equipment often used in the process engineering. The consequences of the discussed issues on the characteristics and assessment of generic inhalation products for inhalation are addressed in Section 3.7. Finally, in Section 3.8, perspectives and suggestions to improve the IVIVC of inhaled drugs by technical (engineering) means are outlined.

3.2 The IVIVC problem for inhaled aerosols

The IVIVC for inhaled aerosols is focused on finding trustworthy relationships between the actual clinical response of inhaled medicines and quantitative data obtained by technical characterization and assessment methods: *in vitro* experiments (e.g., PSD determination, aerosol deposition in anatomical casts), but also by computational analysis of aerosol delivery and deposition in the RS (*in silico* approach). Most often the IVIVC seeks the quantitative translation from the aerosol PSD measured according to the pharmacopeial standards [9] to the real lung deposition [10]. However, the IVIVC can be broadened to the quantitative extrapolation of the results of *in vitro* experiments that are focused on deposition in the anatomical models of the RS (e.g., [11]) or on the kinetics of drug release rate (they include pharmacokinetics/pharmacodynamics [PK/PD] [12]) to the *in vivo* effects of drug delivery to the lungs. The PK/PD issue is essential in the bioequivalence assessment of generic drugs with the originator [13], but also finds its applications in the safety or toxicological studies of inhaled aerosols of various origin [5, 14, 15]. The importance of physiologically based pharmacokinetic (PBPK) modeling for the toxicity assessment that can be directly linked with the prediction of reliable deposited doses of inhaled aerosols is also identified [16]. The IVIVC will be discussed here in this broader sense, by analyzing the relationships between various data that can be acquired using *in vitro* experiments and *in silico* computations with the clinical response recognized as the ultimate *in vivo* effect of aerosol inhalation.

Most *in vitro* studies in the field of pulmonary drug delivery (PDD) provide valuable insights into the formulation properties of inhalation medicines, however, they still have a limited application in predicting the *in vivo* effects of inhaled drugs. Similarly, *in silico* computational fluid dynamics (CFD) analyses predicting aerosol behavior in the respiratory tract can be useful in identifying the fundamental phenomena of particles motion in some structures of the RS. Unfortunately, they can be hardly used to calculate the aerosol deposition process on the larger scale (lung delivery) that would help to predict the *in vivo* effects of inhalation. On the contrary, existing simple reduced-order (0D or 1D) modeling methods predicting the whole-lung aerosol delivery (e.g., NCRP, MPPD [17–19]) are suffering limited multiscale, multiphase and multispecies aerosol dynamics capabilities.

Preceding the more detailed discussion, we list the essential limiting factors currently responsible for the inadequate IVIVC of inhaled aerosols, which are as follows:

(1)   The standard size determination techniques of aerosol particles generated from inhaling devices oversimplify the actual dynamics of aerosol formation and flow both in the inhalers and the RS,

(2) Experimental and computational studies are typically done for healthy lungs, whereas the clinical efficacy of inhaled medicines is usually determined for diseased patients,
(3) The results of direct deposition imaging in the lungs that are used to verify *in vitro* predictions are relatively scarce and available mainly for healthy volunteers due to use of radionuclide contrasting agents [20, 21],
(4) CFD approaches cannot model the whole RS geometry down to the alveoli due to RS complexity and number of bronchial/bronchiolar tubes (up to 3×10^5 in Yeh–Schum morphometric model [22]),
(5) The reduced-order whole-lung models do not provide required aerosol dynamics complexity present in the CFD, while most of the CFD approaches do not deliver validated treatments of multiphase air-particle and particle-particle interactions,
(6) Commonly applied endpoints of the clinical response do not provide the data that can be directly associated with the particle deposition in the RS,
(7) Patient variability (anatomy, respiratory physiology/breathing patterns) does not allow the construction of a "universal" airway model for experimental or *in silico* studies,
(8) Patient adherence to the inhaler is typically neglected in *ex vivo* studies, but it is often critical for *in vivo* results,
(9) Drug delivery and its bioavailability is not the same and universal for different molecules and formulations.

Most of these limitations will be discussed further in more detail starting from the overall characteristics of the technical issues of drug delivery by inhalation.

3.3 Basics of aerosol dynamics in the respiratory system

Airborne particles can enter the RS assuming they are smaller than 10–20 μm in size, as larger objects are suspended in the air only for a short time and they quickly sediment due to the gravitational force [23]. During the flow in the anatomical structures of the RS, inhaled particles are sequentially filtered out in the upper respiratory tract, URT (mouth or nose, throat, pharynx) and then in the lower respiratory tract, LRT (bronchial tree and pulmonary region) [3]. Aerosol separation in the URT and trachea is mainly due to inertial effects (impaction on the walls of the airways) since the local flow velocity is the highest compared to other parts of the RS. Airway narrowing (e.g., in the nose and larynx) and bends (in the nasopharynx and throat) additionally enhance the inertial deposition of the heaviest objects, eliminating particles larger than approximately 5 μm. The efficiency of this process depends not only on the size of particles (diameter, d_p) but also on their density ρ_p, and on the local velocity u, which is proportional to the actual volumetric flow rate Q. The impaction parameter (IP) is often used to analyze particle deposition in the URT due to inertial mechanisms:

$$IP = Q d_p^2 \rho_p \tag{3.1}$$

The inertial interactions can be also described by the Stokes number, Stk, which is a dimensionless number that relates inertial forces acting on a particle to the resistance (viscous) forces of the fluid (in this case, air) with the viscosity μ, acting on the particle in a geometry with the characteristic dimension d_0 (typically, effective diameter of the airway):

$$Stk = \frac{u \rho_p d_p^2}{18 \mu \, d_o} \tag{3.2}$$

In contrast to *IP*, the Stokes number considers the individual anatomical factors of the RS. For cylindrical air channels modeling trachea or bronchi, the relationship between both parameters can be written as:

$$Stk = \frac{2}{9\pi} \frac{IP}{\mu d_o^3} \tag{3.3}$$

Usually, Q and u in equations (3.1)–(3.3) are assumed constant at a given location in the RS, which neglects airflow unsteadiness during the inhalation process. As the most often approximation, either the average or the peak inspiratory flow (PIF), is used in calculations of particle deposition due to the inertial forces [24]. For the adult oral cavity, the following equation describing the aerosol deposition efficiency, E, has been proposed based on the *in vitro* (cast) experiments:

$$E = 1 - \exp(-a\,Stk) \tag{3.4}$$

where $a = 19.2 \pm 1.2$ is valid for Q range of 15–60 dm³/min [25]. Analogous equations can be obtained for pediatric airways and for the nasal deposition in both age groups [24].

In the LRT, which is modeled as consisted of a system of branching (bifurcating) tubes, the consecutive airways become narrower, but their number strongly increases, according to 2^n rule where n denotes airway generation ($n = 0$ for trachea). Accordingly, the total cross-section area of all tubes in each next bronchial generation is larger so the local velocities are smaller than in the URT airways at a given Q. Consequently, the inertial impaction in the LRT becomes ineffective as deposition mechanism. Inertial deposition in the LRT is less important also due to the largest particles (i.e., with $d_p > 5$ μm) have already been removed from the inhaled aerosol in the URT. The primary deposition mechanism of particles smaller than 5 μm flowing at reduced velocity, known as "fine particles", is gravitational sedimentation. This mechanism becomes quite efficient if the LRT where the settling length (i.e., particle distance to the wall) is shortening and particle residence time becomes longer due to a slower flow. Particles that have not been deposited in bronchi and bronchioles penetrate to the alveolar region. They can settle down gravitationally (if $d_p > 1$ μm), deposit by Brownian diffusion (if $d_p \ll 1$ μm), or not

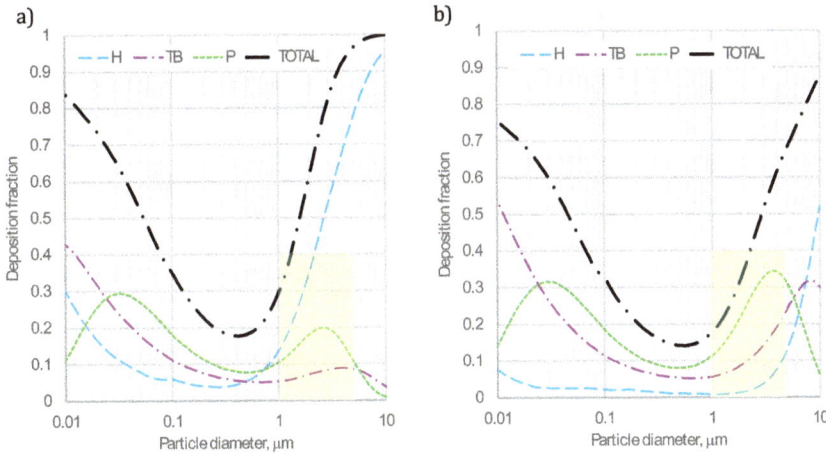

Figure 3.1: Comparison of particle deposition fraction in different regions of the respiratory system for nasal (a) and oral (b) breathing: H – head airways (URT), TB – tracheobronchial tree, P – pulmonary region. Based on the calculations using MPPD model for the symmetrical lung structure, standard RS volumes and tidal breathing [19]. Yellow fields show the particle size-range (1–5 μm) that is most desired in inhalation therapy of the lower respiratory tract.

deposit at all, so eventually many of them can be exhaled. The general description of the fate of inhaled particles in the RS was presented in more detail elsewhere [26]. Representative deposition plots for nasal and oral breathing are presented in Figure 3.1. They show that deposition efficiency of 0.1–1 μm particles in the RS equals only 20–30 %, meaning that these particles are exhaled. This is under assumption that they do not evolve and change their size in the lungs, which is often not the case due to the hygroscopic growth. Since particles smaller than 0.3–0.5 μm either are absent in the aerosols released by the inhalers or the amount of a drug they carry is very low, particles with the aerodynamic size of 1–5 μm are considered as the most useful in PDD.

The most essential information concerning devices used to deliver aerosols to the lungs is highlighted in the next section. This overview provides specific, related issues in prediction of the IVIVC of inhaled drugs.

3.4 Drug delivery devices for inhalation therapies

Currently marketed types of devices used to aerosolize drugs for the lung delivery are listed in Table 3.1, along with their basic technical characteristics and limitations of use.

Nebulizers are the oldest but still important class of devices used in the PDD [27, 28]. From an engineering point of view, these devices are based on the liquid atomization process. Occasionally, they are equipped with pre-separators (baffle system) to separate and recycle the largest particles and allow for the emission of an aerosol with the

Table 3.1: The basic technical characteristics of medical inhalers.

Class of inhalers	Subtype	Form of a medicament	Aerosol generation mechanism	Limitations and other remarks	Typical mode of operation
Nebulizers	Jet (pneumatic)	Liquid (solution or suspension)	Liquid atomization	Not suitable for drug molecules sensitive to high stresses	Constant output during tidal breathing; valved systems for aerosol holding is possible
	Ultrasound	Liquid (solution)		Liquid rheology; not suitable for drug molecules sensitive to heat	Constant output during tidal breathing
	Vibrating mesh (VMN)	Liquid (solution or suspension)		Liquid rheology; size of drug particles in suspension	Constant output during tidal breathing
Dry powder inhalers (DPI)	Single dose (capsule) Multi-dose pre-metered (powder in blisters) Multi-dose metered (powder in a reservoir)	Micronized API with or without lactose as excipient	Powder fluidization and deagglomeration	Humidity, electric charge, flow-dependence; difficult to use properly (compliance)	Dose delivered during single inhalation
Pressurized metered dose inhalers (pMDI)	Manually activated Breath-actuated	Solution or suspension in the liquified carrier gas (HFA)	Liquid atomization and flash evaporation of volatile solvent	Coordination errors (compliance) No coordination errors; more complicated and expansive inhaler	Dose delivered during single inhalation; holding chamber can be used to improve the compliance and reduce URT deposition
Soft mist inhalers (SMI)		Liquid (solution)	Liquid atomization	Less prone to coordination errors (longer puff duration)	Dose delivered during single inhalation

required PSD. Unlike other types of inhaling devices, such as pressurized metered dose inhalers (pMDIs), dry powder inhalers (DPIs), and soft mist inhalers (SMIs) that are available as unique medical products (drug-device combination: the inhaler with the drug formulation of a certain active pharmaceutical ingredient [API] concentration), nebulizers are more universal medical devices that can be used to atomize a variety of liquid drugs. This feature leads to the questions whether aerosol properties remain the same if (i) a given drug is atomized in various nebulizers and (ii) different drugs are atomized in the same nebulizer. Influence of physicochemical properties of atomized liquids, such as surface tension, viscosity, and ionic strength, on the mass output rate and PSD of the aerosol emitted from nebulizers are reported [29–31]. The actual effects depend not only on the nebulization principle which is different for jet, ultrasonic, and vibrating mesh devices, but also on the specific features of each nebulizer (internal design of the nebulizing vessel and mouthpiece, applied air pressure or ultrasound energy/frequency, material of the mesh, etc.) Therefore, despite the wide knowledge gathered from the atomization processes applied in numerous engineering problems, the setting up of general rules describing the relationships between drug properties and aerosol quality for all nebulizers, or even for nebulizers of the same class but with different construction, is impossible. The situation becomes even more complicated for nebulized suspensions, where the size of micronized drug particles present in the liquid phase (typically, in the physiological salt solution) and their tendency to aggregation can be quite different, even for generic drugs with the same API concentration [32].

A possible shift in the PSD of emitted particles caused by different drug properties must be always considered in the performed IVIVC since nebulizers are tested by manufacturers according to the ISO standard, only for the physiological salt or a few other solutions (2.5 % NaF aq. or albuterol sulfate) [33]. Accordingly, the PSD and mass output of aerosol generated in a device using the specific API (e.g., steroid suspensions, mucolytics, antibiotics, etc.) is not known *a priori* and should be determined for each drug-device combination. Reliable data on the PSD are crucial as they are needed to predict the likelihood of regional drug deposition in the RS.

On the other hand, knowing that aerosol properties depend on physicochemical properties of atomized liquid offers a possibility to tune the regional drug deposition, e.g., by adding small amounts of bio-compatible and biologically safe compounds to change viscosity or the surface tension of the aerosolized solution [34, 35]. This strategy can lead to a better drug targeting to specific lung regions in the personalized aerosol therapy.

Table 3.1 lists some factors related to the real-life inhaler use that affect the actual efficacy of inhalation therapy and are important in the further discussion of the IVIVC. Some limitations are expected to be alleviated by the so-called "smart inhalers," which can eliminate basic errors associated with the use of the inhalers. These aspects will be discussed in the next sections.

3.5 Aerosol characterization assessment methods

Inhalation products are tested according to pharmaceutical standards under controlled conditions. These differ from those encountered during actual use of inhalers by the patients. Artificial and reproducible testing conditions ignore the issue of patient-to-patient variability and compliance, i.e., good inhaler use technique. This reduces the accuracy of the IVIVC predictions for the actual translational purpose.

The recommended and most common methods used to assess the quality of aerosols emitted from inhalers or nebulizers are based on standard tests established for the pharmaceutical inhalation products. The pharmaceutical industry typically applies these protocols to evaluate or confirm product stability and reproducibility of API delivery. Consequently, they follow pharmacopeial recommendations [9] or guidelines issued by regulatory agencies such as the FDA (Food and Drug Administration – USA), EMA (European Medicines Agency – EU), MHRA (Medicines and Healthcare Products Regulatory Agency – UK), PMDA (Pharmaceuticals and Medical Devices Agency – Japan), Health Canada, etc (see [36] for more details). These recommendations are predominantly focused on the quality of pharmaceutical products to assure dosing reproducibility rather than addressing the problem of clinical efficiency. The regulations for orally inhaled products (OIP) demand a demonstration of the consistency of the emitted dose (ED) or the delivered dose (DD), and fine particle dose FPD (the dose contained in particles smaller than 5 μm in the aerodynamic diameter) in each aerosol portion released during the product's lifetime. Cascade impactors devices (e.g., Andersen cascade impactor [ACI], next generation impactor [NGI]) are required by the Pharmacopoeia as a standard for the PSD measurements [9]. The inertial separation principle applied in the impactors allows to determine the mass-based PSD at a fixed flow rate for which the cut-off sizes on each impactor stage are known. Such tests are usually done for a single airflow rate, but sometimes different rates are used if the flow-dependency of aerosol release from the inhaler is expected [36]. Consequently, both ED and FPD are determined at the steady flow conditions. Although such results allow assessing the quality of inhalation products, they do not reflect the actual flow conditions during inhalation, which are intrinsically unsteady. As a direct consequence, the standard PSD determination methods may blur the actual process of aerosol entrainment in the inhaler and particles motion in the airways.

Temporal characteristics of respiratory physiology (breathing) and aerosol emission in different types of inhaling devices are schematically shown in Figure 3.2. It is seen, for instance, that nebulizers release the aerosol continuously (unless equipped with systems for holding the aerosol during exhalation [37]) whereas the inhalation flow varies (Figure 3.2a). As already mentioned, the API can enter the body only during the inspiration cycle, so all aerosol emitted during exhalation or breath-hold period is released to the surroundings (so-called, fugitive aerosol). In this way, the drug is not only wasted but potentially contributes to unwanted exposure of bystanders [38].

It also means that nominal dose, emitted dose and delivered dose are not equal although sometimes they are considered as the same. In nebulizers of simple design, ED will be significantly higher than DD [38]. Similarly, in pMDIs, the dose released (ED) will not equal the dose that enters the RS (DD) if inhalation is not properly synchronized with aerosol generation (i.e., pressing the canister), Figures 3.2d,e. In addition, emitted doses

a) Continuously operating nebulizer (without valving system)

c)

b) DPI - Dry Powder Inhaler (passive)

pMDI - pressurized Metered Dose Inhaler (without holding chamber)

d) e)

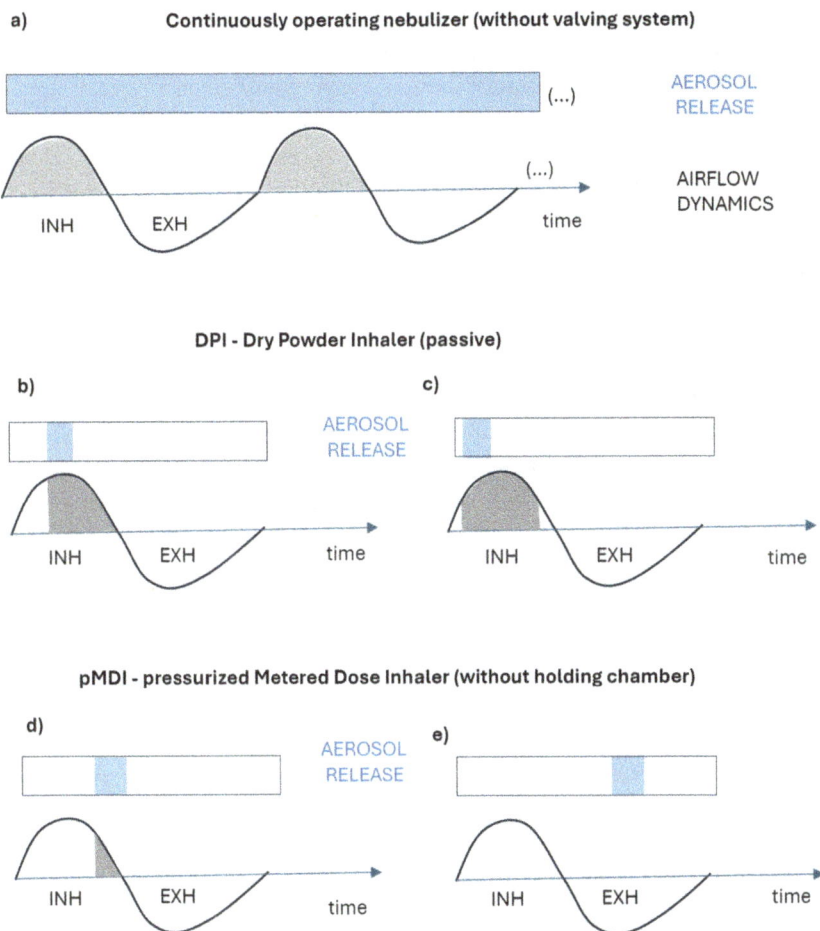

Figure 3.2: Airflow dynamics during inhalation–exhalation (breathing curves) and temporal aerosol release from nebulizers and inhalers (blue areas). Grey areas below the breathing curves show the fraction of the breath where aerosol can enter the organism (delivered dose). The airflow patterns are shown schematically (the actual flow characteristics during the continuous use of nebulizers are different than for single breath through DPIs or pMDIs).

will be lower than the nominal doses due to losses inside of the device and accompanied spacers or holding chambers [39].

Aerosol generation in nebulizers does not depend on the patients' breath, so aerosol quality, characterized by fine particle dose (FPD) or fine particle fraction (FPF), should be the same regardless of the breathing pattern. However, if a patient inhales an additional volume of dry air which is mixed with the aerosol emitted from a nebulizer, particles will encounter modulated hygroscopic growth in the humid mouth atmosphere, leading to a change in the PSD and potential partitioning of the API between the phases, and consequently modulation of the inhaled aerosol distribution and absorption in the RS. Obviously, dry and warm air promotes faster particle evaporation, which will affect the aerosol PSD. According to the *d*-square law of evaporation, smallest particles can completely evaporate leaving only ultrafine residues, whereas the diameter of larger particles will be visibly reduced [40]. Consequently, the aerosol that enters the RS will have a lower MMAD and higher FPD than aerosol that leaves the nebulizer without admixing of ambient air. As the entry conditions will be modulated, these will have impact on the hygroscopic growth of the particles further in the RS. This shows that assessing the IVIVC also should consider the real-life conditions of inhalation using nebulizers and the analysis of possible change in the PSD due to mass and heat exchange with air simultaneously drawn by a patient. Additionally, the particle sizing method itself can be a source of increased particle evaporation causing a bias in the measured PSD. Cascade impactors are made of metal, and when their temperature is higher than for the aerosol emitted from the nebulizer (which is common for jet nebulizers that cool the aerosol liquid due to gas expansion from the nozzles), the particle size is reduced during flow through the impactor, resulting in smaller measured particles than originally emitted. Therefore, cooling the impactor before the measurement is proposed to avoid this problem [41–43], and this procedure was recently added to pharmacopeial recommendations [9], but not the ISO standard [33]. Such situation caused some confusions in the assessment of the quality of aerosols delivered from the nebulizers.

Taking into account that the generated aerosol enters the mouth or nose almost immediately after leaving the nebulizer, it seems more appropriate to determine the PSD directly at the nebulizer outlet instead of aerosol classification in cascade impactors, which is associated with a risk of the ambiguous results. PSD measurements at the nebulizer outlet can be conveniently done using optical methods such as laser diffraction spectrometry [44]. These methods give the exact information about the API mass contained in particles of each size fraction in case of nebulized solutions assuming API concentration in the liquid aerosol is the same regardless of the particle size. Such assumption can be violated for the volatile APIs and nebulized suspensions where the mass of API crystals can be disproportionate to the particle volume. It is also possible that the smallest aerosol particles (1–2 μm) of nebulized suspension do not contain API if crystal sizes in the suspensions [5] are bigger than the particle diameter [32, 45].

Ambient conditions during nebulization can also affect the size of inhaled particles by influencing the atomization process. A specific and convincing example is the influence of the conditions in a subterranean spa in the salt mine (135 m below the ground level) where nebulization is often used as additional treatment for the patients with pulmonary diseases [46]. Jet nebulizers generate larger aerosol particles in such conditions compared to nebulization done on the Earth's surface (i.e., at room temperature and air with a relatively low humidity). This can be attributed to the reduced evaporation of particles during the atomization process. In this case colder and humidified air (13 °C, up to 80 % relative humidity) is drawn into the compressor, which generates a jet of atomizing air that further increases the viscosity of the liquid due to cooling [47]. Interestingly, no effect on the PSD was observed for VMNs, which confirms that observed particle evaporation was mainly due to extensive heat and mass transfer processes between aerosol particles and the ambient air in the jet nebulizer.

Since penetration and deposition of inhaled aerosols depend on the particle size, accurate particle sizing is one of the key factors in IVIVC. However, a widely discussed problem of unsatisfactory IVIVC has been focused on the impactor inlet (known as "USP throat") and the concepts of its substitution by an anatomically correct model of the URT [10]. In our opinion, these concepts can lead to additional uncertainties and confusion. Compendial impactors or impingers (ACI, NGI and others) are particle classifiers and should not be considered as adequate simplifications of the lung models. Therefore, their inlet does not necessarily mimic the oropharynx, as the common name "USP throat" may suggest. This bent metal tube is used to redirect the aerosol flow from the horizontal position, which is characteristic for the standard inhaler usage, to the vertical flow alignment allowing the aerosol to enter the separation stages. Each impactor stage is characterized by a specific cut-off (separation) aerodynamic diameter of aerosol particles for a given airflow rate, whereas no defined cut-off diameter is attributed to the "USP throat" [9]. Adopting a realistic URT model at the impactor inlet can falsify the PSD determined by the particle sizing device. After replacing the "USP throat" with another inlet with better separation efficiency for the large particles, such particles will be collected there instead of in the initial stages of the impactor. As a result, the mass of particles accumulated on the initial stages will be lower, which will result in a biased PSD as confirmed by collected experimental data [48, 49]. Consequently, the mass median aerodynamic diameter (MMAD) derived from the modified impactor cannot be directly compared to MMAD determined by the standard impactors or other particle sizing equipment. Of course, an anatomically correct impactor inlet can be used to reliably assess particle deposition in the URT and the total mass capable of LRT penetration. Simultaneously, it prevents reliable determination of the particle size, so it does not help improve IVIVC based on an the precisely known aerosol PSD.

One should note that nebulizers are easiest to use by the patients because aerosol is produced independently of the breathing effort. They are considered as "active devices". Usually, a patient uses spontaneous tidal breathing, i.e., without applying any specific inhalation maneuver to draw the aerosol to the RS, as shown in Figure 3.2a. As mentioned earlier, since the aerosol can penetrate the RS only during inspiration, approximately half of the emitted dose can be lost, unless a special mechanism/device is applied to prevent aerosol emission during other phases of the breathing. In contrast to the nebulizers, the use of pMDI and DPIs is more demanding and can be troublesome for the patients. Due to different handling and breathing maneuvers required for various inhalation devices, patients often make mistakes that are subcritical (delivered dose is variable and lower than expected) or critical (no dose is delivered to the lungs).

Virtually all DPIs present in the market today are passive, i.e., they require an intense air flow generated by a patient to fluidize and deagglomerate powder particles. The threshold inhalation flow needed to fluidize the powder depends on the DPI, i.e., the design of the aerosolization chamber and the flow arrangement in the DPI. Both design parameters result in the specific internal aerodynamic resistance, R_D, in relation to the DPI flowrate, defined as:

$$R_D = \frac{\sqrt{\Delta P}}{Q} \tag{3.5}$$

where ΔP denotes the pressure drop across the inhaler at the volume airflow Q. According to the R_D value, DPIs can be classified as low-, medium-, and high-resistant devices. Low-resistant DPIs are easier to use since they require less patient's effort to draw air through the device. At the same time, they can be less efficient in releasing aerosols with a high FPD capable of penetrating the LRT. Deagglomeration of powder particles requires large aerodynamic stresses to break-up particle clusters. This is achieved in special flow arrangements with relatively large flowrates. A required deagglomeration can be rarely obtained using small inhalation flowrates through low-resistant devices. These DPIs perform better at high flow rates. On the other hand, large flowrates induce significant velocities of particles entering the URT, which leads to unfavorable enhanced inertial aerosol deposition in this region. Accordingly, there is an optimal range of airflow rates in each DPI allowing to produce large FPD without causing extensive particle separation in the mouth and throat. It must be noted that in addition to the aerodynamic conditions, interparticle adhesion forces strongly affect powder deagglomeration. These interactions depend on the particle surface properties that can be optimized using chemical engineering methods [50–52]. Aerosol formation in DPIs at a particular airflow does not mean that aerosol has the required PSD because deagglomeration process is typically flow-dependent. Compendial recommendations [9] demand testing each DPI at the specific airflow rate that induces 4 kPa (40 hPa) pressure drop across the inhaler. Accordingly, a DPI with $R_D = 0.1\,\text{hPa}^{0.5}\,\text{min/dm}^3$ is tested at $63\,\text{dm}^3/\text{min}$, while a DPI with $R_D = 0.07\,\text{hPa}^{0.5}\,\text{min/dm}^3$ – at $90\,\text{dm}^3$. It helps comparing different DPIs at the airflow conditions corresponding to the same inhalation effort. It may be noted that the maximum inhalation effort corresponds to the time instant of the maximum flow (PIF) through the DPI (see Figure 3.2b). Consequently, when the drug aerosolization starts early during the inhalation cycle, the flow rate is small, and the aerosol will have inadequate properties to penetrate the LRT (small FPD). This scenario is schematically shown in Figure 3.2c. It also means that the PSD obtained at the flowrate equal to PIF (according to the compendial *in vitro* methods of particle sizing) is usually better than the real PSD obtained *in vivo* when the aerosol is generated before the inhalation flowrate achieves its maximum. This discrepancy can contribute to a weak IVIVC calculations, and it is currently under dispute. Inhalation flow dynamics in a selected inhaler used by patients with various health status has been determined in [53], allowing for a more thorough discussion of the above issue [40]. It is seen that DPIs need a special inhalation technique enabling the required flow intensity and duration and it is related to the so-called patient compliance. Children, the elderly, or patients with restricted inhalation flowrate capabilities have the least chance of achieving the required inhalation dynamics. They can obtain suboptimal dose per inhalation. This also contributes to a weak IVIVC estimations because the emitted dose and the particle size distribution determined in the standard laboratory setups neglect these real-life constraints.

When analyzing pMDIs, approximately 45 % of the patients cannot correctly coordinate their breath with the aerosol emission [54]. As schematically shown in Figures 3.2d,e, a delayed start of the inhalation after aerosol emission may lead to a low delivered dose or no dose at all (the critical error). The coordination problem can be overcome in breath-activated devices (see Table 3.1) or by using the holding chambers [55].

The information presented in this section showed that weak IVIVC results can be due to predictions of *in vivo* delivered dose based on the PSD determined by the standard laboratory techniques. These neglect the airflow dynamics and other features of inhalers' performance that are dependent both on the mechanisms of the aerosol generation, and patient inhalation techniques. Adherence (compliance) improvement can be achieved through engineering-based innovations, such as introduction of the so-called "smart inhalers" or add-on devices to existing inhalers [37]. These improved systems can inform the patients (by visual or sound signals) about the performance of the inhalation and allow to use the inhalers more efficiently by avoiding common operational errors. Inhalation devices should also be designed ergonomically to reduce the risk of manual misuse. It is desired that a patient does not have to use different inhalers and remember distinct and specific manual and inhalation maneuvers for each of the device.

In conclusion, the weakness of IVIVC results can be attributed to deficiencies in the standard assessment methods applied to characterize the quality of medical aerosols. These methods do not mimic real-life conditions of aerosol generation, flow, and deposition in the RS. Consequently, they cannot correctly predict the expected *in vivo* effects.

3.6 Inter-patient variability (anatomy, respiratory physiology)

Another factor that limits obtaining satisfactory IVIVC results is a variability between patients regarding the RS anatomy and breathing (respiratory physiology) patterns. Prediction of aerosol flow and deposition in the respiratory tract is typically done assuming an idealized RS geometry, taken as the average for a population. This approach fails to describe the peculiarities of aerosol behavior in the individual lung geometry of a given patient that depends, among others, on the age, gender, body size, and health conditions. An example of the averaged geometry of the URT is the so-called Alberta Idealized Throat (AIT) developed at the University of Alberta in Canada [56, 57] (see Figure 3.3). It approximates the anatomical features of the oro-pharynx by smooth surfaces and simplified geometrical shapes. This geometry also has been proposed as an alternative inlet to the impactors, which was discussed in the previous section. A similar

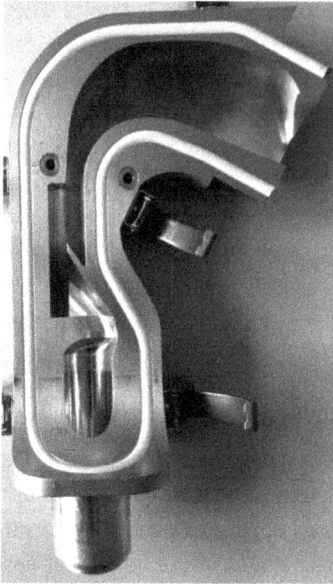

Figure 3.3: Alberta idealized throat – a universal model of adult oropharynx.

model has been developed for pediatric oro-pharynx and the nose [58]. These standard geometries help to obtain reproducible and comparable results for the *in vitro* experiments or CFD simulations performed across laboratories [59]. Both the AIT and Alberta Idealized Nasal Inlet (AINI) have been commercialized for the use in the standardized experiments [60].

In contrast to this approach, the analysis of aerosol flow and deposition can be done in the actual and unique geometries obtained from the patient's computed tomography (CT) or magnetic resonance imaging (MRI) scans [61]. Such simulations help to identify specific details of the realistic flow that can be lost during the analyses performed in the idealized geometries. However, such results are not representative for a population. This reduces their application in the IVIVC calculations. The investigations in such geometries have been done, among others, to study the influence of (i) unsteady flow impact on particle deposition in the oropharynx [62], (ii) spray and liquid parameters on the nasal deposition of drugs [63], (iii) pulmonary disease (COPD) on particle deposition pattern in the RS [11].

Both *in vitro* experiments and CFD simulations help to investigate the fundamental phenomena present in the airways, but they are less useful in calculating aerosol deposition in the deeper airways regions (lobes or functional segments), especially regarding the peripheral parts of RS.

The complex geometry of the LRT, composed of millions of fine bronchioles and alveoli, makes practically impossible to construct the complete lung model for experimental or *in silico* studies. This is why macroscopic computational models such as MPPD [19] have been developed and are often used to predict the whole lung particle deposition. These are applicable in both the exposure to ambient aerosols and PDD conditions. Its origin is dated back to developments in the radiological protection field [17] mentioned in Section 3.2. MPPD model is based on calculations of particle deposition mechanisms in each generation of model RS based on the averaged flowrates data and RS geometry.

Another problem related to IVIVC comes from the specifically defined endpoints of clinical response of individual patients to inhaled drugs. A common way of assessing *in vivo* effects of PDD is monitoring the improvement in respiratory parameters such as FEV1 (forced expiratory volume in 1 s), which is expected to improve after bronchodilator inhalation in asthmatic or COPD patients [64]. This information confirms that the inhaled medicine has clinical benefits but does not inform what locally delivered dose induced the effect. In addition, the reported data are scattered due to the intersubject variability regarding anatomical and functional parameters, and disease severity and patient's susceptibility to a given medicament. Consequently, positive clinical data may do not allow to define the minimum effective dose and can lead to define doses larger than required for obtaining the clinical response, simultaneously neglecting potential unfavorable side effects of the therapy. Interpatient variability may also be responsible for a different response to the same delivered dose, indicating that not only PK but also PD factors are important in the analysis of the IVIVC problem.

3.7 Generic inhalation drug products delivery

Generic drugs contain the same API with the same mass per dose as the reference (the original) drug. They are expected to induce the same pharmacological effect. However, as discussed earlier (Figures 3.1 and 3.2, Table 3.1) aerosolized medicaments – in contrast to injections or tablets – are never delivered in full (nominal) dose to the organisms. This is particular for LRT, which is the most important target for their delivery. Therefore, the therapeutic equivalence assessment must consider not only the chemical composition of the drug (API concentration and purity of the formulation), but also the efficiency of aerosolization and administration [65].

For generic orally inhaled products (OIP), it is required to demonstrate that their technical performance (regarding the PSD and other essential indicators) is similar – with a margin, typically ±15 % – to the original product for which the clinical studies have been done [36]. Sometimes it is problematic, because it requires that generics are no worse, but also no better than the reference original product. One may notice that technologies (e.g., involving powder preparation for DPIs) have evolved since the time when for example the original drug was developed. It can be easier obtaining a product allowing better drug delivery than the reference. Still, such a generic product will not comply with the regulations having better efficiency but being beyond the acceptance limits. Generic development is even more challenging for powder inhalation products which contain two or more API molecules [66], especially if each API should have a different mass in a single dose (e.g., 50 mcg vs. 500 mcg as in case of bronchodilator/ corticosteroid combination product). In this case not only the particle size of each drug, but also the way of powder mixing and aerosolization dynamics in the DPI should be thoroughly elaborated to meet the required criteria [67]. A broader discussion of generic OIPs bioequivalence have been presented by [13], including the PK problems after delivering the similar doses of inhaled drugs.

In case of nebulized generic drugs, particular differences were demonstrated for several generics of a glucocorticosteroid (budesonide) suspensions atomized with a vibrating mesh nebulizer [32]. It was shown that drug suspensions contained budesonide crystals with different sizes did not possess identical physicochemical characteristics (e.g., zeta potential and crystal aggregation, surface tension). This could be attributed to the presence of the functional adjuvants, which – in contrast to API – do not have to be identical as in the original drug. These differences mean that nebulization drugs with the same API concentration can be nebulized to aerosols that may induce modified clinical effects.

In conclusion, both the physicochemical properties and aerodynamic phenomena responsible for the final quality of inhaled aerosol drug need to be analyzed and opti-mized. Undoubtfully, chemical engineering technologies offer appealing and robust scientific methodologies for such analyses.

3.8 Perspectives and final remarks

Today, the IVIVC problem of orally inhaled products remains largely unsolved. However, considering the progress in understanding the key constraints in the processes of aerosol generation, flow and local delivery to distinct regions of the respiratory system, a few suggestions to improve the IVIVC of aerosol inhalation products can be proposed:

(1) Development of "smart inhalers", i.e., new inhalation devices or modifications of existing ones (e.g., by add-on adapters) to improve patient compliance and hence unify the delivered dose regardless of the individual patient's characteristics (age, health condition, etc.) Several devices are already on the market, and more are under development (see [37, 68]). The most useful systems should monitor the inhalation flow/pressure and release the aerosol only when lung penetration can reach desired level. There is also a chance to take the advantage of machine learning algorithms to optimize the operation of smart inhalation systems. Meanwhile, such devices may have built-in optical/sound systems or integrated connectivity with mobile (IoT) applications to help train patients' skills in the proper use of the inhaler.

(2) A deeper understanding of aerosol particle dynamics in the RS: e.g., hygroscopic growth, possible particle coagulation, dependence of particle motion on the

dynamics pattern of inhalation, partitioning of substances between the phases, and deformation of lower airways during breathing. More sophisticated *in silico* modeling (CFD) focused on evaluating specific phenomena is available and should be applied in the PDD analyses [69, 70];

(3) Well-designed *in vitro* experiments using contemporary, more sophisticated experimental techniques (e.g., variable flow for the aerosol generation in the inhalers and measuring the actual PSD at the inhaler outlet) [40].

(4) Deeper understanding of particle fate after deposition on the lung surface, e.g., by analyzing physicochemical interactions with bronchial mucus or pulmonary surfactant to assess drug residence time and mass transport rate to receptors and cells [71, 72].

(5) PK/PD assessment using *in vitro* cell models. Many aspects of this IVIVC problem are analogous to the assessment in the field of toxicology [16]. A promising approach is provided by microfluidic *lung-on-a-chip* methodologies [73, 74]. Selected biophysical methods can be also used to evaluate the safety or potential toxicity of inhaled compounds [75, 76].

These suggestions should be effectively developed in the multidisciplinary context with the use of existing chemical engineering methods. In conclusion, this manuscript highlighted the key limitations and challenges of IVIVC in the aerosol inhalation drug delivery space. It was shown that this problem requires in-depth insight into the dynamics and mechanics of multiphase dispersed systems, which lies within the scope of modern chemical engineering. Both mathematical modeling (*in silico* approach) and technical experiments focused on *in vitro* predictions of the fate of inhaled aerosols in the airways, use methodologies directly adapted from engineering applications. A challenge that substantially complicates accompanied analyses is the dynamic nature of aerosol generation and delivery to the RS. This is due to the unsteady nature of respiration and varying conditions of the flowing aerosol particles during their formation in the inhalers and their transport in the RS. These issues cannot be adequately addressed without extensive input from the physical chemistry field and other scientific sub-disciplines that are widely used and well-known to chemical engineers. Existing chemical engineering methods can provide strong support in solving selected problems of pulmonary medicine. Future perspectives may extend beyond PDD and consider the delivery of aerosolized drugs to treat pathologies inside other body cavities including benefits of minimizing various side effects [77]. Similar study focused on gene therapy in this context has recently started at the Warsaw University of Technology in co-operation with the Warsaw Medical University.

Acknowledgments: The authors would like to thank the editor David Bogle for his guidance and review of this article before its publication. The work has been done under umbrella of the scientific section "Chemical Engineering as Applied to Medicine" (ChemE-Med) of the European Federation of Chemical Engineering (EFCE).

References

1. Newman SP, Chan H-K. *In vitro/In vivo* comparisons in pulmonary drug delivery. J Aerosol Med Pulm Drug Deliv 2008;21:77–84.
2. Langer R, Peppas NA. A bright future in medicine for chemical engineering. Nat Chem Eng 2024;1:10–12.
3. Sosnowski TR. Aerosols and human health – a multiscale problem. Chem Eng Sci 2023;268:118407.
4. Hickey A, Kwok PCL. *In vitro-in vivo* correlation of pharmaceutical aerosols. Adv Drug Deliv Rev 2021;179: 114025.
5. Moreau M, Simms L, Andersen ME, Trelles-Sticken E, Wieczorek R, Pour SJ, et al. Use of quantitative in vitro to in vivo extrapolation (QIVIVE) for the assessment of non-combustible next generation product aerosols. Front Toxicol 2024;6:1373325.
6. Suarez-Sharp S, Li M, Duan J, Shah H, Paul Seo P. Regulatory experience with in vivo in vitro correlations (IVIVC) in new drug applications. AAPS J 2016;18:1379–90.
7. EPA. Exposure assessment tools by routes – inhalation [online]. https://www.epa.gov/expobox/exposure-assessment-tools-routes-inhalation [Accessed 20 Dec 2024].
8. AARC. A guide to aerosol delivery devices for respiratory therapists [online]. https://www.aarc.org/wp-content/uploads/2015/04/aerosol_guide_rt.pdf [Accessed 20 Dec 2024].
9. European Pharmacopeia. Chapter 2.9.18 preparations for inhalation: aerodynamic assessment of fine particles, 10th ed. Strasbourg: European Directorate for the Quality of Medicines and HealthCare (EDQM); 2021.
10. Newman SP, Chan H-K. *In vitro–in vivo* correlations (IVIVCs) of deposition for drugs given by oral inhalation. Adv Drug Deliv Rev 2020;67:135–47.
11. Kadota K, Matsumoto K, Uchiyama H, Tobita S, Maeda M, Maki D, et al. *In silico* evaluation of particle transport and deposition in the airways of individual patients with chronic obstructive pulmonary disease. Eur J Pharm Biopharm 2022;174:10–19.
12. Li J, Zheng H, Qin L, Xu E-Y, Yang L, Zhang L, et al. *In vitro–in vivo* correlation of inhalable budesonide-loaded large porous particles for sustained treatment regimen of asthma. Acta Biomater 2019;96:505–16.
13. Sandell D. Bioequivalence assessment of pharmaceutical aerosol products through IVIVC. Adv Drug Deliv Rev 2021;176:113895.
14. Di Ianni E, Erdem JS, Møller P, Sahlgren NM, Poulsen SS, Knudsen KB, et al. *In vitro–in vivo* correlations of pulmonary inflammogenicity and genotoxicity of MWCNT. Part Fibre Toxicol 2021;18:25.
15. Kreutz A, Chang X, Hogberg HT, Wetmore BA. Advancing understanding of human variability through toxicokinetic modeling, *in vitro–in vivo* extrapolation, and new approach methodologies. Hum Genomics 2024;18:129.
16. Kolli AR, Kuczaj AK, Martin F, Hayes AW, Peitsch MC, Hoeng J. Bridging inhaled aerosol dosimetry to physiologically based pharmacokinetic modeling for toxicological assessment: nicotine delivery systems and beyond. Crit Rev Toxicol 2019;49:725–41.
17. ICRP. Human respiratory tract model for radiological protection, Ottawa: ICRP Publication 66; 1994:1–3 pp, vol. 24.
18. Phalen RF, Cuddihy RG, Fisher GL, Moss OR, Schlesinger RB, Swift DL, et al. Main features of the proposed NCRP respiratory tract model. Radiat Protect Dosim 1991;38:179–84.
19. MPPD, Applied Research Associates, Inc.. Multiple-path particle Dosimetry model (MPPD v 3.04) [Online]. https://www.ara.com/mppd/[Accessed 20 Dec 2024].
20. Laube BL. Imaging aerosol deposition with two-dimensional gamma scintigraphy. J Aerosol Med Pulm Drug Deliv 2022;35:333–41.
21. Darquenne C, Corcoran TE, Lavorini F, Sorano A, Usmani OS. The effects of airway disease on the deposition of inhaled drugs. Expert Opin Drug Deliv 2024;21:1175–90.

22. Yeh HC, Schum GM. Models of the human lung airways and their application to inhaled particle deposition. Bull Math Biol 1980;42:461–80.
23. Byron PA. Factors affecting aerosol sampling 2016 [Online]. https://www.cdc.gov/niosh/docs/2014-151/pdfs/chapters/chapter-ae.pdf [Accessed 20 Dec 2024].
24. Cheng YS. Aerosol deposition in the extrathoracic region. Aerosol Sci Technol 2003;37:659–71.
25. Cheng YS, Zhou Y, Chen BT. Particle deposition in a cast of human oral airways. Aerosol Sci Tech 1999;31: 286–300.
26. Sosnowski TR. Inhaled aerosols: their role in COVID-19 transmission including biophysical interactions in the lungs. Curr Opin Coll Interf Sci 2021;54:101451.
27. Martin AR, Finlay WH. Nebulizers for drug delivery to the lungs. Expert Opin Drug Deliv 2015;12:889–900.
28. Tashkin DP. A review of nebulized drug delivery in COPD. Int J Chronic Obstruct Pulm Dis 2016;11:2585–96.
29. McCallion ON, Taylor KM, Thomas M, Taylor AJ. Nebulization of fluids of different physicochemical properties with air-jet and ultrasonic nebulizers. Pharm Res (N Y) 1995;12:1682–8.
30. Ghazanfari T, Elhissi AMA, Ding Z, Taylor KMG. The influence of fluid physicochemical properties on vibrating-mesh nebulization. Int J Pharmacol 2007;339:103–11.
31. Beck-Broichsitter M, Oesterheld N, Knuedeler M -C, Seeger W, Schmeh IT. On the correlation of output rate and aerodynamic characteristics in vibrating-mesh-based aqueous aerosol delivery. Int J Pharm 2014;461: 34–7.
32. Dobrowolska K, Emeryk A, Janeczek K, Krzosa R, Pirożyński M, Sosnowski TR. Influence of physicochemical properties of budesonide micro-suspensions on their expected lung delivery using a vibrating mesh nebulizer. Pharmaceutics 2023;15:752.
33. ISO. ISO 27427:2023, Anaesthetic and respiratory equipment – nebulizing systems and components, 2023 [Online]. https://www.iso.org/standard/78542.html [Accessed 2024 Dec 2024].
34. Dobrowolska KE, Kinowska M, Sosnowski TR. Nebulization of solutions containing guar gum as a viscosity modifier of natural origin. In: Respiratory drug delivery. Richmond, VA, USA: RDD Online; 2022.
35. Dobrowolska K, Miros M, Sosnowski T. Impact of natural-based viscosity modifiers of inhalation drugs on the dynamic surface properties of the pulmonary surfactant. Materials 2023;16:1975.
36. EMA. CHMP, Guideline on the pharmaceutical quality of inhalation and nasal products, 2005 [Online]. https://www.ema.europa.eu/en/pharmaceutical-quality-inhalation-nasal-products-scientific-guideline [Accessed 20 Dec 2024].
37. Sosnowski TR. Towards more precise targeting of inhaled aerosols to different areas of the respiratory system. Pharmaceutics 2024;16:97.
38. Sosnowski TR, Janeczek K, Grzywna K, Emeryk A. Mass and volume balances of nebulization processes for the determination of the expected dose of liquid medicines delivered by inhalation. Chem Process Eng 2021;42:253–61.
39. Laube BL, Janssens HM, de Jongh FHC, Devadason SG, Dhand R, Diot P, et al. What the pulmonary specialist should know about the new inhalation therapies. Eur Respir J 2011;37:1308–417.
40. Dorosz A, Moskal A, Sosnowski TR. Dynamics of aerosol generation and flow during inhalation for improved *in vitro–in vivo* correlation (IVIVC) of pulmonary medicines. Chem Process Eng: New Front 2023;44:e39.
41. Zhou Y, Ahuja A, Irvin CM, Kracko DA, McDonald JD, Cheng YS. Medical nebulizer performance: effects of cascade impactor temperature. Respir Care 2005;50:1077–82.
42. Berg E, Svensson JO, Asking L. Determination of nebulizer droplet size distribution: a method based on impactor refrigeration. J Aerosol Med 2007;20:97–104.
43. Schuschnig U, Heine B, Knoch M. How cold is cold enough? Refrigeration of the Next-Generation Impactor to prevent aerosol undersizing. J Aerosol Med Pulm Drug Deliv 2022;35:25–31.
44. Mao L, Wilcox D, Kippax P. Laser diffraction particle size analysis: a powerful tool for rapidly screening nebulizer formulations. Drug Deliv Techn 2010;10:64–7.
45. Sosnowski TR. Critical assessment of the quantitative criteria used in the comparison of nebulizers. EC Pulm Respirat Med 2019;8:656–62.

46. Kostrzon M, Sliwka A, Wloch T, Szpunar M, Ankowska D, Nowobilski R. Subterranean pulmonary rehabilitation in chronic obstructive pulmonary disease. Adv Exp Med Biol 2019;1176:35–46.
47. Sosnowski TR, Koprowski M. Nebulization in the subterranean conditions: the influence of ambient conditions on the generation of aerosols for inhalation. In: Chemical and process engineering for environment and health. Current status in 2024. Radom, Poland: Łukasiewicz Institute for Sustainable Technologies; 2024:136–43 pp.
48. Copley M, Mitchell J, Solomon D. Evaluating of Alberta Throat: an innovation to support the acquisition of more clinically applicable aerosol aerodynamic particle size distribution (APSD) data in oral inhaled product (OIP) development. Inhalation 2011;5:12.
49. Copley M, Parry M, Solomon D, Mitchell J. Comparison between in vitro performance of the Child "Alberta" Idealized Throat and Ph.Eur./USP induction port for the delivery of salbutamol sulfate inhalation aerosol by pressurized metered dose inhaler. Inhalation 2015;1:3.
50. Kramek-Romanowska K, Odziomek M, Sosnowski TR, Gradoń L. Effects of process variables on the properties of spray-dried mannitol and mannitol/disodium cromoglycate powders suitable for drug delivery by inhalation. Ind Eng Chem Res 2011;50:13922–31.
51. Gradoń L, Sosnowski TR. Formation of particles for dry powder inhalers. Adv Powder Technol 2014;25: 43–55.
52. Kadota K, Sosnowski TR, Tobita S, Tachibana I, Tse J, Uchiyama K, et al. A particle technology approach toward designing dry-powder inhaler formulations for personalized medicine in respiratory diseases. Adv Powder Technol 2020;31:219–26.
53. Dorosz A, Urbankowski T, Zieliński K, Michnikowski M, Krenke R, Moskal A. Modeling of inhalation profiles through dry powder inhaler in healthy adults and asthma patients as a prerequisite for further in vitro and in silico studies. J Aerosol Med Pulm Drug Delivery 2022;35:91–103.
54. Sanchis J, Gich I, Pedersen S. Systematic review of errors in inhaler use. Has patient technique improved over time? Chest 2016;150:394–406.
55. GINA. The global initiative for asthma [Online]. http://ginasthma.org [Accessed 20 Dec 2024].
56. Stapleton KW, Guntsch E, Hoskinson MK, Finlay WH. On the suitability of k-eps turbulence modeling for aerosol deposition in the mouth and throat: a comparison with experiment. J Aerosol Sci 2000;31:739–49.
57. Heenan AF, Matida E, Pollard A, Finlay WH. Experimental measurements and computational modeling of flow in an idealized extrathoracic airway. Exp Fluids 2003;35:70–84.
58. Carrigy NB, Ruzycki CA, Golshahi L, Finlay WH. Pediatric *in vitro* and *in silico* models of deposition via oral and nasal inhalation. J Aerosol Med Pulm Drug Deliv 2014;27:149–69.
59. Zhang Y, Finlay WH, Matida EA. Particle deposition measurements and numerical simulation in a highly idealized mouth-throat. J Aerosol Sci 2004;35:789–803.
60. Copley Scientific Limited. Realistic throat and nasal cast models [Online]. https://www.copleyscientific.com/inhaler-testing/realistic-throat-and-nasal-models/alberta-idealised-nasal-inlet-aini/[Accessed 20 Dec 2024].
61. Grgic B, Finlay WH, Burnell PKP, Heenan A. In vitro intersubject and intrasubject deposition measurements in realistic mouth-throat geometries. J Aerosol Sci 2004;35:1025–40.
62. Sosnowski TR, Moskal A, Gradoń L. Dynamics of oropharyngeal aerosol transport and deposition with the realistic flow pattern. Inhal Toxicol 2006;18:773–80.
63. Sosnowski TR, Rapiejko P, Sova J, Dobrowolska K. Impact of physicochemical properties of nasal spray products on drug deposition and transport in the pediatric nasal cavity model. Int J Pharm 2020;574:118911.
64. Taube C, Kanniess F, Grönke L, Richter K, Mücke M, Paasch K, et al. Reproducibility of forced inspiratory and expiratory volumes after bronchodilation in patients with COPD or asthma. Respir Med 2003;97:568–77.
65. Pirożyński M, Sosnowski TR. Inhalation devices: from basic science to practical use, innovative vs generic products. Expert Opin Drug Del 2016;13:1559–71.
66. Taki M, Esmaeili F, Martin GP. The scientific basis and challenges of combination inhaled products. J Drug Deliv Sci Technol 2011;21:293–300.

67. Hejduk A, Urbańska A, Osiński A, Łukaszewicz P, Domański M, Sosnowski TR. Technical challenges in obtaining an optimized powder/DPI combination for inhalation delivery of a bi-component generic drug. J Drug Deliv Sci Technol 2018;44:406–14.

68. Kikidis D, Konstantinos V, Tzovaras D, Usmani OS. The digital asthma patient: the history and future of inhaler based health monitoring devices. J Aerosol Med Pulm Drug Deliv 2016;29:219–32.

69. Lucci F, Frederix E, Kuczaj AK. AeroSolved: computational fluid dynamics modeling of multispecies aerosol flows with sectional and moment methods. J Aerosol Sci 2022;159:105854.

70. AeroSolved. CFD software package [Online]. https://github.com/pmpsa-cfd/aerosolved [Accessed 20 Dec 2024].

71. Sosnowski TR. Particles on the lung surface – physicochemical and hydrodynamic effects. Curr Opin Colloid Interface Sci 2018;36:1–9.

72. Odziomek M, Kalinowska M, Płuzińska A, Rożeń A, Sosnowski TR. Bronchial mucus as a complex fluid: molecular interactions and influence of nanostructured particles on rheological and transport properties. Chem Process Eng 2017;38:217–29.

73. Francis I, Shrestha J, Raj Paudel K, Hansbro PM, Ebrahimi-Warkiani M, Saha SC. Recent advances in lung-on-a-chip models. Drug Discov Today 2022;27:2593–602.

74. Zamprogno P, Wüthrich S, Achenbach S, Thoma G, Stucki JD, Hobi N, et al. Second-generation lung-on-a-chip with an array of stretchable alveoli made with a biological membrane. Commun Biol 2021;4:168.

75. Sosnowski TR, Podgórski A. Assessment of the pulmonary toxicity of inhaled gases and particles with physicochemical methods. Int J Occup Saf Ergon. 1999;5:433–49.

76. Sosnowski TR, Jabłczyńska K, Odziomek M, Schlage WK, Kuczaj AK. Physicochemical studies of direct interactions between lung surfactant and components of electronic cigarettes liquid mixtures. Inhal Toxicol 2018;30:159–68.

77. Solass W, Kerb R, Mürdter T, Giger-Pabst U, Strumberg D, Tempfer CZJ, et al. Intraperitoneal chemotherapy of peritoneal carcinomatosis using pressurized aerosol as an alternative to liquid solution: first evidence for efficacy. Ann Surg Oncol 2014;21:553–9.

Daniel Sebastia-Saez, Tao Chen*, Benjamin Deacon and Guoping Lian

4 Modelling drug permeation across the skin: a chemical engineering perspective

Abstract: This review provides insight on how the application of core chemical engineering concepts helps with current challenges in dermal permeation research from a mathematical modelling perspective. The skin fundamentally behaves like a diffusion reactor, where mass conservation featuring Fick's diffusion flux can be applied to obtain the differential equations that govern the permeation of a chemical compound. Advanced phenomena like systemic circulation or complex thermodynamics can be added mathematically into the models to complement the diffusion equation. Depending on research objectives, the reach of these mechanistic continuum mechanics models can: i) consider the skin as a homogeneous compartment, where spatial dependency is overlooked, or ii) include detailed spatio-temporally-discretised geometric descriptions of complex features like the bricks-and-mortar layout of the stratum corneum. The capabilities of this powerful approach to study advanced topics in dermatological research are discussed. These include topics such as the role of the hair follicle as a shortcut to bypass the stratum corneum, the effect of evaporation during the application of multicomponent formulations, and the facilitation of skin permeation by means of external forces (i.e., electromagnetic fields and mechanical action). The chapter closes with a note on current challenges towards the future development of mechanistic skin Digital Twins, which are gaining further importance of late to avoid animal experimentation in dermatological research.

Keywords: dermal drug delivery; mathematical model; skin; compartmental models; mechanistic models; advanced drug delivery

List of symbols

Latin characters

a	Activity coefficient, dimensionless
A	Area, [m^2]
C	Concentration, [$mol\ m^{-3}$]
D	Diffusion coefficient, [$m^2\ s^{-1}$]

*Corresponding author: Tao Chen, School of Chemistry & Chemical Engineering, University of Surrey, Guildford, GU2 7XH, UK, E-mail: t.chen@surrey.ac.uk
Daniel Sebastia-Saez and Benjamin Deacon, School of Chemistry & Chemical Engineering, University of Surrey, Guildford, GU2 7XH, UK
Guoping Lian, School of Chemistry & Chemical Engineering, University of Surrey, Guildford, GU2 7XH, UK; and Unilever R&D Colworth, Bedfordshire, MK44 1LQ, UK

As per De Gruyter's policy this article has previously been published in the journal Physical Sciences Reviews. Please cite as:
D. Sebastia-Saez, T. Chen, B. Deacon and G. Lian "Modelling drug permeation across the skin: a chemical engineering perspective" *Physical Sciences Reviews* [Online] 2024. DOI: 10.1515/psr-2024-0056 | https://doi.org/10.1515/9783111394558-004

e	Elementary charge, [A s]
h	Height of diffusion cell, [m]
J	Molar flux, [mol m^{-2} s^{-1}]
k	Mass transfer coefficient, [m s^{-1}]
K	Clearance rate, [m^3 s^{-1}]
MW	Molecular weight, [g mol^{-1}]
n	Number of cells in computational grid, dimensionless
N	Length parameter, [m]
P	Partition coefficient, dimensionless
Q	Volumetric flow rate, [m^3 s^{-1}]
r	Radius of molecule [m]
R	Source term, [mol m^{-3} s^{-1}]
t	Time, [s]
T	Temperature, [K]
u	Wind speed, [m s^{-1}]
V	Volume, [m^3]
x	Molar fraction, dimensionless
z	Valence of ionic species, dimensionless

Greek characters

δ	Thickness of the stratum corneum, [m]
Δ	Increment
η	Dynamic viscosity, [Pa s]
μ	Permeability, [m s^{-1}]
ρ	Density, [kg m^{-3}]
φ	Volume fraction, dimensionless
ϕ	Electric potential [kg m^2 s^{-3} A^{-1}]

Subscripts

b	Blood
B	Refers to Boltzmann constant k_B.
$closed$	Refers to blocked hair follicles in *in-vitro* tests
d	Dermis
e	Viable epidermis
eq	Equilibrium
$evap$	Evaporative
gas	Denotes gas phase
k	Used as a counter for number of cells in computational mesh
liq	Liquid
lip	Lipid
non	Denotes non-ionised in non-ionised fraction of permeant f_{non}.
o	Octanol

open	Refers to open hair follicles in *in-vitro* tests
pro	Protein
r	Receptor fluid or compartment
s	Skin
se	Sebum
hyp	Short for hypobaric. Denotes area of application of suction on skin
u	Denotes unbound in fraction of permeant unbound to protein f_u
v	Vehicle
vap	Denotes vapour in vapour pressure P_{vap}.
w	Water

Others

∇	Nabla operator

Abbreviations

CFR	Contribution of the follicular route
IVPT	*In-vitro* permeation test
ODE	Ordinary differential equation
PBPK	Physiologically-based pharmacokinetic model
PDE	Partial differential equation.
QSPR	Quantitative structure-property relationship
RF	Receptor Fluid
SC	Stratum Corneum
TEWL	Transepidermal water loss

4.1 Introduction

Skin is the largest organ of the human body, making up about 15 % of the overall body mass [1]. It plays various roles critical to the survival and functioning of the organism, such as temperature regulation, sensation, vitamin D production, and of particular interest here, its barrier function. Skin provides excellent barrier properties, preventing water from being unnecessarily lost to the environment and keeping harmful chemicals and microorganisms out of the body. This barrier function is primarily physical, enacted by the densely packed corneocytes (i.e., dead cells originated from keratinocytes), which are embedded in lipid bilayers forming the topmost layer of the skin (i.e., the stratum corneum). Secondarily, some skin biological functions also play a role in the barrier property. These are: i) the enzymatic transformation of drugs into less toxic substances, and ii) desquamation, which sheds the stratum corneum and any chemicals trapped in it.

This excellent barrier function has created a significant challenge for topical and transdermal drug delivery. Topical delivery is preferred for treating local diseases (over the oral route), as it bypasses the first-pass metabolism of the liver and reduces systemic exposure and toxicity. However, delivery into the skin is often inefficient due to its barrier function. The general knowledge is that molecules with size greater than 500 Da are difficult to passively diffuse into the skin to reach therapeutically meaningful concentrations unless applying external means to weaken the barrier [2]. Some of these external means include iontophoresis, microneedles, and others. Conversely, extracting biomarkers from the skin with no (or minimal) invasion also proves to be a significant engineering challenge.

Fundamentally, chemical transfer across the skin is a mass transfer problem, coupled with phenomena like partitioning between the different phases and layers in the skin. Moreover, the thermodynamics of formulated skin products can be complex due to their multi-phase nature and can undergo dynamic changes due to evaporation of ingredients. This mass transfer/thermodynamics problem can be further complicated by, to name a few, biochemical reactions (e.g., skin metabolism), heat transfer (e.g., elevated temperature can be applied to improve drug delivery), and/or biomechanics (e.g., skin can be mechanically deformed to facilitate drug delivery or biomarker extraction). This creates a multi-faceted challenge to chemical engineers, necessitating a cross-disciplinary approach.

As the largest organ of the human body, the skin plays a crucial role far beyond its surface appearance. The effectiveness of dermatological products hinges on the understanding of how substances interact with and penetrate the skin, which depends on its physiology and health. Understanding the complex physico-chemical phenomena behind dermal absorption is key to enhancing the delivery of therapeutic drugs and skincare formulations. Mechanistic mathematical models are an essential means to achieve this objective from a Chemical Engineering perspective, as will be seen in the subsequent sections of this chapter.

In this chapter, we intend to provide an overview of computational modelling of chemical transfer across the skin. This in-silico approach, while emerging in pharmacology and toxicology, is well appreciated in engineering for its role in enhancing our understanding of the process and mechanisms of complex systems, and in aiding rapid and rational design of products and systems. We will start with short summary on the physiology of the skin in Section 4.2. Then, compartment-based models, which are similar to how continuously stirred tank reactors (CSTRs) are modelled, are discussed in Section 4.3.1. Section 4.3.2 delves deeper into modelling diffusion and partitioning explicitly in a spatial setting, which enables not only predicting the dynamics of chemical distribution at different spatial locations but also making such predictions more mechanistic. Beyond the basic approaches, we discuss a few advanced topics in Section 4.4, demonstrate a few cases in Section 4.5, and conclude the chapter with future perspectives in Section 4.6.

4.2 Skin physiology

The structure of the skin has been thoroughly studied and defined over the past century. The skin consists of three main sections, from the topmost layer to the deepest layer: the epidermis, the dermis, and the hypodermis, as shown in Figure 4.1. The epidermis is further divided into several layers, including the stratum corneum, stratum lucidum, the stratum granulosum, the stratum spinosum the stratum basale. From the standpoint of drug permeation into the skin, the stratum corneum (SC) is considered a separate layer due to its unique structure and contribution to the protective function of the skin. The rest of the layers in the epidermis are usually grouped under the term 'viable epidermis' due to their similar diffusive properties. The SC comprises a network of corneocytes and an extracellular bilipid matrix, commonly referred to as a bricks-and-mortar structure, where the corneocytes make up the bricks and the lipid matrix plays the role of the mortar [3].

The described structure of the SC gives rise to two unique diffusion pathways in the SC, including the lipidic and the transcellular route, which favours the permeation of lipophilic and hydrophilic compounds respectively. The bricks-and-mortar approach is the most popular way to describe the SC in the scientific literature. The barrier function of the skin is primarily attributed to the small permeability of the SC relative to the rest of the skin layers, which is caused by the dead, flattened corneocytes (i.e., the bricks in the bricks-and-mortar layout). The lipid matrix includes ceramides, free fatty acids, and

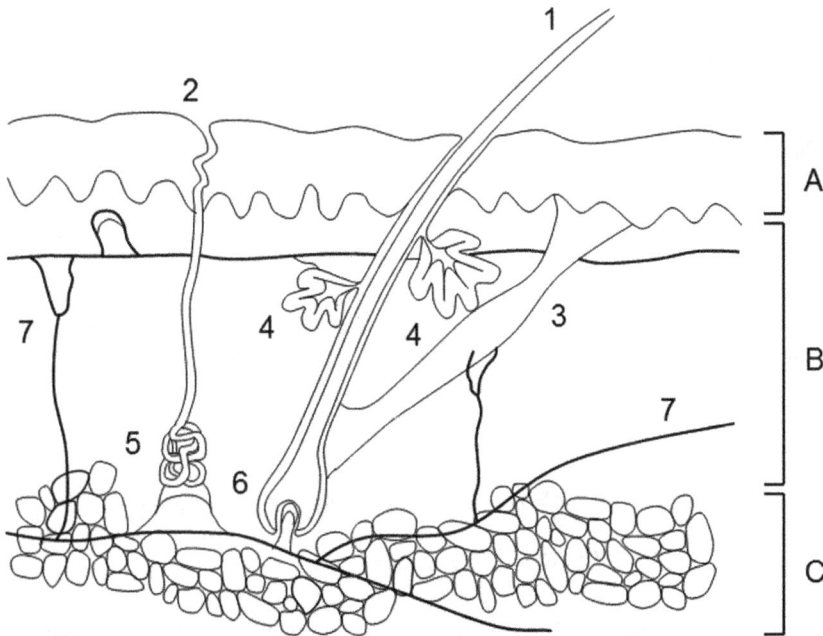

Figure 4.1: A simplified diagram of the skin structure showing the different layers and features of the skin: (A) Epidermis, (B) dermis, and (C) hypodermis. 1 – hair shaft, 2 – pore, 3 – hair erector muscle, 4 – sebaceous gland, 5 – sweat gland, 6 – hair follicle, 7 – blood vessel [4].

cholesterol, which are crucial for maintaining the integrity of the barrier and preventing transepidermal water loss (TEWL). The dynamic nature of the SC involves continuous desquamation (shedding of corneocytes) and renewal from the underlying keratinocytes of the viable epidermis, which become corneocytes on their way up towards the skin surface [5].

The viable epidermis is mainly composed of keratinocyte cells, with a combination of melanocytes, Langerhans cells, and Merkel–Ranvier cells. The dermis consists of collagenous fibres (70 %), providing a scaffold of support and cushioning, and elastic connective tissue in a matrix of mucopolysaccharides. Additionally, the skin immuno-logical functions of the skin are mediated by Langerhans cells in the epidermis and a network of immune cells in the dermis. These cells play a crucial role in detecting and responding to pathogens, making the skin an active component of the immune system [6]. The subcutaneous tissue is comprised of fat cells and connective tissue that protect internal organs and muscles. This tissue is generally termed receptor fluid, an umbrella term to include the subcutaneous tissue, blood, or any other structure below the dermis. Furthermore, the skin hosts an array of important structures, called appendages, which contribute to its functionality. Notable structures include hair follicles, sweat glands, and sebaceous glands. Hair follicles and glandular structures not only serve their specific physiological roles but also provide alternative pathways for drug delivery, helping with overcoming the low-permeability SC. The follicular route can bypass the SC barrier, offering a route for large and hydrophilic as will be seen in this chapter.

The complex structure and diverse functionalities of the skin make it a challenging yet promising target for drug delivery. Understanding the intricacies of skin physiology, including the roles of different layers and structures and their inherent natural vari-ability, is essential to formulate mathematical models to help with the development of efficient therapeutic strategies. The following sections illustrate how mathematical models based on Chemical Engineering principles can help with different aspects of research. It is estimated that 20–33 % of the global population suffers from skin diseases at any given moment, while approximately 54 % of the UK population will develop a skin condition each year [7]. Companies have capitalised on skin health, producing a multitude of products to enhance and protect skin health and cosmetics. Pharmaceutical companies have produced moisturisers, sun creams, anti-pollution creams, and protec-tive barrier creams through research and development. Mathematical models are contributing increasingly to the development of these products.

4.3 Mechanistic mathematical models for drug permeation across the skin

In this section, mechanistic models (i.e., those based on fundamental physical principles) of drug permeation will be discussed. Mechanistic models, as opposed to data-based models, allow the use of mathematical language to describe drug permeation by means of core chemical engineering concepts. As mentioned, drug permeation across the skin is fundamentally a diffusion problem, which can be posed by means of the continuity equation (i.e., conservation of mass), using Fick's laws of diffusion to define flux. There are mainly two types of mechanistic models for drug diffusion across the skin in the literature. These are compartmental models and spatial diffusion models. A description of these two types of models from a chemical engineering perspective follows.

4.3.1 Compartmental models

Compartmentation is a widely used method in pharmacokinetic modelling. This method treats different organs and tissues as individual compartments each having uniform concentration. This is equivalent to assuming each compartment is perfectly mixed, using chemical engineering terminology. In the context of skin, the work in [8] is a typical example, and there are others reviewed by [9]. This essentially takes the form of mass transfer equations:

$$J = k \, \Delta C \tag{4.1}$$

where ΔC denotes the molar concentration difference between two neighbouring compartments, k is the mass transfer coefficient and J the molar flux.

Consider a simple two-compartment representation of the skin as shown in Figure 4.2, where it is assumed that the vehicle is an infinite dose (i.e., neither the vehicle nor its ingredients deplete during dermal absorption) and thus has a constant concentration C_v. The mass balance equation with respect to the skin compartment is thus represented by the following ordinary differential equation (ODE):

$$V_s \frac{dC_s}{dt} = A \, k_{vs} \left(C_v - \frac{C_s}{P_{sv}} \right) + Q_{bs} \left(C_b - \frac{C_s}{P_{sb}} \right) \tag{4.2}$$

where Q_{bs} is the volumetric flow rate of the blood through the skin and A is the application area of the vehicle on the skin. The terms on the right-hand side of Equation (4.2)

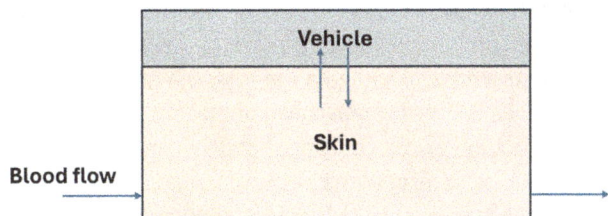

Figure 4.2: A schematic illustration of a two-compartment model featuring the skin as a whole and an additional compartment for the vehicle (i.e., the formulated skin product applied to the skin). Arrows represent flux of chemical compounds in and out of the compartments.

represent the bi-directional exchange of mass between skin and vehicle and between skin and blood flow, each of which is represented by an arrow in Figure 4.2. The balance is equated to the accumulation term $V_s \frac{dC_s}{dt}$. Notice here that we introduce the partition coefficient between the skin and vehicle P_{sv}, and between the skin and the blood compartment P_{sb}, to account for the fact that at equilibrium, the concentration of the chemical at the two sides of the interface between the two compartments accords to the ratio:

$$P_{sv} = \frac{C_{s,eq}}{C_{v,eq}} \tag{4.3}$$

If one is interested in the delivery of the chemical through the skin and into the blood (i.e., systemic circulation), then a similar mass balance equation can be used for the blood compartment. Otherwise, C_b can be assumed to be zero. Figure 4.2 illustrates an *in-vivo* exposure condition. However, it is *in-vitro* lab experiments that are most widely used in product development and risk assessment. In such an *in-vitro* permeation test (IVPT) *in-vitro* permeation test (IVPT) scenario, there is a receptor chamber below the skin membrane filled with liquid to 'receive' the permeants. The mass balance equation needs to be modified to:

$$V_s \frac{dC_s}{dt} = A\, k_{vs} \left(C_v - \frac{C_s}{P_{sv}} \right) - A\, k_{sr} \left(C_s - \frac{C_r}{P_{rs}} \right) \tag{4.4}$$

where C_r is the concentration in the receptor fluid. Normally in IVPT C_r is sufficiently small, because of the large volume of the chamber, so that it is safe to assume that $C_r \approx 0$, to simplify Equation (4.4). The mass transfer coefficients, k_{vs} (from vehicle to the skin) and k_{sr} (from the skin to receptor), can be interpreted as permeability as such. These partition coefficients are typically experimentally measured, or approximated by solubility data, or calculated from chemistry packages which are either based on quantitative structure-property relationships (QSPR) or sometimes molecular dynamics simulation [10]. The balance Equation (4.4) is completed with the appropriate initial condition (e.g., $C_s[t = 0] = 0$) and can be solved using standard ODE solvers.

The above illustrates the relationship between three compartments, including the vehicle, the skin as a whole, and the systemic circulation. This, however, would be one of the simplest definitions for a compartmental model of the drug permeation process into the skin. Compartments can be defined for other layers of the skin, hence introducing as many complexities in the model as needed depending on the research objectives. The common characteristic of the equations defining compartmental models, such as those stated above, is that they do not account for spatial gradients, but only temporal. In fact, only the derivatives of the concentration with respect to time, and not spatial coordinates, appear in Equations (4.2) and (4.4). These results in substantial economy of computer resources and therefore, it is common to find compartmental models in the literature that are not limited to the skin only and the systemic circulation but extend the reach to the effect of drug permeation in other organs of the body or even the entire body, resulting in the so-called whole body PBPK models [11].

4.3.2 Spatial diffusion-based models

A compartmental modelling approach assumes a constant concentration in each layer of the skin and organ considered in the model. Compartmental models can be dynamic or static, which means that they give the user the possibility to solve temporal gradients, but spatial gradients are however neglected within each compartment. Spatial diffusion-based models described in this section offer the user the choice of considering both spatial and temporal changes of concentration in skin layers. Spatial distribution is crucial to obtain a realistic concentration profile of the permeant within the skin. To solve such partial differential equations, both time and space must be discretised (i.e., forming a computational grid, aka computational mesh) to solve the mass balance equations for the chemical species considered, with appropriate initial and boundary conditions.

Including space discretisation offers greater degree of detail than compartmental models in terms of spatial concentration profiles across the skin layers. This is usually at the expense of a more computationally intensive calculation than compartmental models. Loosing detail at the smaller scale means that computational resources can be used to extend the reach of a model when a compartmental approach is used. Thus, compartmental models can be used to link phenomena occurring locally in the skin with phenomena taking place at the full organism scale (e.g., additional compartments can be included in the compartmental model to link diffusion from a vehicle into the skin with liver metabolism).

Both compartmental and spatial diffusion-based approaches are not exclusive. An efficient use of the computational resources available might entail the use of a spatial diffusion-based approach where spatial concentration is key, with a compartmental approach in the rest of the skin layers or organs considered. This mixed approach has been used in the literature on several occasions. For instance [12], used a spatial diffusion-based approach to describe spatial gradients in the stratum corneum, viable epidermis and dermis linked with an additional compartment to describe clearance of nicotine in the human body. A detailed geometry of the stratum corneum including the bricks-and-mortar approach, as well as the hair follicle, were included. This allowed an accurate visualisation of the spatial concentration profiles of nicotine in the skin as well as quantifying the dosage fraction that permeates into the dermis through the keratinocytes and the lipidic layers in the stratum corneum, and also via the sebum pathway in the hair follicle. The model simulated an *in-vivo* experimental situation and therefore, accurate results could only be obtained considering permeation in the skin itself and on to the systemic circulation and clearance by the organism. A visualisation of the concentration profiles obtained can be observed in Figure 4.3. These modelling requirements resulted in the mixed compartmental/spatial diffusion-based approach used by [12].

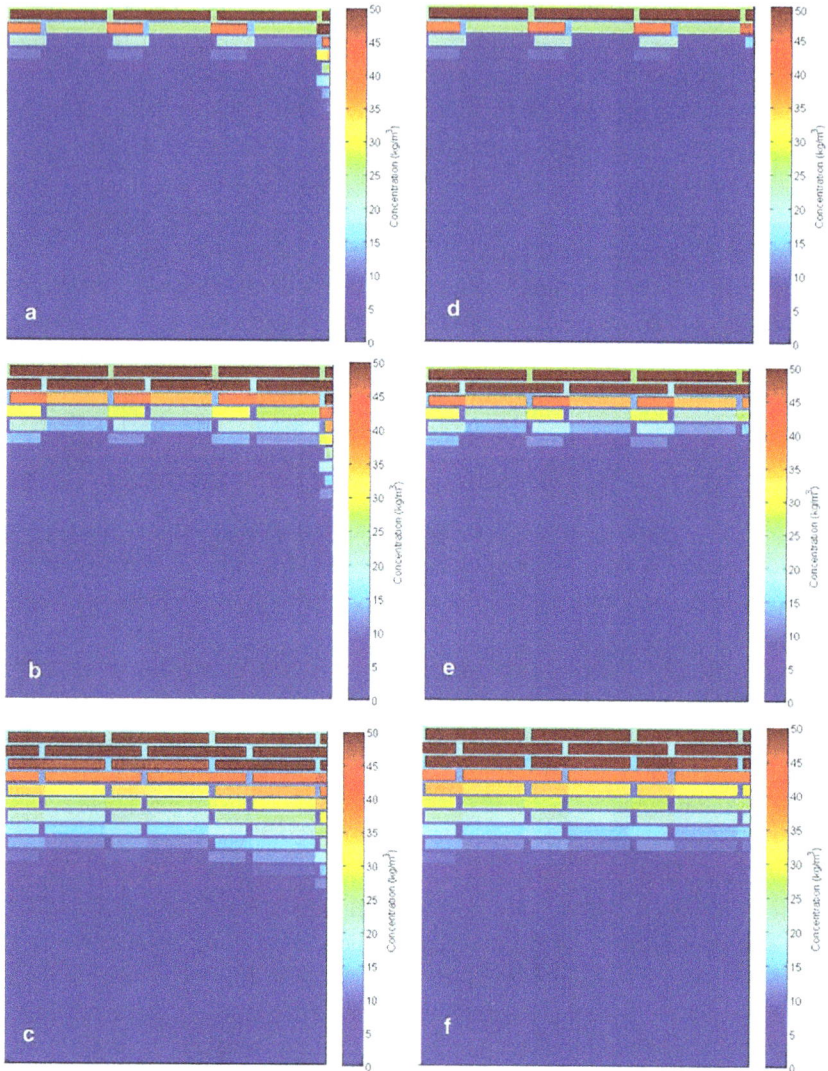

Figure 4.3: Illustration of concentration profiles obtained in the stratum corneum using a diffusion-based model. The simulation replicated an *in-vivo* experiment where a caffeine patch was administered to human volunteers. The description of the stratum corneum included the bricks and mortar model, where keratinocytes and lipidic gaps were modelled explicitly. Image reproduced with permission from [12].

The equation solved in the spatial diffusion-based part of the model was the following partial differential equation (PDE) (i.e., the diffusion equation without convection):

$$\frac{\partial C}{\partial t} + \nabla \bullet \vec{J} = R \tag{4.5}$$

where C is the concentration of caffeine, t denotes time and $\vec{J} = -D\nabla C$ accounts for Fickian diffusion. The term R on the right-hand side of the equation is a source term. The source term can be used to describe the metabolism reaction rate that would result in consumption of the administered drug and production of any metabolism products. In the work of [12], metabolism was neglected, hence $R = 0$. An example of a reported study considering metabolism was published by [13]. In the case of metabolism, it could be assumed that the skin behaves as a reaction-diffusion system, where the mass flux due to convective transport can be neglected, with the rest of the terms in the molar balance Equation (4.5) different from zero. The diffusion equation above includes temporal changes through the accumulation term of the molar balance $\frac{\partial c_i}{\partial t}$, and also spatial gradients ∇c_i by means of Fick's diffusion flux. The model included one such diffusion equation for each layer of the skin where spatial changes were solved. These are denoted in Equation (4.5) by the subscript i and included the stratum corneum (both keratinocytes and lipidic phase), the viable epidermis, the dermis and the follicular sebum pathway.

On the other hand, the compartmental part of the model solved the following molar balance equation:

$$V_b\frac{\partial C_b}{\partial t} = \frac{Q_{b,d}}{V_d}\iiint\left(\frac{C_d(x,y,z)}{P_{db}} - C_b\right)dV - KC_b \tag{4.6}$$

where C_b is the concentration of caffeine in blood, V_b is a constant denoting the volume of blood in the average body, $Q_{b,d}$ is the volumetric flow rate of blood through the dermis (i.e., approximately 5 % of the overall blood outflow from the heart), V_d is the volume of the dermis, K_{db} is the partition coefficient between the dermis and blood, K denotes clearance rate, and C_d is the concentration of caffeine in the dermis, which is space-dependent. This molar balance considers the spatial changes in the concentration in the dermis to calculate the integral (i.e., the average concentration in the dermis), but there is no description of the spatial gradients of caffeine concentration in the blood compartment. Rather, it only changes with time, hence the compartmental nature of this part of the model describing changes in the concentration of caffeine in the systemic circulation.

Equation (4.6) above can be re-written in the following form in a spatio-temporally discretized 2-D skin model (i.e., spatial diffusion-based) like the one published by [12].

$$V_b\frac{\Delta C_b}{\Delta t} = \frac{Q_{b,d}NA_k}{V_d}\sum_{k=1}^{n}\left(\frac{C_{d,k}}{P_{db}} - C_b\right) - KC_b \tag{4.7}$$

where A_k, assumed constant across the geometric domain, is the area of the mesh element with the subscript k used as a counter for the number of elements in the mesh, n is the number of mesh elements, and N is a length parameter that translates the 2-D skin model into the 3-D real case.

Equation (4.7) presents two aspects of spatial diffusion-based modelling worth noting. On the one hand, the need for discretising a 1-D, 2-D, or 3-D geometry of the skin. In general terms, permeation of a chemical through the skin is a 1-D phenomenon, which occurs mainly in the direction perpendicular to the skin surface. An example of such a simulation is the study reported by [13], where a 1-D representation of the skin, plus the source terms describing metabolism, were included. A 2-D geometry would not be needed unless mass transfer on the direction parallel to the skin surface needs consideration. That would be the case where considerable diffusion rate of a permeant through skin appendages such as the hair follicle must be considered. In principle, a 3-D representation of the skin would not be needed to describe diffusion unless some special features need to be considered. The need for 3-D models can be illustrated by means of the study reported in [14], for instance, who used a 3-D description of the skin geometry to describe drug delivery through microporated skin. The asymmetric character of these micropores made necessary the use of a 3-D approach.

Following up with the two aspects of Equation (4.7) worth noting, the second aspect is that an integral appears in the version presented in Equation (4.6), while the integral is substituted by a finite sum in Equation (4.7). The sum represents the spatial discretisation of spatial diffusion-based models. In essence, the term calculates the amount of caffeine being transferred from the dermis and into the blood compartment. While Nature is continuous, hence the integral in Equation (4.6) as per the fundamentals of differential calculus, the simulation is the result of a spatial discretization, hence the finite sum in Equation (4.7). The sum in the input term in Equation (4.7) must therefore be computed over all the mesh elements in which the skin geometry has been discretised. Equation (4.7) can also be understood as the result of adding the molar balances over each one of those mesh elements. Back in its continuous form, one such molar balance over a mesh element would read as follows:

$$\frac{V_b}{n}\frac{\partial C_b}{\partial t} = \frac{Q_b N A_k}{V_d}\left(\frac{C_{d,k}}{P_{db}} - C_b\right) - \frac{KC_b}{n} \tag{4.8}$$

Adding an Equation (4.8) for every mesh element would thus give rise to Equation (4.7). A closer look at Equation (4.8) will tell that each of these molar balances over a mesh element is one of the compartmental equations presented in Section 4.3.1 of this chapter. In summary, it is safe to say that a spatial diffusion-based model is a collection of many small compartments interconnected between them (i.e., one compartment per mesh element). The more compartments, the more detailed the description of the spatial concentration profiles in the skin will be, although the modeller must ponder the minimum degree of detail required according to computational power constraints.

Another example of mixed compartmental/spatial diffusion-based model was presented by [15], who presented a similar description of the skin in the spatial diffusion-based side of the model to the one reported by [12]. Two differences can be noted though between the two models, as the work of [12] dealt with caffeine, a small molecule of 194 Da, while the model reported by [15] was an adaptation of the model to the permeation of large molecules (dextrans between ~30 kDa and ~100 kDa). One difference was the description of the basement membrane, an additional diffusion barrier that can be neglected for the case of small molecules (i.e., and thus grouped in the viable epidermis), but that represents a significant barrier to the permeation of large molecules. The other difference between the two models is that [15] combined the skin diffusion model with hyperelastic deformation of the skin. The reason for this multiscale approach presented by [15] was that permeation of large molecules into the skin must be externally assisted. A large molecule cannot permeate the skin in significant quantities by passive diffusion only. In this case, permeation was assisted by the application of hypobaric pressure on the skin surface, which resulted in a modified geometry of the skin (i.e., the formation of a suction dome), as well as disruption of the diffusion barriers (i.e., smaller values of the diffusion coefficients than in the case of passive diffusion). The reader is referred to article published by [15], for more details on how the hyperelastic deformation of the skin was coupled with the diffusion equations. Multiscale and multiphysics approaches like this have the potential to expand the capabilities of spatial diffusion-based models beyond passive diffusion and follow the general trend reported amongst the modelling community where multiphysics descriptions can give rise to more realistic models with further reach.

In the simulation approach of [15], the compartmental side of the model was an additional differential equation that described the receptor fluid in the simulated *in-vitro* experimental setup (i.e., a Franz's cell) used to validate the calculations. The additional equation was:

$$\frac{dC_r}{dt} = \frac{A_{hyp}}{V_r}\bar{J} \tag{4.9}$$

where C_r is the concentration of dextran in the receptor fluid, A_{hyp} is the suction application area, V_r is the volume of the receptor compartment, and $\bar{J}$ is the average of the molar flux from the dermis and into the receptor compartment. Equation (4.9) shows again that only temporal variations, not spatial, are considered for the receptor fluid, hence the mixed compartmental/spatial diffusion-based character of the model. It is also worth noting that neglecting spatial gradients is an acceptable assumption when the receptor fluid is perfectly mixed.

Another aspect worth noting in spatial diffusion-based models is the setup of the boundary conditions. The flexibility of spatial diffusion-based models in this aspect allows the user to consider different scenarios encountered both *in-vivo* and *in-vitro*. Boundary conditions between the layers of the skin are partition boundaries. Partition coefficients, along with diffusion coefficients must be calculated and introduced into the simulation from QSPR expressions reported in the literature. No flux boundaries can be implemented between the skin layers and the hair shaft and to neglect diffusion in the direction parallel to the skin surface in those areas of the skin without appendages. Boundary type specification where a permeant enters and exits the skin offers the user flexibility to mimic different experimental scenarios. On the top of the stratum corneum, a finite or infinite dose scenario can be established. An infinite dose would be characterized by a constant concentration boundary. A finite dose on the other hand, can be mimicked by adding an additional layer with an initial concentration C_0 to represent the vehicle, with no flux boundaries everywhere but the junction between the vehicle and the stratum corneum, where a partition coefficient must be implemented. At the bottom part of the dermis, where the permeant would abandon the skin, different possibilities exist. One of them is the simulation of a receptor fluid by means of Equation (4.9). Another possibility would be to impose a zero concentration boundary at all times, which mimics an infinite sink and is useful to obtain the value of the permeability of a specific drug *in-vitro*. Ref. [16] used the latter, along with a 2-D geometry that included the hair follicle, to calculate differences in flux and permeability of different drugs between having the follicular route blocked or unblocked, hence obtaining quantification of the overall importance of the follicular route in the permeation process for a wide range of lipophilic and hydrophilic drugs. Finally, the other possibility is the approach used by [12] and commented above, where a no flux boundary was implemented in the bottom boundary

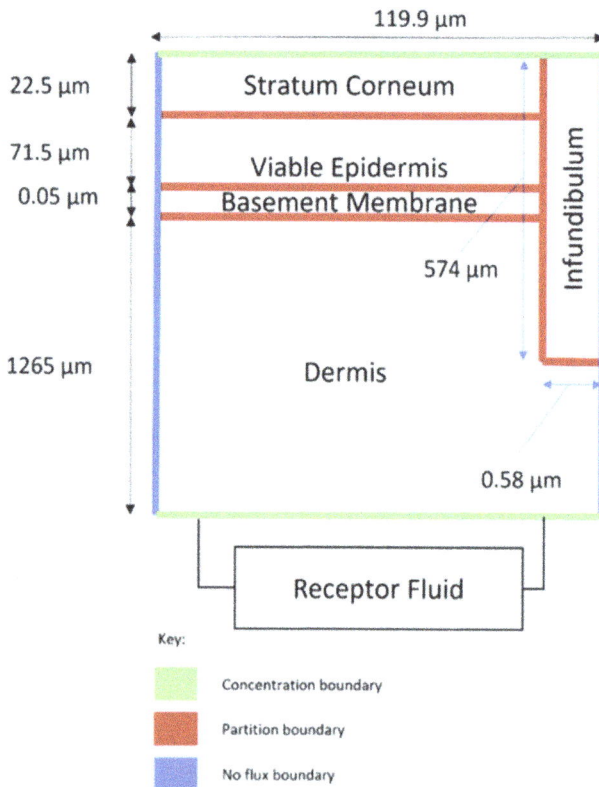

Figure 4.4: Schematic illustration including the skin geometry used by [15]. The schematic includes the boundary conditions used, with partition boundaries between the different layers of the skin, no flux boundaries to neglect diffusion in the direction parallel to the skin's surface except for the follicular route (i.e., infundibulum), and concentration boundaries where the permeant enters or leaves the skin. Image reproduced with permission from [15].

of the dermis *in-vivo* and evacuation of the permeant to the systemic circulation was introduced by means of Equation (4.6). This approach assumes that the drug passes to the systemic circulation only, and there is no permeation into the hypodermis. Figure 4.4 is an illustration of the boundary conditions used in the work of [15]; following the guidelines mentioned in this paragraph.

In conclusion, spatial diffusion-based models are useful when localised phenomena in the skin have to be represented but are somehow limited when it comes to simulate the relationship between said localised phenomena and the rest of the body. In some cases, a mixed compartmental/spatial diffusion-based approach is needed to optimise computational resources at hand.

4.4 Beyond the basics: chemical transfer facilitated by external forces

Chemical transfer across the skin can be further modulated by a number of external physical means, such as iontophoresis, sonophoresis, and mechanical means using microneedles, temporal positive pressure and hypobaric (i.e., negative) pressure. In those cases, the equations shown above must be expanded using a multiphysics approach to represent said external forces. Iontophoresis applies a low electric potential across the skin in order to drive ions across the skin membrane [17]. By modulating the current density this method could provide controlled delivery of active ingredients into the skin, as well as extraction of chemicals from the skin [18]. The governing equation for the transport process is the Nernst–Plank equation:

$$\frac{\partial C}{\partial t} = \nabla \cdot \left(D\nabla C + \frac{Dze}{k_B T} C\nabla\phi \right) \tag{4.10}$$

where in addition to diffusion, the transport of ions is further facilitated by the gradient of the electric potential ϕ. Here D is the diffusivity, z the valence of ionic species, e the elementary charge, k_B the Boltzmann constant and T the absolute temperature.

The complexity of modelling iontophoresis-assisted transport processes is that the electric potential ϕ is a function of space (though its variation over time can be ignored as it is a much faster process than chemical transfer) and needs to be predicted from the voltage equation and the current source applied through electrodes (Figure 4.5). The placement of the electrodes has a significant impact on the effectiveness of the device and is a major design consideration.

While iontophoresis may be limited to polar chemicals, sonophoresis utilises ultrasound to perturb the skin in a way to increase its permeability, thus facilitating chemical transport. Existing modelling efforts could be largely classified into two categories based on the perceived mechanisms: enhanced diffusion due to ultrasound induced structure alterations [20], or ultrasound induced convection [21]. In the former, the same spatial

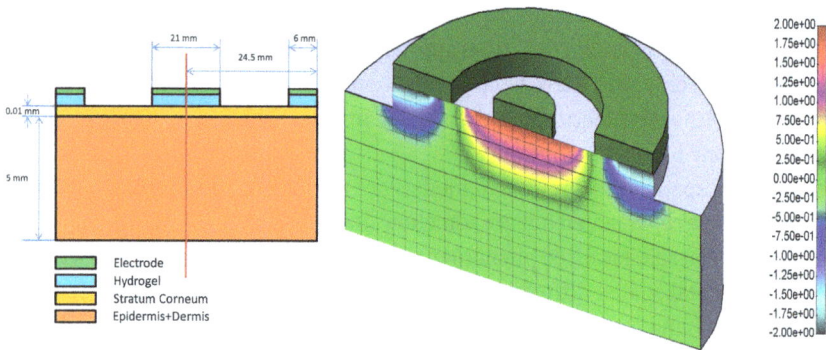

Figure 4.5: Left – geometry used in simulating iontophoresis assisted transdermal delivery system; right – simulated voltage distribution after applying the current source. Image reproduced with permission from [19].

diffusion-based transport equation is used but diffusivity modified based on ultrasound intensity; in the latter, a convective flow term is included in addition to diffusion.

Application of external pressure appears to be a natural way of increasing transdermal delivery. Ref. [22] developed a method to apply temporal positive pressure on the skin surface for this purpose. Interestingly, another study found that applying a negative pressure (i.e. hypobaric pressure), as opposed to a positive one, tends to stretch the skin into a dome formation which opens up the hair follicles and weakens the skin barrier properties [15, 23]. It is worth noting that such models use a multiphysics approach, since it necessarily combines the biomechanics of the skin alongside models for chemical transfer due to the mechanical deformation of the skin when applying hypobaric pressure.

Another useful technique is the use of microneedles [24], which consists in the application of 0.5 mm needles and longer to penetrate the stratum corneum so that the active ingredients loaded onto the needles can be directly released into the dermis. With several decades of development there are many designs available with a variety of materials used (e.g., metals, conventional polymers, biodegradable polymers). In terms of modelling the focus has been on biomechanics [25] – the mechanical interaction between the needles and the skin tissue, while the chemical transfer process can be treated as a typical diffusion process from a source (the needles coated with active ingredients).

4.5 Case studies

The previous sections have presented the fundamentals of *in-silico* models to describe dermal permeation, both in terms of the basic problem of passive diffusion and diffusion assisted by external forces. In this section, two selected case studies of how these models can help with answering specific research questions of application in industry will be presented to the reader. These case studies include i) the evaporation of certain components of formulated skin products and ii) the overall effect of the hair follicle in dermal permeation.

4.5.1 Integrated evaporation and skin permeation for *in-vitro* permeation

Experimental emphasis has shifted towards chaptering finite dose and unoccluded conditions in IVPT studies, recognising the impact of evaporation on dermal absorption. While *in-silico* modelling of dermal absorption has progressed significantly in the past two decades, the incorporation of evaporation is still limited, especially when investigating the impact of volatile permeants on IVPT results.

Several models of evaporation and dermal penetration of volatile permeants have been proposed. In these models, evaporation is described by a mass transfer equation with the evaporation rate represented by a mass transfer coefficient. The mass transfer coefficient is empirically related to the vapour pressure and molecular weight of the ingredients, alongside wind speed in the environment. This empirical equation was originally published by the US Environmental Protection Agency (EPA) for the evaporation of liquid spills [26] in the context of laboratory accidents; however, [27] considered it to be applicable to dermal scenarios if appropriate input values are used.

Achieving satisfactory evaporation predictions often requires further fitting of key parameters in the mass transfer rate equation due to uncertainties in the experimental conditions. Wind speed on the skin surface has a large impact on evaporation [28] but can be difficult to measure accurately. For example, [29] needed to fit the air flow rate to obtain a satisfactory result for the evaporation and skin absorption of N,N-diethyl-*m*-toluamide. The evaporative mass transfer coefficient was calculated as follows:

$$k_{evap} = \frac{1.756e^{-5} \, P \, MW^{\frac{2}{3}} \, u^{0.78}}{RT} \tag{4.11}$$

where u accounts for wind speed.

A second method for consideration of the evaporation of volatile permeants is modelled by the mechanistic diffusion equation driven by the vapour pressure of the permeant at the liquid-air interface [30]. We applied this integrated model to simulate the published IVPT data under finite dose, unoccluded conditions commissioned by the Cosmetics Europe task force [31]. The model presented here [32] investigates evaporation as a passive diffusion process driven by the concentration gradient between the air-vehicle interface and the ambient environment. The model simulates the likely evaporation of all ingredients in the vehicle. Evaporation has a dynamic impact on the vehicle. Solvent evaporation leads to an increasing concentration of the active ingredient, which can even precipitate when it exceeds the solubility. On the other hand, if the active ingredient is volatile its evaporation will decrease the concentration in the vehicle. The complex and dynamic changes in the vehicle creates a non-trivial impact on dermal absorption.

The modelling equations are given below. The evaporative flux of an ingredient from the vehicle J_{evap} is given by the Fick's first law of diffusion in the gas phase above the vehicle:

$$J_{evap} = - D_{evap} \frac{C_{gas} - C_{amb}}{h} \tag{4.12}$$

where C_{gas} is the gas-phase molar concentration of the ingredient at the vehicle surface, C_{amb} is the concentration in the ambient environment beyond the donor chamber of the diffusion cell, and h is the height from the vehicle surface to the top wall of the donor chamber (taken as the height of the diffusion cell). We assume that there are no ingredients in the ambient ($C_{amb} = 0$) except water for which C_{amb} can be calculated using the ideal gas law based on humidity. The same ideal gas law can be used to calculate C_{gas}:

$$C_{gas} = \frac{P_{vap} \, x_{liq} a}{R_{gas} \, T} \tag{4.13}$$

where P_{vap} is the vapour pressure of the pure ingredient, x_{liq} is its mole fraction in the liquid vehicle and a is the activity coefficient to account for non-ideal liquids (all vehicles assumed to be ideal liquids, $a = 1$), T is the temperature and R the gas constant.

The diffusivity of a molecule in the air D_{evap} can be obtained from many physical chemistry manuals or calculated through theoretical equations including Maxwell–Stefan, Chapman–Enskog, and Stokes–Einstein equation. Little variation is seen among the three methods for the chemicals tested in this chapter. The results reported here are based on D_{evap} calculated using the Stokes–Einstein equation below:

$$D_{evap} = \frac{k_b T}{6 \pi \eta r} \tag{4.14}$$

where k_b is the Boltzmann constant, η is the dynamic viscosity of air, and r is the radius of the molecule.

To integrate evaporation into a dermal model, the latest modelling framework developed in our group has been used. The technical details of the model are described in [33]. The integration of evaporation with PBPK modelling considered both solvent and solute volatiles. Volatile evaporation will change the volume of the vehicle V and this is modelled through the following mass balance:

$$\frac{dV}{dt} = -\sum \frac{J_{evap} A}{\rho}$$ (4.15)

where the summation is with respect to all volatile ingredients in the vehicle and ρ the density of that ingredient. A is the application area. Here again, we assume that the vehicle can be approximated well as an ideal solution to calculate its volume change. In addition, the volume change due to skin permeation is considered negligible.

Evaporation of a volatile will lead to the dynamic change of its mass balance in the vehicle. The overall mass balance of a volatile in the vehicle due to both evaporation and skin penetration is thus given by

$$V\frac{dC}{dt} = -J_{evap}A + C\sum \frac{J_{evap} A}{\rho} - J_s A$$ (4.16)

where J_s is the skin permeation flux computed using our existing PBPK model.

Here, the PBPK-E model has been applied to remodel the datasets from Cosmetics Europe ADME [31], focussing on volatile chemicals (n = 23). To determine volatility, we used the mass balances of permeants reported by [31], below 90 % was considered indicative of evaporation occurring in the experiment. The chemicals are listed in Table 4.1, with further details such as experimental mass balance reported in [31].

The PBPK-E model has been applied to simulate the Cosmetics Europe IVPT set of cosmetic relevant chemicals [31]. First, the model prediction of the 23 volatiles was compared with the mass imbalance of the reported data as shown in Figure 4.6. The predicted evaporation results agreed well with the reported mass loss (R^2 = 0.76, n = 23). The data is taken from [32] and reproduced under the creative commons license http://creativecommons.org/licenses/by/4.0/.

Table 4.2 shows the predicted distribution of the permeants in each compartment compared with the Cosmetics Europe data with and without evaporation.

Further details of the predicted kinetic change of cutaneous distribution and receptor fluid in comparison with reported experimental data are plotted in Figure 4.7. 4-tolunitrie, diethylmaleate and vanillin were chosen to represent a range of physiochemical properties and model-data agreement.

The RF kinetics, predicted by models and compared with experimental data, for the remaining 20 chemicals can be found in [32]. The predictions of the PBPK-E model of evaporation of the permeants align well with atmospheric data, producing a high R^2 value (R^2 = 0.76, n = 23). This indicates that the approach to model evaporation through the use of vapour pressure as the main factor is a valid method. The cumulative amounts in the vehicle and the RF are predicted satisfactorily, with an R^2 of 0.55 and 0.68, respectively. However, the amount remaining in the SC is generally overpredicted, and those in the viable epidermis and dermis compartments were poorly predicted. It was well recognised that quantifying the amount of permeant in individual skin layers is challenging and the existing methods (e.g., tape stripping) are subject to significant variabilities. Among the 23 chemicals examined, varying levels of agreement between the model and

Table 4.1: The 23 volatile permeants considered in this chapter and their relevant physico-chemical parameters. A – taken from the EPA dashboard (https://comptox.epa.gov/dashboard), B – taken from [34].

Permeant	CAS number	MW[A]	Log P_{ow}[A]	Vapour pressure [Pa][B]
4-Tolunitrile	104-85-8	117.15	1.58	41.72
Acetophenone	98-86-2	120.15	0.20	52.90
Aminophenol	95-55-6	109.13	0.62	0.011
Benylidene acetone	122-57-6	146.19	2.07	1.65
Benzophenone	119-61-9	182.22	3.18	0.26
Benzophenone	119-61-9	182.22	3.18	0.26
Cinnamaldehyde	14371-10-9	132.16	1.90	5.12
Diethylmaleate	141-05-9	172.18	0.82	14.00
Dimethyl fumarate	624-49-7	144.13	1.74	40.00
Dimethyl phthalate	131-11-3	194.19	1.58	0.41
Ethylhexyl acrylate	103-11-7	184.28	4.20	23.70
Eugenol	97-53-0	164.20	2.27	3.02
Geraniol ethanol	106-24-1	154.25	3.56	4.00
Geraniol PBS	106-24-1	154.25	3.56	4.00
Isoeugenol	97-54-1	164.20	3.04	1.60
Methyl methane sulfonate	66-27-3	110.13	0.74	55.20
Methylisothiazolinone	2682-20-4	115.15	−0.10	4.13
Naphthalene	91-20-3	128.17	3.30	11.30
Nitrobenzene	98-95-3	123.11	1.85	32.70
Propylparaben	94-13-3	180.20	3.04	0.24
Tetramethyl thiuram disulfide	137-26-8	240.42	1.73	0.0023
Thioglycolic acid	68-11-1	92.11	0.09	11.60
Vanillin	121-33-5	152.15	1.19	0.016

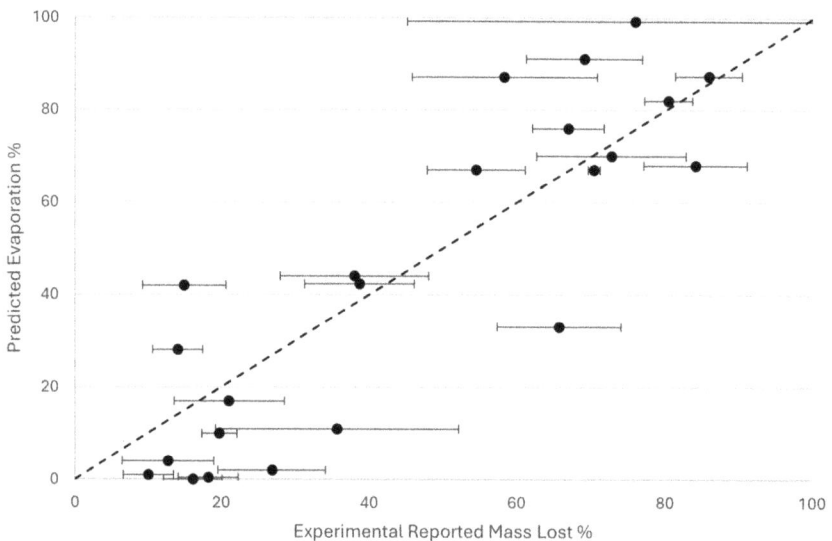

Figure 4.6: Comparison of PBPK-E model predictive evaporation with experimental mass loss and error bars reported by [31]. $R^2 = 0.76$ ($n = 23$). The dashed line indicates perfect agreement. The figure is taken from [32] and reproduced under the Creative Commons license http://creativecommons.org/licenses/by/4.0/.

Table 4.2: Comparison of model prediction with experimental data in terms of percentage accumulated of permeants in each compartment after 24 h' exposure.

Compartment	R^2 PBPK reported by (4.16)	R^2 PBPK-E model [32]
Atmosphere (mass loss)	–	0.76
Vehicle	0.19	0.55
Stratum corneum (SC)	0.15	0.11
Viable epidermis	0.01	0.00
Dermis	0.00	0.01
Receptor fluid (RF)	0.19	0.68
Dermal delivery[a]	0.15	0.60

[a]Dermal delivery refers to the combination of viable epidermis, dermis and receptor fluid. The comparison is taken from [32] and reproduced under the Creative Commons license http://creativecommons.org/licenses/by/4.0/.

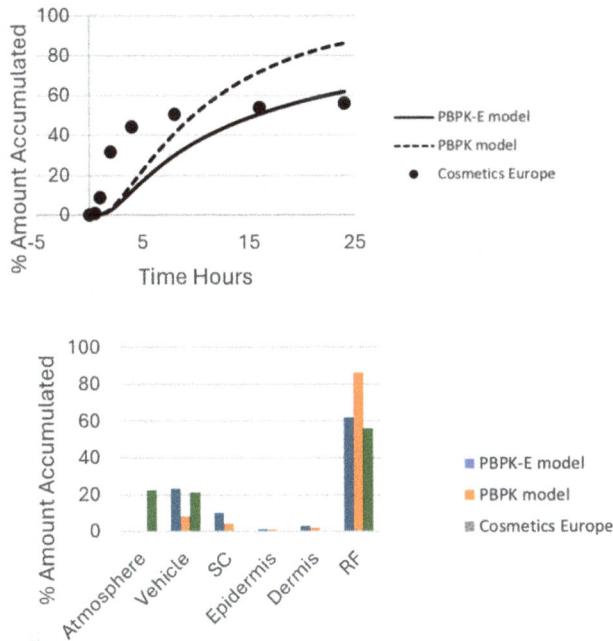

Figure 4.7: Modelling of vanillin for both RF kinetics over 24 h and cutaneous distribution after 24 h, as predicted by the two models against experimental data. The vanillin data is taken from [32] and reproduced under the Creative Commons license http://creativecommons.org/licenses/by/4.0/.

experiment were observed. For both RF kinetics and cutaneous distribution Vanillin demonstrated good agreement, especially for the distribution of the chemical at 24 h post exposure across all compartments. There is a significant improvement of the PBPK-E model over the PBPK model without evaporation. This highlights evaporation is needed to obtain accurate predictions of IVPT dermal absorption data under unoccluded, finite dose conditions.

4.5.2 Dermal permeation and delivery through the follicular pathway

Among the advantages of the use of mathematical models in research, they allow testing hypotheses swiftly by changing the simulation setup only, without the logistic implications that lab work entails. In this case study, a spatial diffusion-based model was utilised to elucidate whether preparation of samples for *in-vitro* dermal permeation studies can end up modifying the composition of the substance filling the follicular gap. The research is summarised in this chapter. The reader can find a fully detailed report in [16]. While, *in-vivo*, the follicular gap is known to be filled with sebum via its secretion by the sebaceous gland, washing and manipulating samples before *in-vitro* studies can result in the follicular gap filled partially with PBS, turning the follicular route from a lipophilic to a hydrophilic shortcut towards the dermis, and hence distorting conclusions drawn experimentally. The follicular route has been proved to have a significant impact on dermal permeation [35], and therefore, a change in its lipophilicity/hydrophilicity can have profound implications in the absorption of dermal permeants. In fact, differences can be seen in the literature between *in-vivo* and *in-vitro* studies regarding whether the follicular route favours the permeation of lipophilic or hydrophilic permeants, hence providing inconclusive results. In this case study, a spatial diffusion-based model of the skin including the follicular route was used to study the contribution of the follicular route to dermal permeation in two cases, including a follicular route filled with sebum and water.

The spatial diffusion-based mathematical model presented in this case study was used to elucidate the reason behind these differences by calculating the percentage of contribution of the follicular route to overall permeation (CFR) for small molecules with a wide range of octanol/water partition coefficients. Figure 4.8 is an illustration of the geometric domain where Equation (4.1) is solved. The concentration boundary conditions are an infinite dose in the vehicle (i.e., constant concentration at the top boundary $C_v = 1$ mol m^{-3}, affected by the corresponding partition coefficient between the stratum corneum and water P_{SCw}), and an infinite sink (i.e., concentration equal to zero) at the bottom boundary. This setup allows reaching a steady state molar flux, and thus the calculation of the skin's permeability to a specific permeant. The permeability μ is calculated as:

$$\mu = \frac{J}{C_v} \tag{4.17}$$

where J is the molar flux across the skin. The parameter *CFR* can be obtained as the difference in skin permeability between a case where the permeant can diffuse freely from the skin surface to the follicular route and a case where the follicular route is blocked (e.g., by using wax as in the experiments reported by [36]). In the present simulations, the same effect can be mimicked by using a no flux boundary on the top part of the follicular route. Thus, the CFR can be calculated using the following formula:

$$CFR = \frac{\mu_{open} - \mu_{closed}}{\mu_{open}} \times 100 \tag{4.18}$$

CFR among the molecules tested is a function of their specific partition and diffusion coefficients, which were calculated using the expressions in Table 4.3. Two simulations were needed to calculate the CFR for a specific compound, including a case with open and another with closed follicular route.

From the expressions included in Table 4.3, it can be concluded that for the case of a follicular route filled with water, the contribution of the follicular route CFR depend on five parameters: the octanol/water partition coefficient $P_{o,w}$, the fraction of permeant unbound to protein f_u, the non-ionised fraction of permeant f_{non} and the molecular weight MW. The partition coefficient between sebum and water was obtained from experimental measurements reported by [39]. To study the effect of these parameters on CFR, simulations were run for virtual compounds including all combinations for 11 values of log $P_{o,w}$ in the range [−3.70, 5.49], two values of molecular weight (i.e., MW = 50 Da and 285 Da), two values of the fraction of permeant unbound to protein and non-ionised fraction f_u, f_{non} = 0, 1.

The results of the test using virtual molecules for a follicular route filled with water are in Figure 4.9, where it is shown that the molecular weight MW and the octanol to water partition coefficient log $P_{o,w}$ have an effect on CFR, while the effect of f_u and f_{non} is negligible. The trend is not modified by the molecular weight MW. Figure 4.9 shows, too,

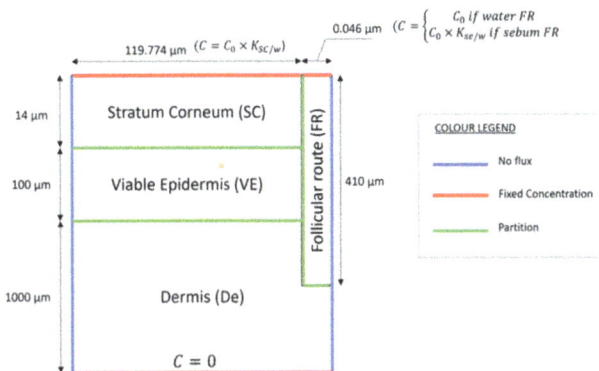

Figure 4.8: Schematic illustration including the skin geometry used by [16] for the study of the contribution of the follicular route to dermal permeation. In this figure C_0 denotes the molar concentration of the infinite dose in the vehicle and $K_{se/w}$ denotes the partition coefficient between sebum and water. Image reproduced with permission from [16].

Table 4.3: Summary of expressions to calculate diffusion and partition coefficients used by [16]. Volume fractions and densities are respectively $\varphi_{pro} = 0.1476$, $\varphi_{lip} = 0.0671$, $\varphi_w = 0.7853$, $\rho_{pro} = 1.37$ g/cm³, $\rho_{lip} = 0.90$ g/cm³, $\rho_w = 1.00$ g/cm³ and $\rho_{SC} = 1.05$ g/cm³. Partition coefficients between protein and water and between lipid and water calculated, respectively, as $P_{pro,w} = 4.2\,K_{o/w}^{0.31}$ and $P_{lip,w} = P_{o,w}^{0.69}$ [37]. The following QSPR was used to calculate the permeability of the SC: $\mu_{SC} = 5.6 \times 10^{-6}\,P_{o,w}^{0.7}\,e^{-0.46\,r^2}$ [38]. Partition coefficient lipid to water was $P_{lip,w} = \frac{\rho_{lip}}{\rho_w}P_{o,w}^{0.69}$. Molecular radius $r = \sqrt{\frac{3}{4\pi} \times 0.9087 \times MW}$. Boltzmann constant $k_b = 1.380649 \times 10^{-23}$ J/K. Temperature $T = 20$ °C. Dynamic viscosity of water $\eta = 1.0016$ mPa s.

Parameter	Expression
Partition coefficient stratum corneum to water $P_{SC,w}$	$P_{SC,w} = \left(\varphi_{pro} \times \frac{\rho_{pro}}{\rho_w} \times P_{pro,w} + \varphi_{lip} \times \frac{\rho_{lip}}{\rho_w} \times P_{lip,w} + \varphi_w\right) \times \frac{\rho_w}{\rho_{SC}}$
Partition coefficient viable epidermis to water P_{ew} and dermis to water $P_{d,w}$	$P_{e,w} = P_{d,w} = 0.7 \times \left(0.68 + \frac{0.32}{f_u} + 0.025 \times f_{non} + P_{ow}^{0.7}\right)$
Diffusion coefficient in stratum corneum D_{SC}	$D_{SC} = \frac{\mu_{SC}\delta}{P_{SCw}}$
Diffusion coefficient in viable epidermis D_e and dermis D_d	$D_e = D_d = \dfrac{10^{-8.15-0.655\times\log MW}}{0.68 + \frac{0.32}{f_u} + 0.025 \times f_{non} \times P_{lipw}}$
Diffusion coefficient in sebum D_{se}	$D_{se} = 2.48 \times 10^{-4}e^{-0.42\,r^2}$
Diffusion coefficient in water D_w (Stokes equation)	$D_w = \frac{k_b T}{6\pi\eta r}$

that the contribution of the follicular route decreases with the lipophilicity of the virtual compound. This is justified by the hydrophilic character of the follicular route in these simulation tests. One can appreciate a similar trend in the *in-vitro* results reported by [36, 40]. The data strongly suggests thus that the follicular route was filled with a hydrophilic substance in the *in-vitro* tests reported in both references. It is hypothesised that the hydrophilic character of the follicular route *in-vitro* should be the result of washing and preparation of samples combined with cessation of sebum secretion *in-vitro*.

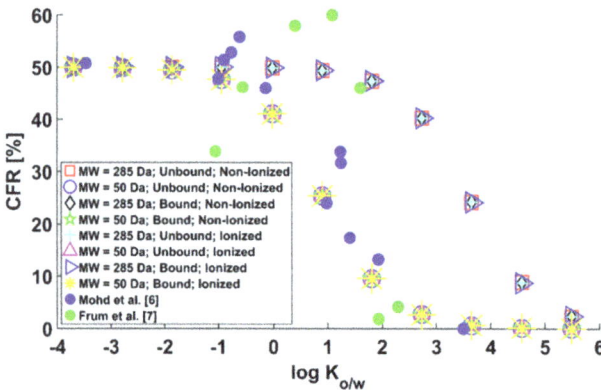

Figure 4.9: Contribution of the follicular route *CFR* to overall dermal permeation as a function of molecular weight *MW*, lipophilicity of the permeant (represented by symbol $K_{o/w}$ in this graph), fraction unbound to protein f_u and non-ionised fraction f_{non}. Image reproduced with permission from [16].

It is worth noting that the maximum *CFR* observed in the simulations is 50 %, which is close the maximum values obtained by [36]. The authors blocked with wax half of the hair follicles in their experimental samples. This was reproduced in the simulations by halving the flux across the top boundary of the follicular route. This is evidence that depending on the lipophilicity/hydrophilicity of the substance being administered, permeation through the stratum corneum may become negligible compared to flux through the follicular route.

The result obtained in Figure 4.9 for a set of virtual compounds was tested on a set of compounds used for therapeutic and cosmetic purposes. The results can be seen in Figure 4.10. The graph includes two series of simulated results: one using experimental measurements of the permeability of the stratum corneum and another using predictions through Mitragotri's QSPR expression. Variations between the two simulated data series were attributed by errors introduced by Mitragotri's QSPR. The two series of simulated data present the same trend though, which provides further evidence that the *in-vitro* experimental results of [36, 40] should have been conducted with the follicular gap filled with a hydrophilic substance.

Additional simulations were conducted changing the setup to accommodate a follicular route filled with sebum. The results can be seen in Figure 4.11, where two conclusions can be drawn. First, that the contribution of the follicular route remains high (>25 %) for all the values of the octanol/water partition coefficient tested. This is evidence that flux through the follicular route *in-vivo* is significant even for mildly hydrophilic permeants. Second, that there is an increasing trend between CFR and octanol/water partition coefficient, hence reinforcing the hypothesis that *in-vitro* results reported in the literature may be distorted by a change in the lipophilicity/hydrophilicity of the follicular route.

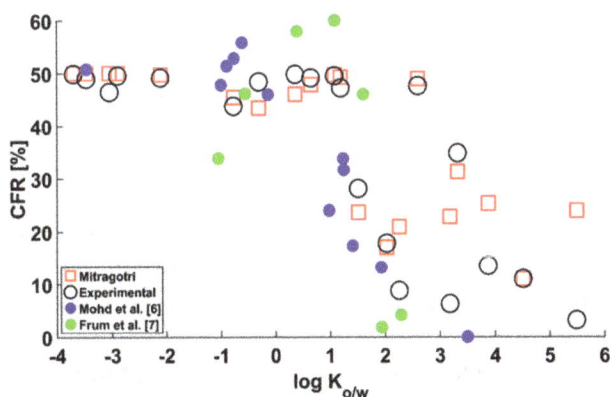

Figure 4.10: CFR calculated for a set of actual compounds used in industry for therapeutic and cosmetic purposes. Follicular route filled with water in the simulations. Octanol-water partition coefficient represented by symbol $K_{o/w}$. Image reproduced with permission from [16].

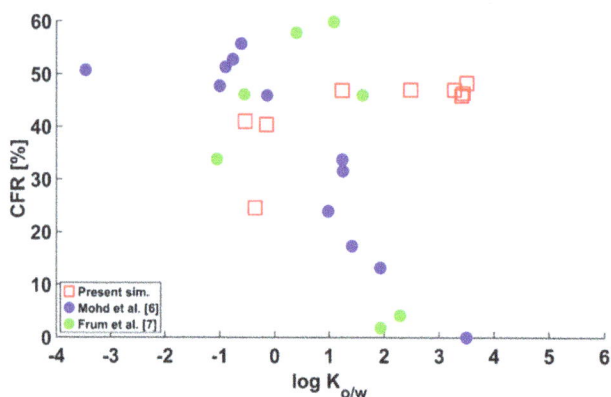

Figure 4.11: CFR calculated for different permeants. The simulation setup was changed to accommodate a follicular route filled with sebum. Octanol-water partition coefficient represented by symbol $K_{o/w}$. Image reproduced with permission from [16].

In summary, this case study provides an example of how a spatial diffusion-based model can help with elucidating a fundamental question, which would otherwise be much more costly should experimental methods only had been used. However, it is important to mention that models suggest only, and experiments are always needed to confirm trends obtained using mathematical models.

4.6 Perspectives and concluding remarks

The application of chemical engineering concepts to drug permeation through the skin opens up the doors towards the development of skin digital twins with the potential to offer companies and academic organisations the possibility to gain valuable insight on the intricacies of dermal permeation.

In chemical engineering terms, drug delivery across the skin is in essence a diffusive mass transfer problem. Some specifics, like externally-assisted drug delivery and consideration of systemic circulation and clearance, may require the application of a multiphysics approach, where mass transfer is complemented with mechanical deformation, electric phenomena, et cetera. The analysis of these phenomena and their expression in mathematical equations gives rise to powerful models based on underlying physical phenomena with the potential for skin Digital Twins that can help companies with the smart skin product development.

With the launch of 3R (Replacement, Reduction and Refinement) principles of animal testing for medical research, modelling has become an increasingly important alternative. Despite significant progress made in mathematical models for dermal permeation and the availability of commercial software packages such as COSMOperm, ESQlabs, GastroPlus and Simcyp to name few, challenges still remain. *In-silico* (i.e., mathematical simulation) methods are still not accepted by regulatory agencies. Much of the challenge is that these models are mostly validated for relatively simple dermal exposure conditions. These include mostly watery vehicles, which do not reflect the complex reality of commercial skin product formulations (e.g., emulsions and dispersions to creams, semi-solids and solids). *In-silico* methods are required to simulate how the critical attributes of topical product formulations impact dermal permeation.

One area of interest is the thermodynamic properties of solute solubility and partition in complex product formulation. Another area of interest is the formulation metamorphosis due to evaporation and phase change of products under nonocclusive condition. It can be envisaged that further advancement in the modelling of meta-morphosis, phase change of thermodynamic properties of complex product formulations will enable better prediction of formulation impact on transdermal absorption and bioavailability.

Acknowledgments: The authors would like to thank the editors David Bogle and Tomasz Sosnowski for their guidance and review of this article before its publication.

References

1. Shah J, McKnight G, Hargest R. Physiology of the skin. Surgery (Oxford) 2024;42:788–92.
2. Bos JD, Meinardi MMHM. The 500 Dalton rule for the skin penetration of chemical compounds and drugs. Exp Dermatol 2000;9:165–9.
3. Bosko CA. Skin barrier insights: from bricks and mortar to molecules and microbes. J Drugs Dermatol 2019; 18:s63–s67.
4. Tsakovska I, Pajeva I, Al Sharif M, Alov P, Fioravanzo E, Kovarich S, et al. Quantitative structure-skin permeability relationships. Toxicol 387:27–42. https://doi.org/10.1016/j.tox.2017.06.008.
5. Fukuda K, Ito Y, Furuichi Y, Matsui T, Horikawa H, Miyano T, et al. Three stepwise pH progressions in stratum corneum for homeostatic maintenance of the skin. Nat Commun 2024;15. https://doi.org/10.1038/s41467-024-48226-z.
6. Clayton K, Vallejo AF, Davies J, Sirvent S, Polak ME. Langerhans cells-programmed by the epidermis. Front Immunol 2017;8. https://doi.org/10.3389/fimmu.2017.01676.
7. Flohr C, Hay R. Putting the burden of skin diseases on the global map. Br J Dermatol 2021;184:189–90.
8. Liu X, Grice JE, Lademann J, Otberg N, Trauer S, Patzelt A, Roberts MS. Hair follicles contribute significantly to penetration through human skin only at times soon after application as a solvent deposited solid in man. Br J Clin Pharmacol 2011;72:768–74.
9. Anissimov YG, Jepps OG, Dancik Y, Roberts MS. Mathematical and pharmacokinetic modelling of epidermal and dermal transport processes. Adv Drug Deliv Rev 2013;65:169–90.
10. Piasentin N, Lian G, Cai Q. In silico prediction of stratum corneum partition coefficients via COSMOmic and molecular dynamics simulations. J Phys Chem B 2023;127:2719–28.
11. Nestorov I. Whole body pharmacokinetic models. Clin Pharmacokinet 2003;42. https://doi.org/10.2165/00003088-200342100-00002.

12. Kattou P, Lian G, Glavin S, Sorrell I, Chen T. Development of a two-dimensional model for predicting transdermal permeation with the follicular pathway: demonstration with a caffeine study. Pharmaceut Res 2017;34:2036–48.
13. Coleman L, Lian G, Glavin S, Sorrell I, Chen T. In silico simulation of simultaneous percutaneous absorption and xenobiotic metabolism: model development and a case study on aromatic amines. Pharmaceut Res 2020;37:1–10.
14. Pavlov AM, Rzhevskiy AS, Anissimov YG. Numerical investigation of analytical models of drug flux through microporated. Skin J Pharm Sci 2019;108:358–63.
15. Sebastia-Saez D, Benaouda F, Lim CH, Lian G, Jones SA, Cui L, Chen T. In-silico modelling of transdermal delivery of macromolecule drugs assisted by a skin stretching hypobaric device. Pharmaceut Res 2023;40: 295–305.
16. Sebastia-Saez D, Lian G, Chen T. In silico study on the contribution of the follicular route to dermal permeability of small molecules. Pharmaceut Res 2024;41:567–76.
17. Kalia YN, Naik A, Garrison J, Guy RH. Iontophoretic drug delivery. Adv Drug Deliv Rev 2004;56:619–58.
18. Moore K, Grégoire S, Eilstein J, Delgado-Charro MB, Guy RH. Reverse iontophoresis: noninvasive assessment of topical drug bioavailability. Mol Pharm 2024;21:234–44.
19. Filipovic N, Saveljic I, Rac V, Graells BO, Bijelic G. Computational and experimental model of transdermal iontophorethic drug delivery system. International Journal of Pharmaceutics 2017;533:383–388.
20. Mitragotri S, Edwards DA, Blankschtein D, Langer R. A mechanistic study of ultrasonically-enhanced transdermal drug delivery. J Pharmaceut Sci 1995;84:697–706.
21. Tang H, Mitragotri S, Blankschtein D, Langer R. Theoretical description of transdermal transport of hydrophilic permeants: application to low-frequency sonophoresis. J Pharmaceut Sci 2001;90:545–68.
22. Chin D, Lio S, Chia RN, Sheng M, Kwek Y, Wiraja C, et al. Temporal pressure enhanced topical drug delivery through micropore formation. Sci Adv 2020;6:eaaz6919.
23. Benaouda F, Inacio R, Hua Lim C, Park H, Pitcher T, Alhnan MA, et al. Needleless administration of advanced therapies into the skin via the appendages using a hypobaric patch. 2022. https://doi.org/10.1073/pnas.
24. Ai X, Yang J, Liu Z, Guo T, Feng N. Recent progress of microneedles in transdermal immunotherapy: a review. Int J Pharm 2024;662. https://doi.org/10.1016/j.ijpharm.2024.124481.
25. Soorani M, Anjani QK, Larrañeta E, Donnelly RF, Das DB. Modelling insertion behaviour of PVP (polyvinylpyrrolidone) and PVA (polyvinyl alcohol) microneedles. Int J Pharm 2024;664. https://doi.org/10.1016/j.ijpharm.2024.124620.
26. Peress J. Estimate evaporative losses from spills. Chem Eng Prog 2003;99:32–4.
27. Gajjar RM, Miller MA, Kasting GB. Evaporation of volatile organic compounds from human skin in vitro. Ann Occup Hyg 2013;57:853–65.
28. Chen L, Lian G, Han L. Modeling transdermal permeation. Part I. Predicting skin permeability of both hydrophobic and hydrophilic solutes. AIChE J 2010;56:1136–46.
29. Kasting GB, Miller MA, Bhatt VD. A spreadsheet-based method for estimating the skin disposition of volatile compounds: application to n, n-diethyl-m-toluamide (deet). J Occup Environ Hyg 2008;5:633–44.
30. Chen L, Lian G, Han L. Use of 'bricks and mortar' model to predict transdermal permeation: model development and initial validation. Ind Eng Chem Res 2008;47:6465–72.
31. Hewitt NJ, Grégoire S, Cubberley R, Duplan H, Eilstein J, Ellison C, et al. Measurement of the penetration of 56 cosmetic relevant chemicals into and through human skin using a standardized protocol. J Appl Toxicol 2020;40:403–15.
32. Deacon B, Silva S, Lian G, Evans M, Chen T. Computational modelling of the impact of evaporation on in-vitro dermal absorption. Pharmaceut Res 2024. https://doi.org/10.1007/s11095-024-03779-y.
33. Chen T, Lian G, Kattou P. In silico modelling of transdermal and systemic kinetics of topically applied solutes: model development and initial validation for transdermal nicotine. Pharmaceut Res 2016;33: 1602–14.

34. Grégoire S, Sorrell I, Lange D, Najjar A, Schepky A, Ellison C, et al. Cosmetics Europe evaluation of 6 in silico skin penetration models. Comput Toxicol 2021;19. https://doi.org/10.1016/j.comtox.2021.100177.

35. Knorr F, Lademann J, Patzelt A, Sterry W, Blume-Peytavi U, Vogt A. Follicular transport route – research progress and future perspectives. Eur J Pharm Biopharm 2009;71:173–80.

36. Mohd F, Todo H, Yoshimoto M, Yusuf E, Sugibayashi K. Contribution of the hair follicular pathway to total skin permeation of topically applied and exposed chemicals. Pharmaceutics 2016;8:32.

37. Wang L, Chen L, Lian G, Han L. Determination of partition and binding properties of solutes to stratum corneum. Int J Pharm 2010;398:114–122.

38. Chen L, Han L, Lian G. Recent advances in predicting skin permeability of hydrophilic solutes. Adv Drug Deliv Rev 2013;65:295–305.

39. Yang S, Li L, Chen T, Han L, Lian G. Determining the effect of pH on the partitioning of neutral, cationic and anionic chemicals to artificial sebum: new physicochemical insight and QSPR model. Pharmaceut Res 2018; 35. https://doi.org/10.1007/s11095-018-2411-8.

40. Frum Y, Bonner MC, Eccleston GM, Meidan VM. The influence of drug partition coefficient on follicular penetration: in vitro human skin studies. Eur J Pharmaceut Sci 2007;30:280–7.

Maryam Zarghami Dehaghani, Thomas Fabiani and
Maria Grazia De Angelis*

5 Chemical engineering contribution to hemodialysis innovation: achieving the wearable artificial kidneys with nanomaterial-based dialysate regeneration

Abstract: Hemodialysis (HD) has long been a cornerstone in the renal replacement therapy for end-stage kidney disease (ESKD), primarily through conventional in-center HD. Current HD systems in hospitals are bulky, water-demanding, and constrain the mobility and quality of life of ESKD patients. Home HD (HHD) offers the chance of delivering more frequent treatments close to the patient, reducing vascular stress and post-treatment hangover and improving patients' lifestyles. However, current HHD devices are analogous to hospital machines, requiring significant space, costly renovations, and they are energy and water intensive. Miniaturisation of HD systems depends on the reduction of water consumption, requiring the introduction of a dialysate regeneration unit, that purifies the spent dialysate of uremic toxins (UTs) and recirculates it, cutting down the amount of dialysate needed. This represents a crucial step for the development of a wearable artificial kidney. However, regenerating dialysate poses significant technical challenges as it involves separating a complex mixture under strict biomedical safety and stability requirements. This paper provides an engineering perspective into current research on using nanomaterials for adsorbing UTs from spent dialysate.

Keywords: hemodialysis; wearable artificial kidney; uremic toxins; nanomaterials; adsorption

5.1 Introduction

5.1.1 Kidney functionality and uremic toxins

Kidney functionality is classified into four primary categories:

---

*Corresponding author: Maria Grazia De Angelis, School of Engineering, Institute for Materials and Processes, University of Edinburgh, King's Buildings, Robert Stevenson Road, EH9 3FB, Edinburgh, SCO, UK, E-mail: grazia.deangelis@ed.ac.uk. https://orcid.org/0000-0002-1435-4251
Maryam Zarghami Dehaghani and Thomas Fabiani, School of Engineering, Institute for Materials and Processes, University of Edinburgh, King's Buildings, Robert Stevenson Road, EH9 3FB, Edinburgh, SCO, UK, E-mail: mzargham@ed.ac.uk (M. Zarghami Dehaghani), T.Fabiani@sms.ed.ac.uk (T. Fabiani)

As per De Gruyter's policy this article has previously been published in the journal Physical Sciences Reviews. Please cite as: M. Zarghami Dehaghani, T. Fabiani and M. G. De Angelis "Chemical engineering contribution to hemodialysis innovation: achieving the wearable artificial kidneys with nanomaterial-based dialysate regeneration" *Physical Sciences Reviews* [Online] 2024. DOI: 10.1515/psr-2024-0055 | https://doi.org/10.1515/9783111394558-005

- excretory, namely the elimination of waste products of protein metabolism (such as urea, creatinine, and ammonia), drugs and their metabolites.
- regulatory, involving the control of body fluid volume and its composition, maintaining electrolyte balance and acid-based balance.
- endocrine, related to the production of hormones including erythropoietin, renin and prostaglandins to regulate various physiological processes.
- metabolic: the kidney converts inactive vitamin D (second hydroxylation of vitamin D, calcidiol) into its active form (calcitriol or 1,25 di-hydroxycholecalciferol) which is essential for calcium homeostasis [1].

A kidney receives one-quarter of the blood cardiac output every minute and approximately consists of one million of functional units, named nephrons. Each nephron operates as an independent entity, consisting of the glomerulus (the actual filtration unit) and the renal tubule. Blood flows from the heart to the kidneys through the renal arteries, and is filtered in the glomerulus, where an ultrafiltration process is propelled by hydrostatic pressure gradient of approximately 10 mmHg (1.33 kPa) so that small molecules, water, and ions pass through the filtration barrier and enter the Bowman's capsule, while larger molecules like blood proteins and cells are retained [2]. The permeate flows through the renal tubule, where water, electrolytes, glucose, and amino acids are reabsorbed into the bloodstream, while waste products are secreted to form urine [3].

Factors such as diabetes mellitus, hypertension, inflammation of the glomeruli (glomerulonephritis), urinary reflux and infections (pyelonephritis), and polycystic kidney disease can cause the gradual loss of functioning nephrons over time, leading to lower filtration activity. As a result, solutes accumulate and they are designated as uremic toxins (UTs) when they disrupt normal biological functions causing the so-called uremic syndrome [4, 5], which is of growing interest in the biological and clinical research. There are three main categories of UTs associated with chronic kidney disease (CKD) [4, 6] as reported below:

1) Small, free water-soluble UTs (<500 Da) such as uric acid, urea, creatinine, oxalate, guanidine, hyaluronic acid.
2) Small molecular weight (<500 Da), protein-bound UTs (PBUTs): these UTs may bind on proteins present in blood, therefore the low UTs concentration in blood makes the clearance challenging. Examples include indoxyl sulfate, and p-cresyl sulfate (p-CS).
3) Middle and large-size (>500 Da) such as cystatin C, leptin, β2-microglobulin.

UTs can be classified based on other parameters such as chemical similarities, metabolic pathway, or toxicity as summarised in the minireview by Myjak et al. [4]. In the review paper by Vandholder et al. [7] it is reported that the most toxic UTs, in descending order, include: p-cresyl sulfate, beta-2 microglobulin, asymmetric dimethylarginine (ADMA), kynurenines, carbamylated compounds, fibroblast growth factor-23 (FGF-23), interleukin-6 (IL-6), tumor necrosis factor-α (TNF-α), and symmetric dimethylarginine (SDMA).

5.1.2 Chronic kidney disease and hemodialysis design

Chronic kidney disease is defined as the decline of the glomerular filtration rate (GFR) to less than 60 mL/min per 1.73 m^2 of body surface, or by detection of albuminuria, haematuria (>30 mg g^{-1}), or abnormalities in urine sediment for at least three months [1]. Annually, CKD is responsible for approximately 1.2 million fatalities globally, underscoring its significant impact on individual health and healthcare systems [8]. CKD is classified into five phases, with the most severe stage referred to as end-stage kidney disease (ESKD) associated with GFR less than 15 mL/min per 1.73 m^2, which requires a renal replacement therapy (RRT), such as hemodialysis (HD) or transplantation [9, 10]. According to the European Renal Registry [11], only 4 % of the patients in RRT had the chance to receive a transplant due to the scarcity of kidneys. According to the Global Kidney Health Atlas published in 2019, approximately 14.5 million people around the world will have developed ESKD by 2030 [12]. Therefore, developing and updating HD systems still remains a topic of research so that individuals with ESKD can maintain a more stable health status, alleviate symptoms, and prolong survival.

5.2 Basic equipment of conventional hemodialysis

HD involves the exchange of UTs, ions and excess fluids between the blood stream and a fluid, called dialysate, through a semipermeable membrane embedded in a housing unit, named dialyser [13]. Figure 5.1a and b demonstrate the equipment of the HD machine and configuration of the dialyser, respectively. Figure 5.1a shows that the patient's blood is drawn from a vascular access and passes through a series of controls, including an arterial pressure meter and a heparin pump to prevent clotting. The blood pump then propels the blood with a rate between 200 and 500 mL/min through the dialyser. In the dialyzer, UTs and excess fluids pass from the blood into the dialysate solution [14]. The dialyser is a module formed by a bundle of hollow fiber membranes designed to mimic glomerular filtration, namely retaining serum proteins, e.g., human serum albumin [15], and blood cells, but able to maximize the clearance of UTs ranging from a few tens of Daltons to 11 kDa. The dialyzer consists of approximately 10,000 to 20,000 thin fibers running longitudinally through the device (as shown in Figure 5.1b), each with an inner dimension ranging from 150 to 250 μm, and thickness between 7 μm and 50 μm and a length of 150 mm. It employs a countercurrent flow mechanism, where blood flows inside the fibres and dialysate flows on the outside [14, 16]. Considering the pore size determining the hydraulic permeability (volume passing through the membrane per unit surface area, time, and pressure), dialysers are classified into **low-flux** (pore radius between 2 and 3 nm, permeability in the range of 10–20 mL m^{-2} h^{-1} mmHg^{-1}) and **high-flux** (pore radius between 3.5 and 5.5 nm and permeability in the range of 200–400 mL m^{-2} h^{-1} mmHg^{-1}) membrane [17].

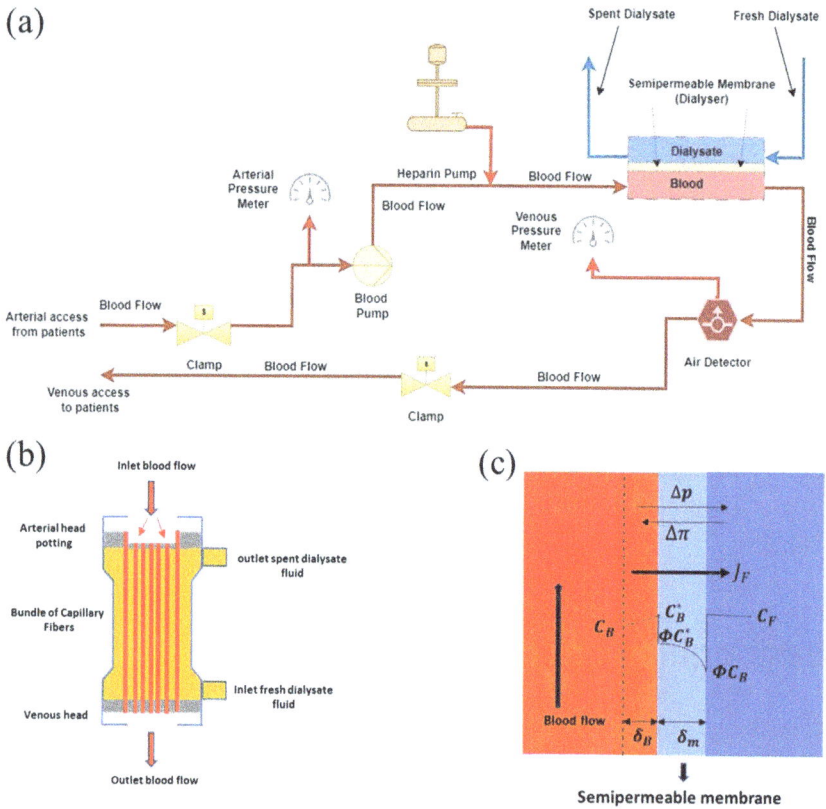

Figure 5.1: Conventional HD equipments. (a) The diagram of conventional HD, (b) the schematic of dialyser having hollow fibres, (c) convective solute transport across a semipermeable membrane in a hemodiafiltration process. Symbols are defined in the text.

Dialysate flows in the whole system with the rate of 600–800 mL min^{-1}. Dialysate is the solution that interacts across a membrane with a patient's blood during dialysis, carrying away waste products and excess fluids from blood without mixing with it. It plays a dual role: removing UTs while adding essential ions, such as calcium and bicarbonate, to maintain pH balance and electrolyte levels. Tailored to match the patient's required solute concentrations, dialysate prevents unwanted fluid shifts by closely matching blood osmolality, and specific concentration gradients drive the diffusion of solutes across the membrane. Key components, such as sodium and bicarbonate, may enter the blood, balancing the patient's electrolyte levels. Modern HD systems precisely regulate the dialysate's composition, temperature, and flow rate to optimise treatment and control fluid removal. Table 5.1 shows the composition of commercial dialysate.

The major components of the conventional dialysate circuit, shown in Figure 5.2, include: 1) water treatment section, 2) heating and deaeration component to warm the

Table 5.1: Dialysate commercial composition [18].

Compound	Concentration in dialysate
Sodium (Na$^+$)	134–145 mM
Potassium (K$^+$)	0–4 mM
Calcium (Ca^{2+})	1.25–1.75 mM
Magnesium (Mg^{2+})	0.5–0.75 mM
Acetate/Citrate	2–4
Chloride (Cl$^-$)	98–124 mM
Bicarbonate (HCO$_3^-$)	30–40 mM
Dextrose	11
Glucose	0–2 gL^{-1}
PH	7.1–7.3
P$_{CO2}$(mmHg)	400–110

dialysate to body temperature and removing bubbles, 3) proportioning section to mix the concentrate solutions (acid and bicarbonate) with ultrapure water to create the fresh dialysate with the correct chemical composition to maintain the proper electrolyte balance, 4) monitoring system to check the composition, temperature, and flow rate of the dialysate, 5) volumetric control component to adjust the transmembrane pressure to ensure that the appropriate amount of fluid is extracted as ultrafiltrate (UF), the fluid permeated through the membrane during the dialysis session [19]. Every session approximately demands 120 L of the dialysate [20, 21].

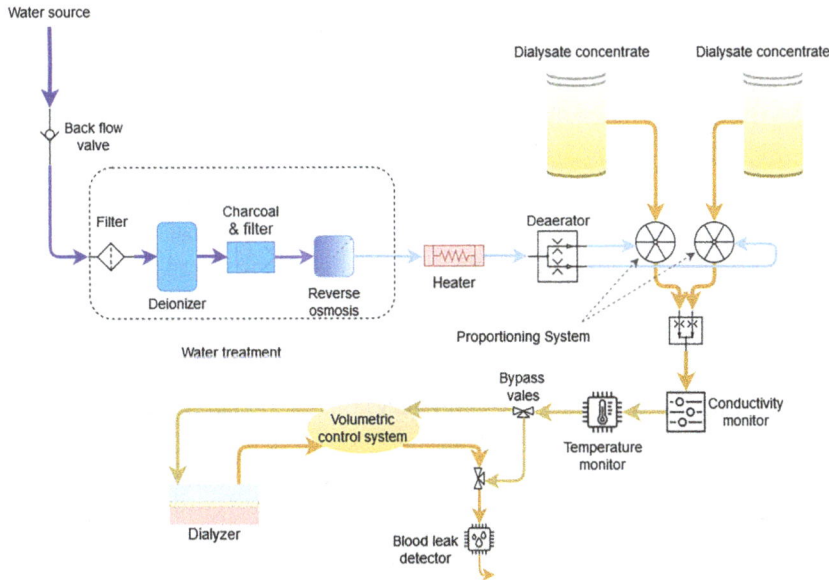

Figure 5.2: Conventional dialysate circuit.

Dialyser **clearance**, a parameter to evaluate the performance of dialyser, is defined as the amount of blood cleared in a minute $\left(K = \frac{Q_{B,in}C_{B,in} - Q_{B,out}C_{B,out}}{C_{B,in}} \right)$ where Q_B refers to the blood flow rate at the inlet $Q_{B,in}$ and outlet $Q_{B,out}$ of the dialyser and C_B gives the corresponding concentration [22]. Urea concentration decreases over time during the session using the principle of exponential decay. The dimensionless parameter Kt/V, derived from a single-compartment kinetic model ($C_t = C_0 e^{Kt/V}$), is used as an index of HD adequacy or dosing. K is the urea dialyser clearance, t is the time of the session, and V refers to the distribution volume [23].

The movement of UTs across a semipermeable membrane is controlled by the physiochemical properties of the molecule, the permeability of the membrane and the operational conditions such as blood flow and dialysate flow rates [14].

Notably, increasing flow rates mainly enhances the clearance of small UTs by minimising boundary layer effects, but it has little impact on larger solutes (e.g., myoglobin, molecular mass 17 kDa), where the membrane is the primary resistance to mass transfer [16].

Standard membrane dialysers with small pores, known as low-flux membranes, rely mainly on diffusion-based mass transfer and are limited in their ability to remove middle molecules due to their restricted pore size. To address this issue, **high-flux** dialysers are used, which have higher **membrane pore size** that facilitate the removal of the larger "middle" molecules such as the beta-2 microglobulin which leads to the dialysis-related amyloidosis.

In **hemodiafiltration**, a novel therapeutic strategy, concentration gradient-driven diffusion is augmented by **convection**, as depicted in Figure 5.1c, that is driven by a net pressure gradient ($\Delta p - \Delta \pi$) where Δp and $\Delta \pi$ correspond to **hydrostatic** and **osmotic** pressure difference across the membrane, respectively. The flow associated to this mechanism (J_F), called ultrafiltration rate, is equal to the net pressure difference multiplied by the **hydraulic permeability** L_p of the semipermeable membrane, that is related to the membrane thickness, pore geometry and fluid properties [24].

Osmotic pressure $\Delta \pi$ depends on the concentration of impermeable solutes in blood and dialysate. At a section of dialyser close to the blood inlet, due to the high concentration of solutes in the blood, the osmotic pressure difference may balance the hydrostatic pressure difference, leading to a reversal of the pressure gradient across the membrane, resulting in flow from dialysate to blood (**back filtration**) [16]. This may cause re-entry of contaminants from the dialysate into the bloodstream [25–27].

According to **stagnant film theory**, the blood concentration of larger solutes close to the membrane interface, in the so-called "**boundary layer**" δ_B becomes larger than in the bulk, reaching a maximum close to the membrane interface ($C_B^* > C_B$). The phenomenon is called **concentration-polarisation** and is exacerbated at high ultrafiltration rates. The equilibrium **partition coefficient** (Φ) describes how substances distribute between the membrane and surrounding fluids.

A **sieving coefficient** $SC = C_F/C_B$, representing the ratio of solute concentration in the filtrate, C_F, versus the same molecule concentration in the blood, C_B, measures the fraction of solute passing through the membrane, and depends on the relative size between the molecule and the pore. Solutes like urea and creatinine, which are much smaller than the membrane pores, have SC values near 1, indicating efficient permeation. Larger solutes with sizes exceeding pore dimensions have SC values close to zero. For solutes near the membrane's molecular mass cut-off, SC values are typically below 0.1. Manufacturers aim for SC values above 0.6 for β2-microglobulin and below 0.008 for albumin (66.5 kDa) [28]. As depicted in Figure 5.1c, SC is affected by concentration polarisation: indeed, the actual sieving coefficient ($SC_a = C_F/C_B^*$) which accounts for middle-size solute accumulation near the membrane ($C_B^* > C_B$) becomes lower than the nominal value especially at high ultrafiltration rates, reducing the membrane's selective filtering and increase useful protein (e.g. albumin) loss. Careful management of ultra-filtration rates through tuning the membrane pore size, alongside blood flow rates, is crucial in balancing toxin clearance and preventing albumin loss in HDF [16].

5.3 Developing dialysate regeneration techniques for the wearable artificial kidney

Conventional HD is generally delivered in three sessions per week, requiring the patient to be in hospital for three or 4 h per session. Moreover, commercial HD machines limit patients' mobility and daily activities, having a detrimental impact on the quality of life [29]. Exploring alternatives to this traditional schedule could potentially enhance patient survival, reduce treatment burden, and elevate overall well-being. Extended or more frequent dialysis sessions have been shown to lessen cardiac stress, regulate blood pressure, and boost metabolic health, underscoring the potential benefits of portable HD devices in improving patient lifestyle [30].

The process of regenerating spent dialysate is critical for the development of portable or wearable HD devices, as it enables the reduction of water use and the downsizing of equipment, eliminating the need for a direct water supply. The primary task of a regeneration unit is to keep uremic toxin concentrations low in the dialysate to ensure effective dialysis. While small, water-soluble uremic toxins like urea are readily removed during HD, making them the most concentrated solutes in the dialysate, certain UTs prove challenging to eliminate. Factors such as larger molecular size or strong protein binding can hinder their removal; these toxins typically appear in lower concentrations in the dialysate and are more difficult to clear efficiently. Amino acids including proline, valine, glycine, glutamate, alanine, leucine and other non-toxic compounds, such as glucose, L-lactate, and glycerol, are also present and can affect the separation process. The details on the amount of each solute removed during HD and their presence in spent dialysate are reported in a review paper by Shao et al. [31]. Efficient dialysate regeneration requires addressing these complexities to ensure effective UTs removal while maintaining essential physiological compounds.

5.3.1 Regeneration of spent dialysate: technologies for uremic toxins elimination

Urea, uric acid, and creatinine are small, water-soluble toxins are easily removed during HD and, as a result, are present in higher concentrations in the spent dialysate. Therefore, most researches focused on optimizing the removal of these molecules from spent dialysate. It must be noticed, however, that other toxins, e.g. protein-bound uremic toxins, present in smaller quantities in blood, are hard to eliminate with standard dialysers due to their larger size but they may be even more toxic. Such substances are believed to cause the uremic syndrome which is observed only in HD patients and not in transplanted ones, due to the incomplete removal of UTs of the HD membrane compared to a working kidney, and are associated to worse health status and higher mortality of HD patients. This requires for an interdisciplinary effort where chemical engineers work in close cooperation with nephrologists and biologists to identify and remove all harmful substances from the blood of the patients and, consequently, from the regenerated dialysis fluid.

Enzymatic conversion of urea. Urease has been used to oxidize urea into ammonium and carbon dioxide with high selectivity. The first portable HD device, the recirculating dialysis (REDY) sorbent system marketed from 1973 to 1993, performed dialysate regeneration through a multi-cartridge technology and weighed 5 kg (including dialysate) [20]. In the REDY system, in the first layer, non-urea organic compounds such as heavy metals, oxidants, chloramines, and other organic molecules were adsorbed by activated carbon. In the second layer, urea was enzymatically converted to ammonium and carbonate ions by immobilized urease. Ammonium was then captured by a cation exchanger of zirconium phosphate, which also removed calcium, magnesium, potassium, and other metal cations, releasing sodium and hydrogen. In the final layer, anions like phosphates and fluoride were absorbed by zirconium oxide and zirconium carbonate, through exchanging bicarbonate and acetate. The issue of leachate of aluminium used to immobilize urease, that was deemed responsible for severe side effects, led to its removal from the market. A similar device based on sorbent layers and immobilized urease named WAK (Wearable Artificial Kidney) was fabricated by Gura et al. [32]: this device underwent clinical trials but encountered issues with CO_2 bubble formation, due to the chemical decomposition of urea by urease, and flow control. Other prototypes similar to the REDY devices have been summarized in the review paper by Gelder et al. [20].

Integration of HD with FO. Another technique proposed to purify part of the dialysate and reduce the water demand of HD is forward osmosis (FO). Although strictly not employed to produce wearable dialysis devices, such technique can be used to regenerate dialysate and is thus included in the present review. Figure 5.3 shows the

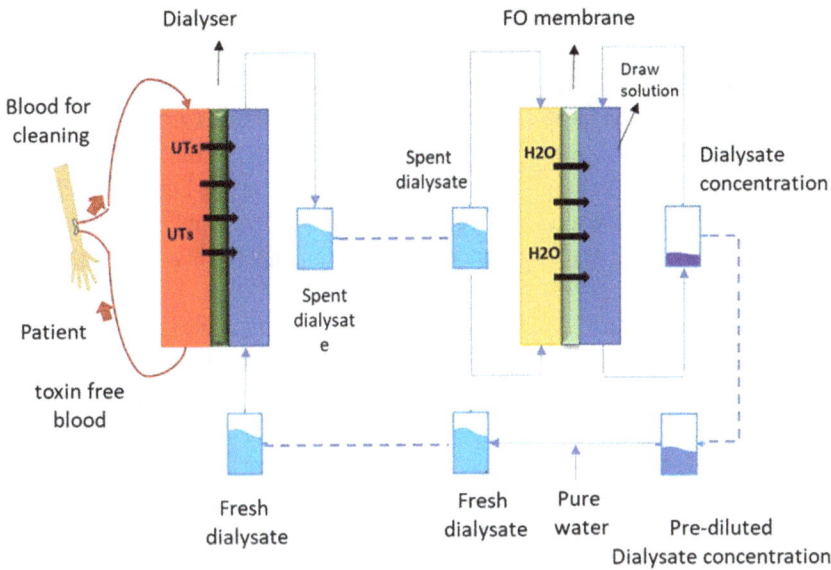

Figure 5.3: Diagram of the integration of HD with spent dialysate recovery through FO process.

schematic of the integration of HD with spent dialysate recovery through FO process. In such a process, water permeates through a semipermeable membrane to reach a draw solution, at higher osmolarity.

Commercially available dialysate concentrates can be used as a draw solution to recover clean water from the spent dialysate. Initial urea concentrations in spent dialysate and blood are 5 mM and 23 mM, respectively. The performance of FO process for regeneration of spent dialysate has two limiting cases: ideal conditions with complete urea rejection, or complete water recovery and minimal urea rejection, which is undesirable since it indicates that almost all urea remains in the dialysate [33]. FO membranes demonstrate a high rejection rate for compounds found in significant concentrations in the dialysate, including ions, glucose, and charged molecules. However, the rejection rate for urea remains comparatively low and is heavily affected by its concentration [34].

Photo-electrocatalytic oxidation. Such a technique leverages light and catalytic materials to facilitate chemical reactions, specifically for oxidizing urea into molecular nitrogen and carbon dioxide. This approach offers the advantages of low power consumption by using LED technology and disadvantages of by-products and low selectivity of oxidation [35, 36].

Adsorbents. One of the most studied strategies uses adsorbents to capture UTs from the dialysate. Porous materials, characterized by their elevated specific surface area, represent an excellent option as sorbents, due to their ability to maximize adsorption capacity, by presenting a high number of adsorption sites to the liquid phase. The dimensions and configurations of the pores, as well as the surface functionalization, play significant roles in influencing adsorption phenomena within the material, providing diverse binding sites for adsorbates [37]. UTs accumulates onto the solid surface of the adsorbent through dispersion forces, hydrogen bonding, electrostatic interactions, polarization, and covalent bonding [38]. The efficacy of the process is given by the static binding capacity, defined as the amount of adsorbate adsorbed per unit mass of adsorbent in equilibrium with a certain concentration of the solute in the liquid. Adsorbents used for UTs adsorption include nanoporous materials and dense polymers (chitosan, starch, and cellulose), as well as mixed matrix membranes composed of a polymer matrix embedding adsorbent particles [39]. The review paper by Gelder et al. [40] provides a summary of urea removal strategies for the regeneration of spent dialysate. Urea is the most abundant toxin in spent dialysate, and the harder to abate with conventional adsorbents: therefore, traditional adsorbent materials have too low binding capacity towards urea to be used in a wearable dialysis device. However, thanks to the advances in nanotechnology, new materials to be employed as adsorbed have been synthesized, such as metal organic frameworks and covalent organic frameworks, with great structural tunability, that could potentially be designed to remove hard-to-abate molecules like urea. A classification of different adsorbent nanoporous materials and their binding capacity towards urea at the typical average concentration in the dialysate is reported in the following section.

5.3.2 Adsorption materials for UT removal

Activated carbon (AC) is widely studied for its UTs adsorption capacity, but achieving the adsorption of the daily production of urea requires a large quantity of material [36, 41]. As a result, research has shifted towards exploring materials with controlled and/or ordered porosity such as zeolites, mesoporous silica, metal-organic frameworks (MOFs), MXenes, and molybdenum disulfide (MoS$_2$), which have shown potential for enhanced physisorption of UTs. Additionally, these sorbents can be incorporated into mixed matrix membranes (MMM), where they effectively adsorb UTs while allowing water to pass through the membrane [42].

5.3.2.1 Experimental studies

Experimental investigation often targets the measurement of the static binding capacity q_{eq}, measured through the variation of the initial concentrations (C_0) and the equilibrium concentrations (C_e) of the adsorbate in the liquid, where the adsorbent is suspended. The amount of uremic toxin adsorbed at equilibrium (q_{eq}) is calculated as:

$$q_{eq} = \frac{(C_0 - C_e)V}{W} \tag{5.1}$$

where V refers to the volume of the solution, and W is the weight of the dry adsorbent.

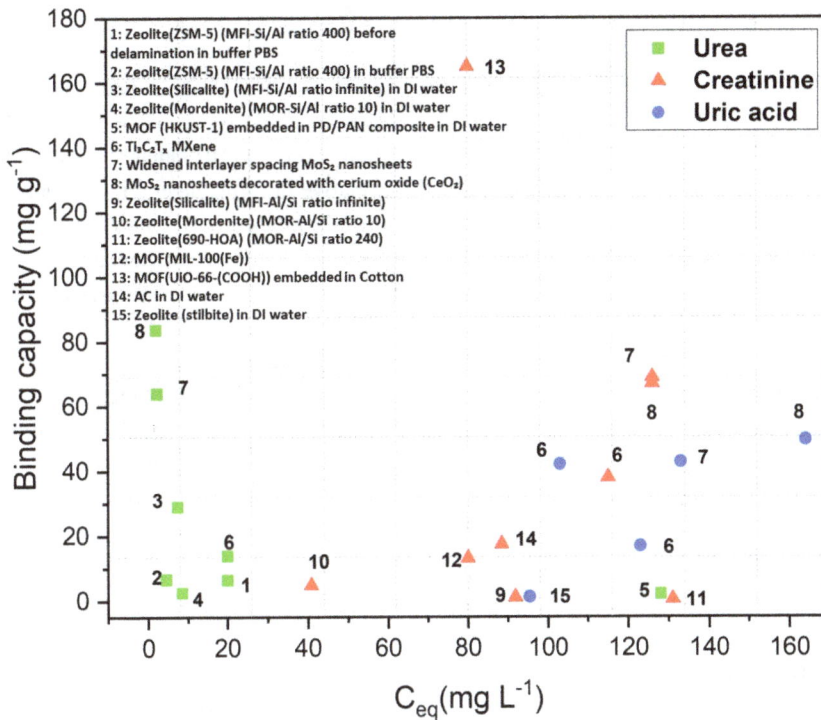

Figure 5.4: Experimentally measured UTs static binding capacity in several adsorbent materials. **Urea** for ZSM-5 before dealumination [42], ZSM-5 [43], silicalite [44], mordenite [44], HUKST-1 [24], Ti$_3$C$_2$Tx MXene [45], widened interlayer spacing MoS$_2$ nanosheets [46], (MoS$_2$) nanosheets decorated cerium oxide (CeO$_2$) ([47], p. 2), SBA-15 NH$_2$ [48], SBA-15 [48], **Creatinine** for silicalite [44], mordenite [44], 690-HOA [49], MIL-100(Fe) [50], UiO-66-(COOH)$_2$ [51], AC [41], Ti$_3$C$_2$Tx MXene [52], widened interlayer spacing MoS$_2$ nanosheets [46], (MoS$_2$) nanosheets decorated cerium oxide (CeO$_2$) ([47], p. 2), and **Uric acid** for stilbite [44], Ti$_3$C$_2$Tx MXene [52], widened interlayer spacing MoS$_2$ nanosheets [46], (MoS$_2$) nanosheets decorated cerium oxide (CeO$_2$) ([47], p. 2), at equilibrium concentration (Ceq), based on literature data.

Considering experimental studies, UTs binding capacities of the aforementioned nanoporous materials at equilibrium concentration for urea, creatinine, uric acid, and hippuric acid (HA) were investigated. Figure 5.4 summarizes the obtained q_{eq} at specific C_e for adsorption of urea, creatinine, and uric acid on various nanoporous materials.

Considering the experimental studies of urea adsorption, Fabiani et al. [53] calculated the static binding capacity of urea adsorption on nanoporous materials at C_{eq} = 5 mM, a typical concentration of urea expected in the spent dialysate. It was reported that the best performing adsorbents are nanomaterials of HKUST-1 embedded in polydopamine/poly-acrylonitrile (PAN/PD) composite [24], MoS$_2$ with widened interlayer spacing [37], SBA-15 NH$_2$ [19], SBA-15 [19], silicalite (MFI) [10], AC [3], MXene (Ti$_3$C$_2$Tx) [33], ZSM-5 (Si/Al ratio 400) [6], mordenite (MOR) [10] showed the binding capacity of 320, 138.9, 50.5, 29.8, 19.6, 4.4, 3.5, 1.6, and 1.47 mg g^{-1}, respectively.

5.3.2.2 Computational modelling

In the study of UTs adsorption by nanoporous materials for dialysate regeneration, computational modelling plays a crucial role in exploring underlying mechanisms and optimizing material performances. In molecular simulations atoms are modelled as spheres interacting according to a force field, dictating their relative movements and interactions. The main methods used involve either MonteCarlo (MC), molecular dynamics (MD), or density functional theory (DFT) methodologies. The detailed discussion and introduction of these methodologies is out of the scope of the present review and we address the reader to other reviews [54, 55].

The adsorption of urea, creatinine, uric acid, indoxyl sulfate, and *p*-cresol on nano-materials has been investigated by several authors using molecular modelling. Table 5.2 summarises the computational researches utilizing the MD, MC, and DFT calculations to study the UTs adsorption by nanomaterials. Jokar et al. [56] explored the adsorption of urea on various nanomaterials such as boron-carbon-nitride (BCN) nanolayers, BCN–nanotubes, graphene, carbon nanotubes (CNTs), and zeolite nanoparticles, finding that BCN nano-materials exhibited the highest urea adsorption due to strong van der Waals (VDW) and electrostatic interactions with urea molecules, along with favorable Gibbs free energy. In a study by Wernert et al. [57], silicalite zeolites demonstrated significant adsorption potential for para-cresol, with 12 molecules adsorbed per unit cell, amounting to 112.8 mg g^{-1}. Palabıyık et al. [58] examined bio-compatible MOFs and identified OREZES, a carboxylate-based MOF, as highly selective for urea/water separation, while BEPPIX, an amino-based MOF, showed strong selectivity for creatinine/water separation with an exceptionally high separation factor. Yıldız et al. [59] further evaluated MOFs, identifying adenine-based bio-MOFs, spe-cifically bio-MOF-11 (YUVSUE) and bio-MOF-12 (BEYSEF), and a dicyanamide-based MOF (KEXDIB) as promising for both urea and creatinine separations due to their molecular properties. Fabiani et al. [60] studied a broad range of 560 nanoporous materials, finding that the excess chemical potential for urea adsorption increased markedly with fluorine content, highlighting a potential design principle for improving urea adsorption in COFs. Li et al. [61] demonstrated that MOFs with aromatic ligands and carboxylic acid groups exhibit excellent adsorption capabilities for indoxyl sulfate, surpassing 2,100 mg g^{-1}. Investigating the adsorption of urea on doped graphene, Karimi et al. [62] found that nitrogen-doped graphene nanosheets (10 % nitrogen) achieved the best adsorption performance based on total and adsorption energy metrics. Meanwhile, Bergé-Lefranc et al. [63] observed a high adsorption rate of both urea and indoxyl sulfate in silicalite zeolite under maximum site occupancy, achieving 1.034 mmol g^{-1}. Jahromi et al. [64, 65] evaluated N- and P-doped fullerenes and specific COFs, revealing that N-doped fullerenes (8 % nitrogen) enhanced hydrogen bonding and adsorption energy for urea, while the TPA-COF modified with–OH functional groups exhibited improved urea adsorption. Skorane et al. [66] investigated azacalix [*n*]arenes (ACAs)-COFs for uric acid and creatinine adsorption, reporting consistent performance even in saline conditions, making it suitable for biofiltration applications. Lastly, Zandi et al. [67] explored MXene nanosheets and found that Cd$_2$C-based MXene exhibited the best stability

Table 5.2: Summary of the computational researches on UTs adsorption by nanomaterials.

	Method	UTs	Nanomaterial
Jokar et al. [56]	MD	Urea	Boron-carbon-nitride (BCN) nanolayer, BCN–nanotube, graphene, carbon nanotube (CNT), zeolite Y, zeolite Z, and zeolite ZSM5 nanoparticles having various surface areas.
Wernert et al. [57]	GCMC	*para*-Cresol	Silicalite zeolite
Palabıyık et al. [58]	GCMC MD	Urea, Creatinine	60 bio-compatible MOFs
Yıldız et al. [59]	GCMC	Urea, Creatinine	122 bio-MOFs
Fabiani et al. [60]	MC and MD	Urea	560 nanoporous material comprising COFs, some siliceous zeolites, MOFs and graphitic materials.
Li et al. [61]	GCMC	Indoxyl sulfate	Biocompatible MoFs
Karimi et al. [62]	MD	Urea	Nitrogen-doped and phosphorus-doped graphene
Bergé-lefranc [63] et al.	GCMC	Urea, Indoxyl Sulfate	Silicalite zeolite (MFI,Si/Al = 30)
Jahromi et al. [64]	MD	Urea	N- and P-doped fullerenes
Jahromi et al. [65]	MD DFT	Urea	TPA-COF, DAAQ-TFP, DAPHTFP, Tp-PaSO3Li–COF, PHOS–COF
Skorane et al. [66]	MD	Uric acid, creatinine	Azacalix [*n*]arenes (ACAs)-CoF
Zandi et al. [67]	MD	Urea	MXene nanosheets including Mn_2C, Cd_2C, Cu_2C, Ti_2C, W_2C, Ta_2C,

and adsorption properties for urea, demonstrating potential for further exploration in practical adsorption applications.

Machine Learning (ML) methods. The continuous expansion of databases for nanoporous materials, particularly COFs and MOFs, has introduced challenges in computational screening due to high computational costs and slower processing times. ML offers a solution by significantly reducing calculation time, thus enhancing the efficiency of large-scale screenings. Recent advancements in ML methods have accelerated the discovery and rational design of new materials by predicting the behaviour of adsorbate-nanoporous systems. By analysing large datasets of nanoporous materials descriptors and computational results, ML can uncover relationships between material composition, structure as features, and performance as target, ultimately helping identify the best-performing nanomaterials [68, 69]. Figure 5.5 represents a flowchart outlining the application of ML techniques to predict adsorption performance in nanomaterials. A typical ML-based study on adsorption processes begins with obtaining parameters defining the adsorption performance from simulations, which serve as targets for the ML model. Next, specific descriptors (features) related to nanomaterials, such as structural and chemical properties, are selected to form the dataset. The dataset is then split into training and test sets, followed by applying a scaling technique to standardize the data. The model is trained on the training set, with hyperparameters optimized to improve performance. The accuracy of the model is evaluated using metrics like R^2 (coefficient of determination) and RMSE (root mean square error). The values of R^2 and RMSE can be calculated using the equations shown below [70].

$$R^2 = 1 - \frac{\sum_{i=1}^{n} (y_i - y_i^*)^2}{\sum_{i=1}^{n} (y_i - \bar{y})^2}, \tag{5.2}$$

$$RMSE = \sqrt{\frac{\sum_{i=1}^{n} (y_i - y_i^*)^2}{n}}, \tag{5.3}$$

where $\bar{y}$ refers to the mean value of the actual responses, and y_i^*, y_i relate to predicted and actual values of the ith sample response, respectively. The value of n corresponds to the number of samples in the dataset.

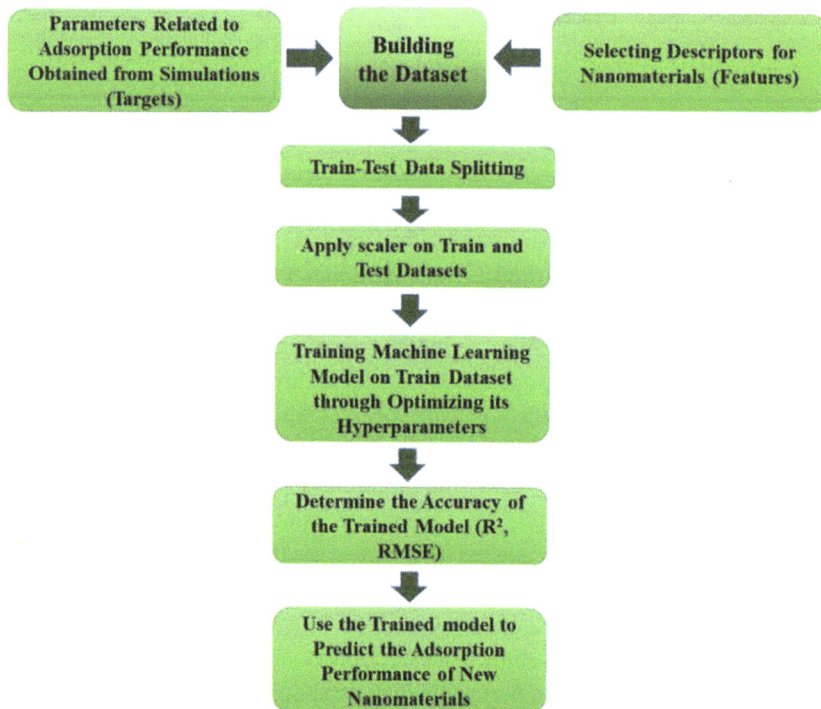

Figure 5.5: Flow chart representing the steps involved in training machine learning models.

Once the model is validated, it can be used to predict the adsorption performance of new nanomaterials, facilitating faster discovery of optimal adsorbents.

Despite the lack of specific studies applying ML to the adsorption of UTs from water solutions, there is a growing body of research on the use of ML in water treatment. For instance, Malloum et al. [54] reviewed the computational research and ML approaches targeting the adsorption process for water treatment. Lowe et al. [71] reviewed the application of ML in adsorption-based water treatment. ML models, such as random forest (RF), artificial neural networks (ANN), and support vector machines (SVM), have been extensively trained to predict the adsorption efficiency of pollutants onto adsorbents like attapulgite clay [72], nickel (II) oxide nanocomposites [73], activated carbon [74], and encapsulated nanoscale zero-valent iron [75], often achieving R^2 values greater than 0.9.

It is worth noting that, given the extensive data screening on the adsorption of UTs using large databases of MOFs and covalent organic COFs, ML can be effectively combined with simulation techniques to uncover correlations between material features (descriptors of porous materials) and target properties (such as the calculated binding capacity of adsorbents).

Our group developed for the first time a method to assess, using ML, the urea removal performance of a set of COFs based on a set of structural descriptors such as the largest included sphere (LIS), available surface area (ASA), and probe-occupiable volume accessible (POVA) along with chemical features like atomic composition percentages. The excess chemical potential of adsorption for urea and water molecules by COFs, estimated by Fabiani et al. from atomistic simulations, was used as target [53].

RF regressor is an "ensemble learning" method that combines a large number of decision trees, effectively reducing variance when compared to using individual decision trees [76]. RF algorithm constructs K regression trees and computes the average of their outputs. Once K trees $\{T(x)\}_1^K$ are generated, the RF regression predictor is expressed as [77]:

$$\hat{f}_{RF}^K(x) = \frac{1}{k} \sum_{k=1}^{K} T(x) \tag{5.4}$$

The performance of the Random Forest model was assessed using R^2 scores on both training and testing datasets, indicating the model's capacity to capture the relationships between descriptors and target properties. Specifically, the training R^2 scores were 0.88 for excess chemical potential of urea and 0.92 for excess chemical potential of water, suggesting strong predictive performance on the training data. The testing R^2 scores, at 0.58 excess chemical potential of urea and 0.650 for excess chemical potential of water, indicate moderate generalizability on unseen data, with potential for further model refinement to enhance predictive accuracy on new samples. Figure 5.6 shows the predicted performance versus the one obtained via atomistic simulations.

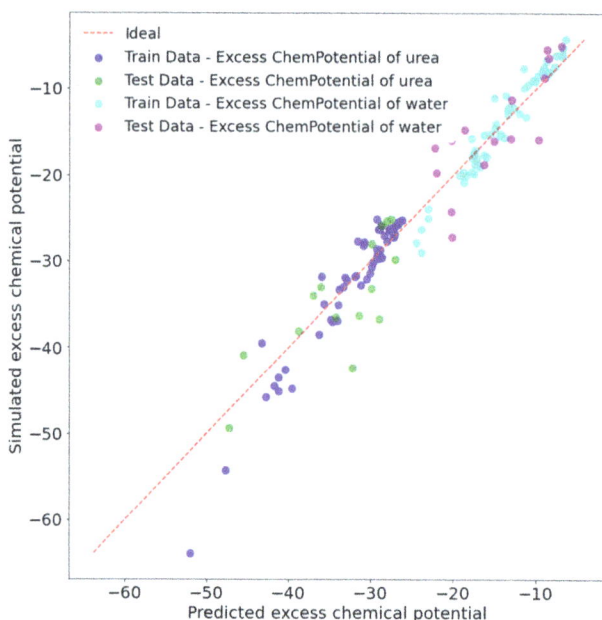

Figure 5.6: Simulated values of excess chemical potential versus predicted excess chemical potential obtained from RF model training (this work).

5.4 Conclusions

The creation of a wearable hemodialysis device could significantly boost patient outcomes and enhance their quality of life, while also easing pressures on healthcare facilities and decreasing water consumption. However, a key technical obstacle is the necessity for effective regeneration of spent dialysate, particularly achieving the complete removal of urea and other harmful toxins.

Historically, the management of urea in wearable dialysis prototypes has utilised chemical methods like oxidation and enzymatic conversion, key features in prototype models. These techniques, however, have considerable limitations due to the creation of toxic by-products such as ammonia and carbon dioxide. On the other hand, physical methods like adsorption and forward osmosis-enhanced HD offer a safer alternative but still do not achieve complete urea removal in a compact and efficient manner.

Recent advances in nanoporous materials and improved computational design tools have reignited interest and made strides in sorbent technologies for dialysate purification and in developing wearable kidney devices. Innovative experimental research has revealed various promising new porous materials for cleansing spent dialysate, though these initial findings require further verification through extended studies to confirm reproducibility and effectiveness under clinically relevant conditions. Concurrently, advancements in computational techniques, including molecular simulations and machine learning, have greatly extended the scope of material testing beyond standard lab methods, accelerating the development and optimisation of materials for toxin elimination. Additionally, molecular techniques may enable the identification of sorbent materials capable of selectively capturing not just standard uremic toxins like urea and creatinine but also more harmful substances with less effort than traditional trial-and-error methods. These techniques facilitate the screening of material families such as covalent organic frameworks (COFs), known for their high tunability and water stability and the absence of potentially harmful metals.

Machine learning, when properly trained with experimental or simulated data, can screen broader arrays of nanoporous crystalline sorbents than atomistic simulations alone, extending performance predictions to novel, yet-to-be-synthesized materials. This opens avenues for efficient reverse material design and we have applied this method to the screening of a family of COFs for the removal of urea from water.

Chemical engineers, with their comprehensive skills in computational modelling, physics, chemistry, and process design, and their ability to collaborate across disciplines, are ideally suited to lead these innovations. Such technological advances are propelling us toward the realisation of wearable artificial kidneys – a significant leap forward that promises to markedly improve patient health and stands as a groundbreaking field in chemical engineering applied to medicine.

Acknowledgments: The authors would like to thank the editors David Bogle and Tomasz Sosnowski for their guidance and review of this article before its publication.

References

1. Kirwan C, Frankel A. The artificial kidney. In: Hakim NS, editor. Artificial Organs. London: Springer; 2009: 39–55 pp.
2. Chronic kidney disease – the lancet. [Online]. https://www.thelancet.com/article/S0140-6736(16)32064-5/abstract [Accessed 23 Jul 2024].
3. Finco DR. Chapter 17 – kidney function. In: Kaneko JJ, Harvey JW, Bruss ML, editors. Clinical Biochemistry of Domestic Animals, 5th ed. San Diego: Academic Press; 1997:441–84 pp.
4. Lisowska-Myjak B. Uremic toxins and their effects on multiple organ systems. Nephron Clin Pract 2014;128: 303–11.
5. Neirynck N, de Smet R, Schepers E, Vanholder R, Glorieux G. Classification and a list of uremic toxins. In: Uremic Toxins. Hoboken, NJ, USA: John Wiley & Sons, Inc; 2012:13–33 pp.
6. Eutox. The European uremic toxins (EUTox) database. [Online]. www.uremic-toxins.org [Accessed 09 Sep 2024].
7. Vanholder R, Pletinck A, Schepers E, Glorieux G. Biochemical and clinical impact of organic uremic retention solutes: a comprehensive update. Toxins (Basel) 2018;10:33.
8. Kalantar-Zadeh K, Jafar TH, Nitsch D, Neuen BL, Perkovic V. Chronic kidney disease. Lancet 2021;398: 786–802.

9. National kidney foundation practice guidelines for chronic kidney disease: evaluation, classification, and stratification. [Online]. https://www.acpjournals.org/doi/epdf/10.7326/0003-4819-139-2-200307150-00013.[Accessed 15 May 2024].

10. Couser WG, Remuzzi G, Mendis S, Tonelli M. The contribution of chronic kidney disease to the global burden of major noncommunicable diseases. Kidney Int 2011;80:1258–70.

11. Astley ME, Boenink R, Abd ElHafeez S, Trujillo-Alemán S, Arribas F, Åsberg A, et al. The ERA Registry annual report 2020: a summary. Clin Kidney J 2023;16:1330–54.

12. Bello AK, Johnson DW, Feehally J, Harris D, Jindal K, Lunney M, et al. Global kidney health atlas (GKHA): design and methods. Kidney Int Suppl 2017;7:145–53.

13. Ledebo I, Blankestijn PJ. Haemodiafiltration – optimal efficiency and safety. NDT Plus 2010;3:8–16.

14. Azar AT, Canaud B. Hemodialysis system. In: Azar AT, editor. Modelling and control of dialysis systems: volume 1: modeling techniques of hemodialysis systems. Berlin, Heidelberg: Springer; 2013:99–166 pp.

15. Ronco C and Clark WR. Haemodialysis membranes. Nat Rev Nephrol 2018;14. https://doi.org/10.1038/s41581-018-0002-x.

16. Mohajerani F, Clark WR, Ronco C, Narsimhan V. Mass transport in high-flux hemodialysis: application of engineering principles to clinical prescription. Clin J Am Soc Nephrol 2022;17:749.

17. Influence of dialysis membranes on clinical outcomes: from history to innovation. [Online]. https://www.mdpi.com/2077-0375/12/2/152.[Accessed 20 Dec 2024].

18. Azar AT, Canaud B. Hemodialysis system. In: Modelling and control of dialysis systems, in studies in computational intelligence. Berlin, Heidelberg: Springer Berlin Heidelberg; 2013:99–166 pp.1

19. Ahmad S. Manual of clinical dialysis, 2nd ed. 2009 edition US, New York: Springer; 2014.

20. van Gelder MK, Mihaila SM, Jansen J, Wester M, Verhaar MC, Joles JA, et al. From portable dialysis to a bioengineered kidney. Expet Rev Med Dev 2018;15:323–36.

21. Geremia I, Jong JAW, van Nostrum CF, Hennink WE, Gerritsen KGF, Stamatialis D. New mixed matrix membrane for the removal of urea from dialysate solution. Sep Purif Technol 2021;277:119408.

22. Jaffrin MY, Ding LH, Laurent JM. Simultaneous convective and diffusive mass transfers in a hemodialyser. J Biomech Eng 1990;112:212–19.

23. Daugirdas JT. Simplified equations for monitoring Kt/V, PCRn, eKt/V, and ePCRn. Adv Ren Replace Ther 1995;2:295–304.

24. Fiore GB, Guadagni G, Lupi A, Ricci Z, Ronco C. A new semiempirical mathematical model for prediction of internal filtration in hollow fiber hemodialyzers. Blood Purif 2006;24:555–68.

25. Oshvandi K, Kavyannejad R, Borzuo SR, Gholyaf M. High-flux and low-flux membranes: efficacy in hemodialysis. Nurs Midwifery Stud 2014;3:e21764.

26. Leypoldt JK, Cheung AK. Removal of high-molecular-weight solutes during high-efficiency and high-flux haemodialysis. Nephrol Dial Transplant 1996;11:329–35.

27. Vienken J. Membranes for haemodialysis. What is more important, sieving coefficient or flux? Probl Eksploat 2013:7–16.

28. Hulko M, Haug U, Gauss J, Boschetti-de-Fierro A, Beck W, Krause B. Requirements and pitfalls of dialyzer sieving coefficients comparisons. Artif Organs 2018;42:1164–73.

29. A wearable artificial kidney for patients with end-stage renal disease – PMC. [Online]. https://www.ncbi.nlm.nih.gov/pmc/articles/PMC4936831/.[Accessed 29 Jul 2024].

30. Chiu Y-W, Teitelbaum I, Misra M, de Leon EM, Adzize T, Mehrotra R. Pill burden, adherence, hyperphosphatemia, and quality of life in maintenance dialysis patients. Clin J Am Soc Nephrol 2009;4:1089.

31. Shao G, Himmelfarb J, Hinds BJ. Strategies for optimizing urea removal to enable portable kidney dialysis: a reappraisal. Artif Organs 2022;46:997–1011.

32. Gura V, Rivara MB, Bieber S, Munshi R, Smith NC, Linke L, et al. A wearable artificial kidney for patients with end-stage renal disease. JCI Insight 2016;1:e86397.

33. Dou P, Donato D, Guo H, Zhao S, He T. Recycling water from spent dialysate by osmotic dilution: impact of urea rejection of forward osmosis membrane on hemodialysis duration. Desalination 2020;496:114605.

34. Shaffer DL, Werber JR, Jaramillo H, Lin S, Elimelech M. Forward osmosis: where are we now? Desalination 2015;356:271–84.

35. Vollenbroek JC, Rodriguez AP, Mei BT, Mul G, Verhaar MC, Odijk M, et al. Light-driven urea oxidation for a wearable artificial kidney. Catal Today 2023:114163. https://doi.org/10.1016/j.cattod.2023.114163.

36. Shao G, et al. Dialysate regeneration via urea photodecomposition with TiO2 nanowires at therapeutic rates. Artif Organs 2023. https://doi.org/10.1111/aor.14514.

37. Wu D, Xu F, Sun B, Fu R, He H, Matyjaszewski K. Design and preparation of porous polymers. Chem Rev 2012;112:3959–4015.

38. Grassi M, Kaykioglu G, Belgiorno V, Lofrano G. Removal of emerging contaminants from water and wastewater by adsorption process. In: Lofrano G, editor. Emerging Compounds Removal from Wastewater: Natural and Solar Based Treatments. Dordrecht: Springer Netherlands; 2012:15–37 pp. in SpringerBriefs in Molecular Science.

39. Ma Y, Li S, Tonelli M, Unsworth LD. Adsorption-based strategies for removing uremic toxins from blood. Microporous Mesoporous Mater 2021;319:111035.

40. van Gelder MK, Jong JA, Folkertsma L, Guo Y, Blüchel C, Verhaar MC, et al. Urea removal strategies for dialysate regeneration in a wearable artificial kidney. Biomaterials 2020;234:119735.

41. Kameda T, Horikoshi K, Kumagai S, Saito Y, Yoshioka T. Adsorption of urea, creatinine, and uric acid onto spherical activated carbon. Separ Purif Technol 2020;237:116367.

42. De Pascale M, De Angelis MG, Boi C. Mixed matrix membranes adsorbers (MMMAs) for the removal of uremic toxins from dialysate. Membranes 2022;12. https://doi.org/10.3390/membranes12020203.

43. Cheng Y-C, Fu C-C, Hsiao Y-S, Chien C-C, Juang R-S. Clearance of low molecular-weight uremic toxins p-cresol, creatinine, and urea from simulated serum by adsorption. J Mol Liq 2018;252:203–10.

44. Wernert V, Schäf O, Ghobarkar H, Denoyel R. Adsorption properties of zeolites for artificial kidney applications. Microporous Mesoporous Mater 2005;83:101–13.

45. Meng F, Seredych M, Chen C, Gura V, Mikhalovsky S, Sandeman S, et al. MXene sorbents for removal of urea from dialysate: a step toward the wearable artificial kidney. ACS Nano 2018;12:10518–28.

46. Zhao H, Huang J, Miao L, Yang Y, Xiao Z, Chen Q, et al. Toward urease-free wearable artificial kidney: widened interlayer spacing MoS2 nanosheets with highly effective adsorption for uremic toxins. Chem Eng J 2022;438:135583.

47. Zhao H, Huang J, Huang L, Yang Y, Xiao Z, Chen Q, et al. Surface control approach for growth of cerium oxide on flower-like molybdenum disulfide nanosheets enables superior removal of uremic toxins. J Colloid Interface Sci 2023;630:855–65.

48. Nguyen CH, Fu C-C, Chen Z-H, Tran TTV, Liu S-H, Juang R-S. Enhanced and selective adsorption of urea and creatinine on amine-functionalized mesoporous silica SBA-15 via hydrogen bonding. Microporous Mesoporous Mater 2021;311:110733.

49. Sasaki M, Liu Y, Ebara M. Zeolite composite nanofiber mesh for indoxyl sulfate adsorption toward wearable blood purification devices. Fibers 2021;9. https://doi.org/10.3390/fib9060037.

50. Yang C-X, Liu C, Cao Y-M, Yan X-P. Metal–organic framework MIL-100(Fe) for artificial kidney application. RSC Adv 2014;4:40824–7.

51. Abdelhameed RM, Rehan M, Emam HE. Figuration of Zr-based MOF@cotton fabric composite for potential kidney application. Carbohydr Polym 2018;195:460–7.

52. Zhao Q, Seredych M, Precetti E, Shuck CE, Harhay M, Pang R, et al. Adsorption of uremic toxins using Ti3C2Tx MXene for dialysate regeneration. ACS Nano 2020;14:11787–98.

53. Fabiani T, Zarghamidehaghani M, Boi C, Dimartino S, Kentish S, De Angelis MG. Sorbent-based dialysate regeneration for the wearable artificial kidney: advancing material innovation via experimental and computational studies. Separ Purif Technol 2025;360:130776.

54. Malloum A, Adegoke KA, Ighalo JO, Conradie J, Ohoro CR, Amaku JF, et al. Computational methods for adsorption study in wastewater treatment. J Mol Liq 2023;390:123008.

55. Chen J. The development and comparison of molecular dynamics simulation and Monte Carlo simulation. IOP Conf Ser Earth Environ Sci 2018;128:012110.

56. Jokar Z, Khademiyan A, Fallah M-A, Smida K, Sajadi SM, Inc M. Molecular dynamics simulation of urea adsorption on various nanoparticles in a spiral microfluidic system. Eng Anal Bound Elem 2022;145:271–85.

57. Wernert V, Schäf O, Faure V, Brunet P, Dou L, Berland Y, et al. Adsorption of the uremic toxin p-cresol onto hemodialysis membranes and microporous adsorbent zeolite silicalite. J Biotechnol 2006;123:164–73.

58. Akkoca Palabıyık B, Batyrow M, Erucar I. Computational investigations of Bio-MOF membranes for uremic toxin separation. Separ Purif Technol 2022;281:119852.

59. Yıldız T, Erucar I. Revealing the performance of bio-MOFs for adsorption-based uremic toxin separation using molecular simulations. Chem Eng J 2022;431:134263.

60. Fabiani T, Ricci E, Boi C, Dimartino S, Angelis MGD. In silico screening of nanoporous materials for urea removal in hemodialysis applications. Phys Chem Chem Phys 2023;25:24069–80.

61. Li B, Gong S, Cao P, Gao W, Zheng W, Sun W, et al. Screening of biocompatible MOFs for the clearance of indoxyl sulfate using GCMC simulations. Ind Eng Chem Res 2022;61:6618–27.

62. Karimi K, Rahsepar M. Optimization of the urea removal in a wearable dialysis device using nitrogen-doped and phosphorus-doped graphene. ACS Omega 2022;7:4083–94.

63. Bergé-Lefranc D, Pizzala H, Paillaud JL, Schäf O, Vagner C, Boulet P, et al. Adsorption of small uremic toxin molecules on MFI type zeolites from aqueous solution. Adsorption 2008;14:377–87.

64. Miri Jahromi A, Zandi P, Khedri M, Ghasemy E, Maleki R, Tayebi L. Molecular insight into optimizing the N- and P-doped fullerenes for urea removal in wearable artificial kidneys. J Mater Sci Mater Med 2021;32:49.

65. Jahromi AM, Khedri M, Ghasemi M, Omrani S, Maleki R, and Rezaei N. Molecular insight into COF monolayers for urea sorption in artificial kidneys. Sci Rep 2021;11. https://doi.org/10.1038/s41598-021-91617-1.

66. Skorjanc T, Shetty D, Gándara F, Pascal S, Naleem N, Abubakar S, et al. Covalent organic framework based on azacalix[4]arene for the efficient capture of dialysis waste products. ACS Appl Mater Interfaces 2022;14:39293–8.

67. Zandi P, Ghasemy E, Khedri M, Rashidi A, Maleki R, Miri Jahromi A. Shedding light on miniaturized dialysis using MXene 2D materials: a computational chemistry approach. ACS Omega 2021;6:6312–25.

68. Yan Y, Zhang L, Li S, Liang H, Qiao Z. Adsorption behavior of metal-organic frameworks: from single simulation, high-throughput computational screening to machine learning. Comput Mater Sci 2021;193:110383.

69. Nagasubramanian S. The future of the artificial kidney. Indian J Urol 2021;37:310.

70. Hamed Mashhadzadeh A, Zarghami Dehaghani M, Kadyr A, Golman B, Spitas C, et al. Machine Learning-Assisted design of boron and nitrogen doped graphene nanosheets with tailored thermomechanical properties. Comput Mater Sci 2024;240:112998.

71. Lowe M, Qin R, Mao X. A review on machine learning, artificial intelligence, and smart technology in water treatment and monitoring. Water 2022;14. https://doi.org/10.3390/w14091384.

72. Bhagat SK, Pyrgaki K, Salih SQ, Tiyasha T, Beyaztas U, Shahid S, et al. Prediction of copper ions adsorption by attapulgite adsorbent using tuned-artificial intelligence model. Chemosphere 2021;276:130162.

73. Mazloom MS, Rezaei F, Hemmati-Sarapardeh A, Husein MM, Zendehboudi S, Bemani A. Artificial intelligence based methods for asphaltenes adsorption by nanocomposites: application of group method of data handling, least squares support vector machine, and artificial neural networks. Nanomaterials 2020;10. https://doi.org/10.3390/nano10050890.

74. Mesellem Y, Hadj AAE, Laidi M, Hanini S, Hentabli M. Computational intelligence techniques for modeling of dynamic adsorption of organic pollutants on activated carbon. Neural Comput Applic 2021;33:12493–512.

75. Mahmoud AS, Mostafa MK, Nasr M. Regression model, artificial intelligence, and cost estimation for phosphate adsorption using encapsulated nanoscale zero-valent iron. Separ Sci Technol 2019;54:13–26.

76. Couronné R, Probst P, Boulesteix A-L. Random forest versus logistic regression: a large-scale benchmark experiment. BMC Bioinf 2018;19:270.
77. Machine learning predictive models for mineral prospectivity: an evaluation of neural networks, random forest, regression trees and support vector machines – ScienceDirect. [Online]. https://www.sciencedirect.com/science/article/pii/S0169136815000037.[Accessed 20 Dec 2024].

Part III: **Disease and treatment**

Davide Manca*

6 Precision medicine in hypothyroidism: an engineering approach to individualized levothyroxine dosing

Abstract: This chapter presents an innovative engineering approach to precision medicine in the treatment of hypothyroidism. By leveraging mathematical modeling of the hypothalamic-pituitary-thyroid (HPT) axis, a novel algorithm, PzeroT, is developed for individualized optimization of levothyroxine dosing. The chapter explores the HPT axis physiology and pathology and the current state-of-the-art in hypothyroidism treatment. The core contribution lies in implementing a compartmental model of the HPT axis, which is the foundation for the PzeroT algorithm. This model-based approach enables the prediction of the optimal levothyroxine dose tailored to individual patient characteristics. The chapter further validates the PzeroT algorithm using real patient case studies, demonstrating its potential to improve hypothyroidism management by reducing treatment times and enhancing dose accuracy compared to standard clinical practices. This work, at the intersection of chemical engineering and medicine, exemplifies how engineering principles can advance precision medicine and paves the way for more personalized and effective treatment of thyroid disorders.

Keywords: thyroid disorders; endocrine system modeling; hormone replacement therapy; dose optimization algorithm; multi-compartmental approach; patient-specific treatment

6.1 Introduction

The foundation of this work rests on the premise that biological processes within the human body can be described through mathematical models, given an adequate amount of biological information and an understanding of complex physiological interactions. The reproducibility of various mechanisms allows for the simulation and study of normal organ functions, their interactions within the organism, and the chains of events that contribute to physiological equilibria. An additional opportunity, arising from the *in-silico* reproducibility of biological mechanisms, lies in the ability to study and observe the metabolic responses of organs and tissues to specific medications.

*Corresponding author: Davide Manca, PSE-Lab, Process Systems Engineering Laboratory, Dipartimento di Chimica, Materiali e Ingegneria Chimica "Giulio Natta", Politecnico di Milano, Piazza Leonardo da Vinci 32, 20133 Milano, Italy, E-mail: davide.manca@polimi.it. https://orcid.org/0000-0003-2055-9752

As per De Gruyter's policy this article has previously been published in the journal Physical Sciences Reviews. Please cite as: D. Manca "Precision medicine in hypothyroidism: an engineering approach to individualized levothyroxine dosing" *Physical Sciences Reviews* [Online] 2024. DOI: 10.1515/psr-2024-0060 | https://doi.org/10.1515/9783111394558-006

The concept of organs dates back to ancient times, with the first studies on human anatomy conducted by Hippocrates in the 4th century BC. However, it was first considered a distinct functional unit of the body by Andreas Vesalius in his 1543 book *"De Humani Corporis Fabrica"*. The idea of an organ as a well-defined, delineated, and highly functionalized anatomical structure laid the groundwork for modern medicine and the study of physiology. The latter describes the organism's functioning and is used to understand physiological processes and diagnose diseases [1, 2].

The first research works, enabling the mathematical modeling of human body processes, emerged from this modern concept of organs, which divides the human body into distinct yet interdependent functional parts. Historically, there are two main types of models: PK (PharmacoKinetic models) and PBPK (Physiologically Based Pharmacokinetic models). Both variants are based on the concept of ADME (Administration, Distribution, Metabolism, Excretion), which describes the metabolism of a drug's active ingredient in the human body, considering the entire process from administration to excretion.

Additionally, the aforementioned pharmacokinetic models are primarily based on the concept of compartments that, through engineering analogy, are described as control volumes within which specific chemical reactions involving the drug's active ingredient, enzymes, proteins, and biological tissues occur. Thus, the organism can be divided into anatomical and physiological subsystems such as blood flow, intestine, stomach, tissues, kidneys, and others, each characterized by specific variables like the inflow and outflow of critical components such as hormones, enzymes, and proteins that regulate biological mechanisms.

On the one hand, the circulatory system can be considered the compartment designated for transporting substances throughout the human body; on the other hand, the liver and intestine can be regarded as chemical reactors, given their function of metabolic processing and elimination of substances. These considerations recall a vital analogy that has allowed finding similarities and affinities between these compartments and typical chemical engineering processes and equipment. Therefore, the result is a mathematical description of the dynamic behavior over time of quantities, such as the concentration of an active ingredient or a protein within various compartments. In particular, PK and PBPK models consist of systems of differential equations and related initial conditions, containing, for each compartment, terms of reaction and diffusion of the drug within and through the control volume [3, 4].

6.2 The thyroid gland

The thyroid gland is located in the anterior lower neck region at the level of the fifth cervical vertebra. It consists of two cone-shaped lobes typically connected by an isthmus, which may sometimes be anatomically absent. The thyroid is the largest endocrine gland in the human body, weighing between 15 and 25 g, with lobes averaging 5 cm long and an isthmus about 1.25 cm wide. This organ performs a unique function, concentrating high amounts of dietary iodine internally (more than 40 times higher than average plasma concentration), enabling the development of the metabolic chain involved in thyroid hormone production.

Iodine is essential for producing triiodothyronine (T_3) and thyroxine (T_4), containing three and four iodine atoms formed by the union of two amino acids called tyrosines. These hormones, secreted by the thyroid gland, are responsible for increasing metabolic activity, proper development of body structure, thermoregulation, regulation of heart and respiratory rates, and other fundamental mechanisms for the human body [1].

6.2.1 Microstructure

The thyroid is equipped with a connective tissue capsule responsible for the internal separation of the glandular parenchyma into irregular areas called lobules, which are active elements in thyroid metabolism. This subdivision is necessary to allow the passage of a dense network of blood vessels, lymphatics, and nerves between the lobules. Follicles represent a further level of glandular microstructure, the functional units of the thyroid and structural constituents of the lobules, which are responsible for synthesizing thyroid hormones T_3 and T_4.

More precisely, follicles have a spherical shape with a diameter between 0.02 mm and 0.9 mm and consist of a central nucleus with a colloidal consistency. The latter is surrounded externally by a wall of follicular cells called thyrocytes, whose shape and size change depending on the thyroid's state of activity, varying between cuboidal, laminar, and squamous cells. The colloid is the substance inside the follicle in which high quantities of thyroglobulin are immersed. Thyroglobulin is a complex protein with two main functions: to act as a precursor in the production of thyroid hormones T_3 and T_4 and to serve as a reserve of iodine stored in the protein itself. Thanks to the action of this protein, the thyroid can accumulate reserves of iodine in an organic form that can compensate for sudden deficiencies or shortages deriving from diet or physiological reasons [5].

The primary function of thyroglobulin is to act as a precursor for the synthesis of monoiodotyrosine and diiodotyrosine, which, in turn, combine within the colloid to allow the production of triiodothyronine and thyroxine, respectively, the T_3 and T_4 hormones [6].

6.2.2 Synthesis of thyroid hormones

Thyroid hormones originate from the union of two tyrosines, amino acids constituting thyroglobulin, to which one or two iodine atoms are added. The union of two diiodotyrosines produces the T_4 hormone through a chemical reaction in the colloid, while the union of a monoiodotyrosine and a diiodotyrosine forms the T_3 hormone. Within the follicular cells, the metabolism is markedly biased towards the production of thyroxine (T_4), synthesized for 93 % of the total, while the remaining fraction consists of only triiodothyronine (T_3). The daily secretion of T_4 is about 110 nmol (85 µg) per day, while that of T_3 is about 50 nmol. The latter is differentiated into 10 nmol from thyroid secretion and 40 nmol derived from removing an iodine atom from the outer ring of T_4 in peripheral tissues. This mechanism is called deiodination and is carried out by specific enzymes on the tissues and target organs of thyroid hormones.

To describe the synthesis of thyroid hormones, it is necessary to start with the metabolism of iodine, a chemical element introduced into the body through diet (*e.g.*, through iodized salt or supplements) in the form of the binary salt NaI. Within the digestive system, this element, in the form I^-, is absorbed and released into the bloodstream, through which it will reach the thyroid. At the level of the latter, iodine is absorbed into the follicular cells thanks to specific transporters called NIS (Na-I Symporter), which allow the passage of the ion thanks to the simultaneous work of the sodium-potassium pump (Na+/K+ ATPase). Thanks to this mechanism, the thyroid can store an iodine concentration varying from 30 to 250 times what is usually present in plasma.

The iodine contained in the follicular cells must then be transported into the colloid, thanks to a protein called pendrin. Working similarly to the sodium-potassium pump, this protein moves a chlorine ion toward the cytoplasm of the follicular cell for each iodine ion poured into the colloid. Subsequently, thyroglobulin (TG) undergoes the halogenation process starting from the iodine oxidation mechanism so that the latter can bind more effectively to the tyrosines present in TG. With the aid of the peroxidase enzyme and a hydrogen peroxide molecule, both produced autonomously by the thyroid, the iodination mechanism of tyrosines is promoted, obtaining thyroglobulin that consists of about one-sixth iodinated tyrosines [1].

Finally, the thyroglobulin that has undergone the halogenation process faces the pinocytosis mechanism, thanks to which part of the apical membrane of the follicular cells extends into the colloid to include a portion in a vesicle. The latter, within the follicular cytoplasm, is then attacked and digested by proteolysis enzymes to release T_3 and T_4 hormones from the protein structure of TG. Subsequently, the produced hormones will diffuse into the plasma thanks to specific transporters inside the cytoplasm [1, 7].

To continue the path toward the target organs, thyroid hormones form a chemical bond with specific blood transport proteins because, being hydrophobic, they cannot bind with the water molecules that make up the plasma. The secreted hormones released into the bloodstream are almost totally bound to transport proteins; T_4 present in the bound form is about 99.98 %, while T_3 is about 99.7 %. The hormone-transport protein complex is biologically inactive due to the high affinity that binds the two constituents. For this reason, it slows the process of communicating hormonal information to target cells, as it will first be necessary to break the chemical bond with the transporter to obtain the free and active hormone. This mechanism is generally very slow; in fact, the time in which half of the amount of thyroxine (T_4) present in the blood penetrates the target tissues is about six days, while triiodothyronine (T_3), being less affine to transport proteins, takes about a day to halve the concentration of the original inactive form [8, 9].

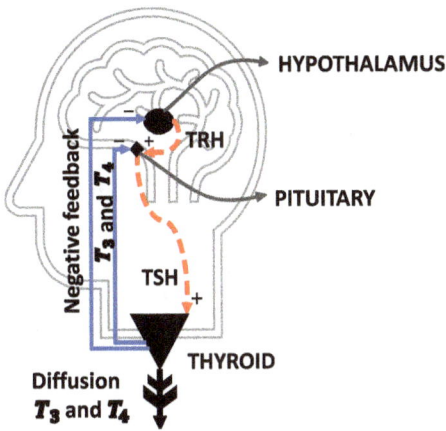

HYPOTHALAMUS

TRH

PITUITARY

TSH

THYROID

Negative feedback

T_3 and T_4

Diffusion
T_3 and T_4

Figure 6.1: Schematic representation of the HPT axis interactions. The "plus" and "minus" symbols identify the stimulating and suppressing effects on hormone secretion within the biological mechanism of the HPT axis.

6.2.3 Regulation of thyroid hormone secretion

The interaction of the hypothalamus, pituitary, and thyroid mainly controls the complex levels of thyroid hormones in plasma and tissue (see Figure 6.1). The interconnection of these three organs constitutes the HPT axis (hypothalamic–pituitary–thyroid axis), thanks to which our body regulates the hormonal levels of T_3 and T_4 in response to endogenous and exogenous stimuli. The set of processes constituting the hormonal regulation of T_3 and T_4 is extraordinarily complex but can be summarized by considering the main actors composing it.

The hypothalamus is the first link in the chain that forms the HPT axis and is located in a small region at the base of the brain below the thalamus. Although its modest size, it plays a fundamental role in the regulation center of the autonomic nervous and endocrine systems. The task of the hypothalamus lies in controlling various processes that intervene in regulating body temperature, sleep, appetite, and other physiological mechanisms. Among the various metabolic substances secreted, the hypothalamus synthesizes TRH (Thyrotropin-releasing hormone), which induces the release of thyrotropin (TSH). TRH is responsible for the pituitary endocrine stimulation.

Once secreted, the TRH hormone passes through the hypothalamic-pituitary portal system to the pituitary, with which it interacts for further endocrine regulation of the organism. The pituitary (also known as the pituitary gland) is located at the base of the brain, posterior to the nose, and comprises neurohypophysis and adenohypophysis. The adenohypophysis is active in hormonal regulation as it secretes different types of hormones, such as thyrotropin, better known as TSH (Thyroid-stimulating hormone), and promotes various mechanisms of regulation and stabilization of the body's homeostasis. Hypothalamic TRH, therefore, interacts with receptors placed on the pituitary, stimulating the production of thyrotropin (TSH), which is subsequently released into the bloodstream. Consequently, TSH interacts with the thyroid gland by binding to the respective receptors and promoting the stimulation of T_3 and T_4 secretion [10].

Having described the process of thyroid gland stimulation, it is now possible to introduce the concept of negative feedback regulation that allows the control of homeostasis, that is, the maintenance of correct hormonal concentrations in the organism. In particular, this mechanism is guaranteed by the retroactive interaction of T_3 and T_4 hormones with the hypothalamus and pituitary. Through systemic circulation, thyroid hormones in the plasma reach the abovementioned organs, interacting with specific receptors placed on hypothalamic and pituitary cells, inhibiting TRH and TSH secretion. More precisely, when high plasma concentrations of thyroid hormones occur, there will be an inhibitory action on hypothalamic and pituitary secretion. At this point, the suppression of TRH and TSH secretion will decrease their plasma concentrations, stimulating the thyroid gland less.

Therefore, we observe how the described feedback mechanism falls into the "negative feedback" type since the output of the process has the effect of obtaining a change opposite to the direction of the initial stimulus. In this case, the increase in the concentration of thyroid hormones produces the suppression of stimuli that promote the secretion of T_3 and T_4. All this allows dynamically responding to fluctuations in hormonal plasma levels in perfect analogy with the functioning of a negative feedback controller, from which this peculiar metabolic regulation mechanism takes its name. This allows for regulating the levels of TSH and TRH in the body if the plasma concentrations of T_3 and T_4 are outside the correct ranges of endocrine functioning [11]. In a healthy individual, during regular physiological activity, T_3, T_4, and TSH hormonal levels define a subject's euthyroid state. On the contrary, when HPT axis pathologies occur, the circulating hormonal quantities are altered [1, 12, 13].

The daily trend of T_4, T_3, and TSH concentrations is vital in regulating HPT axis hormones. Like numerous other hormones, TSH follows a circadian rhythm that repeats daily. The characteristic pattern of TSH can be approximated to a sinusoid with an oscillation period of 24 h, with a minimum between 10 am and 4 pm and a maximum between midnight and 4 am. This peculiarity of TSH is fundamental for deriving correct hormonal values from blood tests, which must be carried out at predetermined times so that the influence of oscillations does not affect the measurement. Typically, it is recommended to perform blood tests in the morning, around 8–8:30 am, when TSH, in a healthy individual, stands at an intermediate point between the maximum and minimum reached during the day. Since TSH is the hormone responsible for thyroid hormonal stimulation, T_3 and T_4 also show a circadian pattern similar to thyrotropin (TSH). However, they show a lower average percentage variation [14].

6.2.4 Pathologies of the HPT axis

Thyroid-related pathologies can be classified into two main groups: hyperthyroidism and hypothyroidism, which indicate the excess or deficiency of thyroid hormones in the blood and peripheral tissues. Hypothyroidism has a more significant clinical relevance compared to hyperthyroidism, with a prevalence ranging from 0.2 % to 5.3 % in the European population and from 0.3 % to 3.7 % in the United States [15]. Instead, hyperthyroidism has a prevalence that stands between 0.2 % and 1.3 % in developed nations that have easy access to sufficient quantities of iodine in the diet. The significant breadth of the reference intervals depends on the criteria used in the study, the population, and the region of origin [16].

For example, the UK population appears to have a particular predisposition for hypothyroidism, which manifests in pathologies such as iodine deficiency hypothyroidism and Hashimoto's autoimmune thyroiditis, with an incidence of the disease that stands at 3.5–5.0 per 1,000 in women and 0.6–1.0 per 1,000 in men. Moreover, in the European population, a high prevalence rate is observed in Spain, with percentages of the population affected by treated and untreated subclinical hypothyroidism of 4.2 % and 4.6 %, respectively. These differences are linked to genetic predispositions together with possible endemic iodine deficiencies, where in specific locations, hypothyroidism prevalence of up to 2.9 % has occurred and where food fortification with iodine is mandatory. Finally, ethnic differences also influence the prevalence and incidence data of this pathology, as in the case of the United States where, thanks to the heterogeneous population, it has been found that African American citizenship shows a halved risk of developing hypothyroid pathologies compared to that composed of white Americans [17].

Regarding hypothyroidism, the pathology can originate from dysfunctions related to the thyroid gland (primary hypothyroidism) or related to the hypothalamus and pituitary, going, in this case, to affect the hormonal interaction of the entire HPT axis (central hypothyroidism). Primary hypothyroidism comprises 99 % of the total cases [18]. It has an incidence of 4–5 cases per 1,000 people per year in women and about 0.9 for men, with a prevalence that stands between 1 % and 2 % for females and about 0.1 % for males [19, 20].

This type of hypothyroidism is characterized by a malfunction directly correlated to the thyroid and, therefore, to hormonal secretion. Among the most widespread pathologies, cases of autoimmune thyroiditis and thyroid cancer are found. Furthermore, primary hypothyroidism is always accompanied by circulating TSH levels higher than usual and plasma T_4 concentrations lower than euthyroid ranges. Instead, in the case of central hypothyroidism, the axis imbalance is due to insufficient thyroid stimulation deriving from a pituitary or hypothalamic pathology that leads to reduced production of TRH or TSH. The latter are much less frequent pathologies and are not always accompanied by increased plasma TSH values. Therefore, they are also challenging to identify and resolve [13, 21, 22].

It is now essential to define the normal levels that allow for determining a patient's thyroid status. The marker considered as a reference for diagnosing thyroid pathologies is the concentration of plasma TSH, together with the free and total concentrations of thyroid hormones fT_4, fT_3 and tT_4, tT_3 [23]. TSH is crucial for diagnosis as it indicates the health status of the HPT axis and overall hormonal balance. The total reliance on plasma thyrotropin (TSH) level as a diagnostic tool represents the standard practice in clinical settings, and it is essential to analyze the reasons for this. 99 % of hypothyroidism cases are of the primary type, so it is possible to pay greater attention to the TSH value since the dysfunction will be directly related to the thyroid gland and not to other organs of the axis. In fact, in this specific case, the interaction of the HPT axis works at a steady state. Still, the levels of T_3 and T_4 do not allow the suppression of TSH production, causing the elevation mentioned above in plasma. Under these premises, in the case of primary hypothyroidism, in response to a deficiency of T_3 and T_4, an increase in TSH levels occurs in the HPT axis to stimulate the production of thyroid hormones. Therefore, in the absence of symptoms or evidence of a particular thyroid pathology, an elevated thyrotropin (TSH) level is a clear sign of a primary hypothyroid state. Furthermore, the plasma concentration value of thyroxine is considered an additional indicator to be used alongside the control of the thyrotropin level to verify the type of thyroid pathology and the degree of hypothyroidism (*i.e.*, overt or subclinical) [24].

The analysis of any symptoms also accompanies the measurement of hormonal concentrations in the blood. In hypothyroid patients, the most common symptomatic manifestations include weakness, dry and rough skin, lethargy, weight gain, and eyelid swelling. The symptoms just mentioned have an incidence between 54 % and 76 % of hypothyroid patients, particularly in cases of overt hypothyroidism [25, 26]. Diagnosing thyroid pathologies consists of symptomatological observation combined with blood chemistry analysis and the observation of non-thyroid pathologies already in progress that could alter the hormonal balance. The diagnosis of hypothyroidism is easy to identify in cases where the patient presents to the endocrinologist with the typical symptoms of the pathology, which are often accompanied by TSH and fT_4 values above and below the normal ranges, respectively (Table 6.1: overt hypothyroidism).

In other cases, however, the symptomatic manifestation could be mild, and a careful analysis of blood test reports can reveal a low or average fT_4 level with a TSH value slightly above normal values (Table 6.1). However, in both cases, if the symptoms are disabling for the patient, it is necessary to determine the replacement dose of thyroid hormones.

The diagnosis is not always immediate; typical TSH values vary according to many parameters, including age, ethnicity, and sex. A study conducted by the National Health and Nutrition Examination Survey [27] highlights the critical differences in TSH values in a very diverse population such as that of the United States. Based on the statistical analysis of data from over 17,000 subjects, TSH's upper and lower limit values show two reference limits within which TSH concentration measurements in healthy individuals must fall. For the upper limit, a value of 4.12 mIU/l was established, rounded to 4.5 mIU/l, while for the lower limit, a value of 0.45 mIU/l was rounded to 0.4 mIU/l [27]. Based on these reference values, a patient is considered to have subclinical hypothyroidism when

Table 6.1: Characteristics of types of hypothyroidism: overt and subclinical.

Type	Symptoms	T_4	T_3	TSH
Overt	Evident	Low	Low	Elevated
Subclinical	Absent or mild	Normal or low	Normal	Slightly above normal

TSH values are below 10 mIU/l but above 4.5 mIU/l; conversely, for values above 10 mIU/l, the diagnosis is that of overt hypothyroidism [22].

6.3 State of the art in hypothyroidism treatment

A subject is defined as hypothyroid when hormonal levels fall outside the reference intervals. Specifically, the most common case is primary hypothyroidism, where the patient shows elevated TSH levels concurrently with low fT_4 levels. Regardless of the causes that induce the onset of the disease, the patient needs to undergo replacement therapy that administers the missing amount of thyroid hormone to restore the correct levels of endogenous fT_4 and TSH.

Historically, the first approaches to treating the symptoms of then-unknown hypothyroidism date back to seventh-century China, where evidence reports the use of animal thyroid gland extracts to treat goiter (*i.e.*, a condition that leads to noticeable thyroid enlargement) [23]. Furthermore, other historically reliable information on treating the condition dates to the nineteenth century, when the scientific literature of the time produced extensive descriptions of subcutaneous injections of sheep thyroid gland extracts to treat symptoms such as lethargy or chronic fatigue [28, 29].

The bioactive substance present in the extracts, later named thyroxine, was first isolated in 1914, and its first use for treating various forms of hypothyroidism began around 1927 [30]. Only in the 1950s was the chemical compound called levothyroxine (LT_4) first synthesized. The sodium salt of the levorotatory isomer of thyroxine would replace the T_4 hormone due to its better absorption within the gastrointestinal tract [31].

Since the 70's of the last century, animal thyroid gland extracts have gradually disappeared, and levothyroxine tablets have become the universally used method for treating hypothyroidism. Regarding the ADME (absorption, distribution, metabolism, and excretion) processes of the drug, the active ingredient is absorbed in the small intestine, reaching peak blood concentration in about 2 h, with a bioavailability between 60 % and 80 % of the administered amount [32].

In clinical practice, a drug equivalent to T_4 instead of T_3 is dictated by the higher biological stability of levothyroxine, which is a long-lasting and constantly circulating reserve in the plasma through binding with blood transport proteins. Treatment can be conducted either with the sole use of LT_4 (monotherapy) or with the addition of restricted amounts of T_3 hormone to the base therapy (combined therapy) to exploit the high biological activity of triiodothyronine to decrease the amount of LT_4 needed and more rapidly mitigate the symptoms of hypothyroidism. However, there is still an ongoing intense debate about the actual better effectiveness of the second type of treatment, and multiple studies on this have often reached conflicting conclusions, indicating the need for further clinical investigations on this type of practice.

To date, the treatment of hypothyroidism through monotherapy is the most widespread in clinical practice due to the characteristics of the drug itself, which allow it to be chemically stable, deteriorate very limitedly during storage, and allow a single daily intake thanks to its half-life of about one week [33]. Monotherapy with levothyroxine is effective thanks to the fundamental deiodination mechanism promoted by the D_2 enzyme and, to a lesser extent, by the D_1 enzyme, thanks to which the synthesis of triiodothyronine is possible at the level of peripheral tissues and target organs.

The fundamental parameter in replacement therapy with LT_4 is the amount of drug that must be prescribed to restore correct hormonal levels in the patient. It is worth mentioning that the drug dosage may need to be adjusted based on the patient's response and follow-up TSH levels. Indeed, the calculation and control of dosage assume a central role in the treatment of hypothyroidism since levothyroxine is a drug that has a highly narrow interval in which its properties are therapeutic for patient care (narrow therapeutic index drug), highlighting the concrete possibility of falling into situations of under or overdosage that can be harmful [17, 34, 35].

In the first instance, the most influential factors in modulating the dosage of LT_4 for hypothyroid patients are the final TSH value to be reached through therapy and the weight of the patient who must undertake the treatment. It is common clinical practice to calculate the levothyroxine dose using correlations that propose an LT_4 value per kilogram of the patient's body mass. Several studies show that achieving TSH values in the euthyroid reference range can be obtained using values between 1.6 µg/kg and 2.1 µg/kg [36]. Instead, for complete suppression of TSH (values below 0.1 mIU/l), necessary in patients affected by thyroid cancer to prevent further growth of tumor masses [37], the micrograms per unit of body mass tend to increase up to reference values between 2.2 µg/kg and 2.7 µg/kg [38]. However, as reported by [39]; it emerges that the lean mass of the subject is a parameter that predicts the dose more reliably and sensitively than the actual body mass of the patient, although, in clinical practice, this precaution is often neglected. In any case, monitoring the patient's weight variations is necessary to obtain a precise and optimal drug dosage. In addition, it is essential to verify the effectiveness of the therapy through periodic measurement of TSH to adapt/correct the amount based on the body's response.

Another critical element for the correct dosage of LT_4 is the sex of the patient who must undertake the treatment. Sex influences the dosage choice by calculating the patient's ideal weight and BMI (body mass index) since the equations for estimating these quantities are specific for men and women. It should be emphasized that the hormone production mechanism is identical for subjects of different sexes; what is different is the individual requirement for thyroid hormones [39, 40].

A matter of debate within the scientific community and among endocrinologists is the influence of age on TSH levels and the doses to be administered to elderly patients. Several studies have determined how TSH values increase in healthy individuals with age by analyzing large population samples. In particular, the value that increases over the years is the upper limit of the TSH reference range, which in those over 70 can exceed 5 mIU/l [27, 41]. The reason for this increase lies in the loss of thyroid secretion efficiency in the elderly. Therefore, to counteract this phenomenon, the HPT axis implements an overstimulation of the thyroid gland by TSH to produce the correct amounts of T_3 and T_4

hormones. This translates into thyrotropin (TSH) values slightly above the upper limit of the euthyroid range and normal T_4 levels, determining cases similar to subclinical hypothyroidism [42, 43].

The problem with this correlation is determining whether it is necessary or not in the case of hypothyroidism in the elderly, to bring their thyrotropin value back to the conventional levels of the adult population between 0.4 and 4.5 mIU/l or whether it is appropriate to define and assign TSH limit levels that are a function of their age. Recent studies suggest that it is relevant to re-examine therapeutic protocols, especially in older patients, because the incidence rate of levothyroxine overdose is very high in this age group. Eligar et al. [44] report that between 30 % and 50 % of cases of patients treated for hypothyroidism have been subjected to either an overdose or an underdose of the treatment. Moreover, up to 50 % of cases of hyperthyroidism turn out to be caused by excessive administration of levothyroxine in subclinical hypothyroid patients. It is, therefore, necessary to consider that normal TSH levels are higher in the elderly and consequently consider them healthy compared to younger patients otherwise considered mild or subclinical hypothyroid.

A further determining factor in the dosage of levothyroxine lies in the maximum amount that a patient can absorb compared to the administration of the drug. The absorption of the active ingredient mainly occurs in the intestine, between the two consecutive portions of jejunum and ileum [45], and the maximum concentration that can be acquired stands at a value between 70 % and 80 % of the amount of active ingredient, under conditions of complete fasting from food [46]. The possible decrease in the absorbable amount derives from several factors: the patient's diet type, interfering drugs, gastrointestinal tract pathologies, and the time of drug intake during the day (an optimal timing for drug intake is 30–60 min before breakfast).

6.3.1 Treatment of hypothyroidism

During the treatment of hypothyroidism, two objectives need to be pursued to define the patient as euthyroid: eliminate the symptoms of the pathology and bring TSH back within the correct reference range. It is, therefore, necessary to measure the patient's TSH value at the beginning of therapy and subsequently at regular intervals to obtain a clear view of the progress of the pathology. The choice of the first dose to prescribe to the patient is extremely important to reduce the time needed to achieve euthyroidism and decrease periodic checks. The literature reports several approaches that can be adopted to calculate the starting dose of treatment.

A first possibility lies in administering an intermediate dosage of LT_4, equal to 100 µg, independent of the patient's body mass, age, and sex, and only at the subsequent check verifying the effectiveness of the treatment and possible adjustments [47]. However, such an approach has several limits, not being able to consider individual differences in patients and presenting the concrete possibility of causing an overdose. It is common clinical practice to evaluate the patient's initial TSH and body mass on the day of the visit to obtain information on the severity of the pathology and the amount of LT_4 that the subject needs [48].

Based on the information acquired during the visit, the endocrinologist uses the reference correlations for LT_4 dosage according to body mass, indicating a weekly intake scheme that allows progressively increasing the dose up to the prescribed value to limit/ zero possible undesired effects (*e.g.*, cardiac decompensation, arrhythmias, fibrillations) during the first phase of treatment. At the next follow-up visit, usually scheduled after 6– 8 weeks, the endocrinologist will view the blood chemistry tests, check the new TSH and fT_4 values, and possibly correct the dosage based on the preset objectives for the two markers of hypothyroidism and the patient's symptomatology [48].

Currently, clinical practice is primarily based on the described methods, mainly focused on the endocrinologist's sensitivity and experience with the dose calculation based on the patient's body mass. It can be noted that little space is dedicated to possible mathematical or algorithmic approaches in clinical practice, even though, over the years, various researchers have worked on formulating more or less complex models for predicting the dose or the functioning of the HPT axis. Among the mathematical relationships most frequently used in the literature for calculating the amount of LT_4 to prescribe, we can find:

- Dose per kilogram of body mass: the formula varies based on the sensitivity of the treating physician, who imposes a multiplication factor of body mass appropriate to the patient. The most frequently used values are 1.6, 1.8, or 2.1 µg/kg.
- Popoian's correlation: determines the multiplication factor of weight to determine the LT_4 dose based on BMI (body mass index):

BMI < 25   1.76 µg/kg
BMI < 30   1.47 µg/kg
BMI < 35   1.42 µg/kg
BMI < 40   1.27 µg/kg
BM ≥ 40   1.28 µg/kg

- Poisson's formula: based on BMI, body mass, age, sex, height, iron, multivitamin supplements:

$$LT_4 = e^X \tag{6.3.1}$$
$$X = 2.02 + 0.01W - 0.0037A - 0.098F - 0.01B + 0.007T + \ldots\ldots +0.108I - 0.014M \tag{6.3.2}$$

Where:
 W: body mass [kg]
 A: age [y]
 F: sex (0 female patient, 1 male patient)
 B: body mass index (BMI)
 T: initial TSH [mIU/l]
 I: iron supplementation (1 for presence, 0 for absence)
 M: multivitamin/mineral supplementation (1 for presence, 0 for absence)

The models that allow simulating the dynamics of thyroid hormone, including external inputs of LT4, are worth mentioning. In particular, according to an in-depth literature review, the *p-Thyrosim* [49] and SimThyr [50] models are the most advanced models. They were developed respectively by DiStefano [51–53] and Dietrich [50]. The *p-Thyrosim* model was used in the present study, given the open-source nature of the base calculation code and its detailed publications.

6.4 A compartmental model of the HPT axis

The mathematical model in this study is derived from the work of DiStefano's research group, whose seminal activity for developing a mathematical model capable of describing the physiology of the HPT axis began in 1968 [54]. That research has continued over the years [49, 51–53], leading to an individualized model capable of simulating the entire HPT axis for both euthyroid subjects and those affected by thyroid pathologies.

The model is of the PBPK (Physiologically Based Pharmacokinetic model) type and describes the interaction of the HPT axis operating based on the aforementioned "feedback control system" (FBCS) [55]. The role played by a chemical engineer in this modeling activity is, first of all, that of adopting a first principles approach that grounds on material balances to lump organs and tissues into dedicated compartments while respecting the anatomy and physiology of the human body. The resulting system of ordinary differential equations with initial conditions is a straightforward numerical activity for a chemical engineer. Again, the numerical identification of adaptive parameters (*i.e.* coefficients and constants) through nonlinear regression procedures is intrinsic to the skills of a chemical engineer. Indeed, the control and regulation of thyroid hormone homeostasis are closely analogous to the dynamics of a typical feedback controller in the process industry. The similarities in the physiological dynamics of the axis compared to a feedback controller have further facilitated the modeling of the axis, dividing it into six main compartments that describe the biological mechanism of hormonal regulation: three of them are dedicated to the hypothalamus, pituitary, and thyroid glands, while the remaining three are devoted to the processes of hormone diffusion and excretion in plasma and tissues/organs. Each compartment is described by a control volume characterized by material flows in and out, to which possible molecular diffusion phenomena (intra and extra compartment) and biological or chemical reactions are added. The mathematical modeling of the HPT axis translates into a set of ordinary differential equations describing the biological functioning of each compartment and the hormonal connections between them. For each compartment, the model takes into account two contributions for the description of the ADME process of the drug and endogenous hormones:

– Secretion
– Distribution and elimination (D&E)

Each compartment is thus described by an equation formulated as follows:

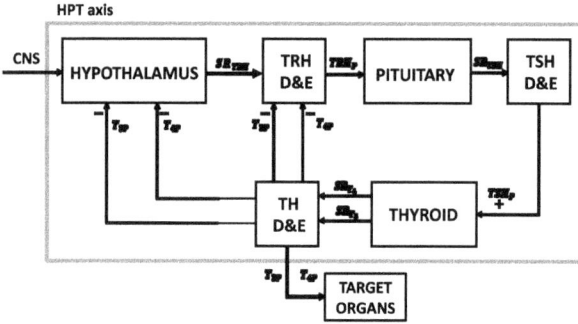

Figure 6.2: Diagram of the negative feedback control scheme of the HPT axis. The "plus" and "minus" symbols identify respectively the effect of stimulation and suppression of hormone secretion within the biological mechanism of the HPT axis. SR$_i$: secretion rate of the corresponding hormone; TRH$_P$, TSH$_P$, T_{3P}, T_{4P}: plasma concentrations of hormones, where the subscript P indicates the plasma compartment; CNS: input from the central nervous system. D&E: distribution and excretion contributions in the body of TRH, TSH and TH (*i.e.*, T_3 and T_4) hormones.

$$\frac{dq_i}{dt} = \dot{q}_i^{in} - \dot{q}_i^{out} \pm r_i \tag{6.4.1}$$

The term dq_i/dt indicates the dynamics over time of the variation of the quantity (either mass or molar) of i-th substance within the compartment, $\dot{q}_i$ indicates the inflow or outflow while r_i is the term of formation or disappearance of the species i.

The *p-Thyrosim* model [49] describes the evolutionary dynamics of circulating hormones in plasma and peripheral tissues according to the structure shown in Figure 6.2 and described in the following paragraphs.

6.4.1 BRAIN submodel

The BRAIN submodel [49] in Figure 6.3 describes the processes of biological interaction of the pituitary and hypothalamus with the T_3 and T_4 hormones present therein. This submodel describes the dynamics of TRH and TSH's endogenous production. It receives as input the plasma concentrations of T_3 and T_4 and returns as output the secretion rate of TSH and, in addition, the conversion rate of T_4 to T_3 at the cerebral level by the deiodinase enzymes D_1 and D_2.

$$\dot{TSH}_P(t) = \left[SR_{TSH}(t) - f_{deg}^{TSH}TSH_P(t)\right]PVR \tag{6.4.2}$$

$$\dot{T}_{3B}(t) = \frac{f_4}{T_{4P}^{EU}}T_{4P}(t) + \frac{k_3}{T_{3P}^{EU}}T_{3P}(t) - k_{deg}^{T_{3B}}T_{3B}(t) \tag{6.4.3}$$

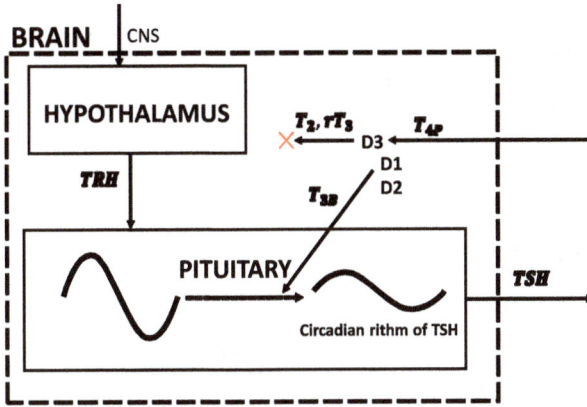

Figure 6.3: Diagram of the BRAIN subsystem leading to TSH secretion. The red cross signifies the elimination or deactivation of thyroid hormones.

$$\dot{T}_{3B}^{\text{LAG}}(t) = f_{\text{LAG}}\left(T_{3B}(t) - T_{3B}^{\text{LAG}}(t)\right) \tag{6.4.4}$$

The LAG suffix identifies a more prolonged permanence of the hormone in the tissues compared to a state of euthyroidism due to the delay in the disappearance of the hormone and an increase in its production in the presence of a hypothyroid state.

The PVR parameter considers the scaling effects of the subject's anthropometric characteristics. In particular, in the case of patients whose height and weight correspond to average reference values for their respective sex, the PVR value is unitary. As it deviates from the reference values, the parameter considers the variation of the average volumes of the compartments, larger for taller subjects and with greater body mass or vice versa.

6.4.2 TH submodel

The TH submodel [49] describes the mechanisms of endogenous production, enzymatic reaction, transport, and elimination of thyroid hormones at the plasma and tissue levels. Regarding the processes of enzymatic reaction, transport, and elimination of thyroid hormones, it is appropriate to introduce the TH D&E subsystem. The latter allows for defining the temporal trend of circulating quantities of T_3 and T_4 hormones in plasma and tissues. The process of conversion from T_4 to T_3 is defined through type 1 (D_1) and type 2 (D_2) deiodinase enzymes, together with the simultaneous mechanism of deactivation of a part of thyroid hormones by type 3 deiodinase (D_3). Figure 6.4 shows how the elimination and distribution processes are divided between slow and fast tissues to distinguish peripheral tissues that differ in speed of absorption and metabolism of T_3 and T_4.

TH SUBMODEL

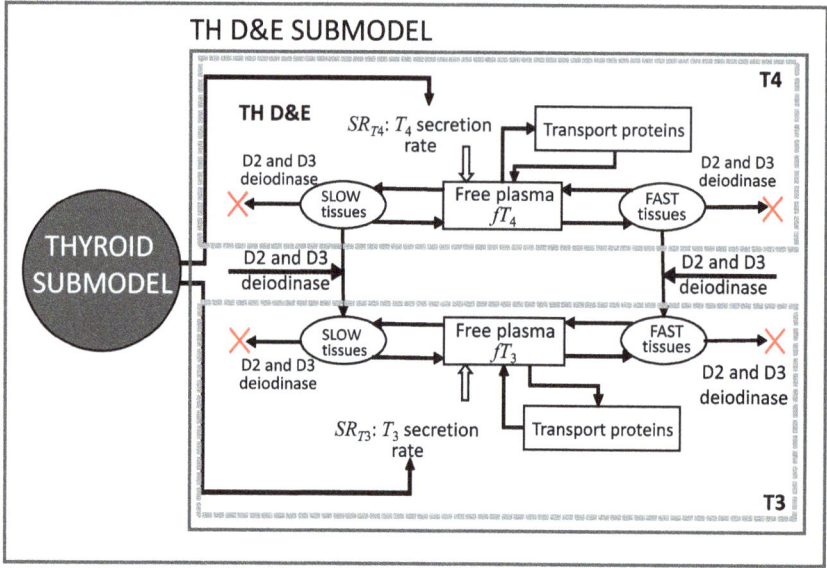

Figure 6.4: Schematic representation of the TH submodel subsystem divided into its TH D&E and thyroid submodel subsystems. Distribution system in plasma and fast and slow tissues of T_3 and T_4 hormones, starting from thyroid secretion to their elimination by the deiodinase enzymes D_2 and D_3 identified by red crosses. The upper part of the TH submodel is related to the T_4 hormone, which is then converted in the tissues into T_3 and described in the lower part of the figure.

The equations below describe the mechanisms just mentioned. In particular, Equations (6.4.5), (6.4.6) and (6.4.7) describe the dynamics of the variation of the amount of T_4 present in the plasma, fast, and slow compartments, while Equations (6.4.8), (6.4.9) and (6.4.10) represent the same dynamics, this time, for the T_3 hormone in the same compartments.

$$\dot{T}_{4P}(t) = \left(\text{SR}_4(t) + k_{12}q_2(t) + k_{13}q_3(t) - \left(k_{31}^{\text{free}} + k_{21}^{\text{free}}\right)FT_{4P}(t)\right)\text{PVR} + \dots$$
$$\dots + k_4^{\text{absorb}}\, T_4^{\text{GUT}}(t) + u_1(t) \tag{6.4.5}$$

$$\dot{T}_{4\text{Fast}}(t) = \left[k_{21}^{\text{free}}FT_{4P}(t) - \left(k_{12} + k_{02} + \frac{v_{\max}^{D_1\,\text{fast}}}{K_m^{D1\,\text{fast}} + q_2(t)}\right)q_2(t)\right]\text{FVR} \tag{6.4.6}$$

$$\dot{T}_{4\text{Slow}}(t) = k_{31}^{\text{free}}FT_{4P}(t)\text{SVR} + \dots$$
$$\dots - \left[\left(k_{13} + k_{03} + \frac{v_{\max}^{D_1\,\text{slow}}}{K_m^{D1\,\text{slow}} + q_3(t)} + \frac{v_{\max}^{D_2\,\text{slow}}}{K_m^{D2\,\text{slow}} + q_3(t)}\right)q_3(t)\right]\text{SVR} \tag{6.4.7}$$

$$\dot{T}_{3P}(t) = \left[\text{SR}_3(t) + k_{45}q_5(t) + k_{46}q_6(t) - \left(k_{64}^{\text{free}} + k_{54}^{\text{free}}\right)FT_{3P}(t)\right]\text{PVR} + \dots$$
$$\dots + k_3^{\text{absorb}}\, T_3^{\text{GUT}}(t) + u_4(t) \tag{6.4.8}$$

$$\dot{T}_{3Fast}(t) = \left[k_{54}^{free} FT_{3P}(t) + \frac{v_{max}^{D_1 fast} q_2(t)}{K_m^{D_1 fast} + q_2(t)} - (k_{45} + k_{05})q_5(t) \right] FVR \qquad (6.4.9)$$

$$\dot{T}_{3Slow}(t) = \left[k_{64}^{free} FT_{3P}(t) + \frac{v_{max}^{D_1 slow} q_3(t)}{K_m^{D_1 slow} + q_3(t)} + \frac{v_{max}^{D_2 slow} q_3(t)}{K_m^{D_2 slow} + q_3(t)} \right] SVR + \dots$$

$$\dots - (k_{46} + k_{06})q_6(t) \qquad (6.4.10)$$

In particular, the terms k_{ij} [h^{-1}] indicate the diffusion rates from compartment j to compartment i where, in this case, subscripts 1, 2, and 3 represent the plasma, fast tissues and slow tissues subsystems in the case of a specific exchange of the T_4 hormone while the k_{ij}^{free} describe the exchange of fT_4 (e.g., k_{12} describes the diffusion from fast tissues to plasma while k_{21} describes the diffusion from plasma to fast tissues). Subsequently, subscripts 4, 5, and 6 always refer to the plasma and fast and slow tissue compartments, but in the case of T_3 diffusion, while for fT_3, the superscript "free" is indicated. Finally, the subscript "0" describes the elimination process that can occur only in the fast and slow compartments by type 3 deiodinase. Regarding the possibility of transformation of T_4 into T_3, the two contributions of deiodinase enzymes described through Michaelis–Menten kinetics [56] are considered, in which the speed of enzyme-substrate interaction (deiodinase-T_4) is here described:

$$v = v_{max}[S] \big/ (K_m + [S]) \equiv v_{max}^{D_{1,i}} T_{4i} \big/ \left(K_m^{D_{1,i}} + T_{4i} \right) \qquad (6.4.11)$$

Subscript i represents the compartment in which the T_4 hormone is present and in which the D_1 enzyme acts. In addition, the term $v_{max}^{D_{1,i}}$ indicates the maximum speed of transformation of T_4 while the term K_m indicates the substrate concentration (T_4) for which the deiodination speed is halved. Equations (6.4.5) to (6.4.8) feature two additional terms that are representative of the contribution of drug absorbed in the gastrointestinal tract described by $k_3^{absorb} T_3^{GUT}(t)$ and $k_4^{absorb} T_4^{GUT}(t)$ where k^{absorb} defines the absorption rate while the terms T_3^{GUT} and T_4^{GUT} describe the dynamics of the absorbable quantity at the level of the jejunum and ileum.

6.4.2.1 Thyroid submodel

The thyroid submodel [49] describes the endogenous secretion of T_3 and T_4 within the TH submodel compartment. Specifically, Equations (6.4.12) and (6.4.13) reported below describe the complex physiological mechanism of T_3 and T_4 hormone production, including the processes that go from the stimulation of the thyroid gland by plasma TSH to the release of secreted hormones into the bloodstream.

$$SR_3(t) = S_3 RTF_{T_3} TSH_{delay_6} \qquad (6.4.12)$$

$$SR_4(t) = S_4 RTF_{T_4} TSH_{delay_6} \qquad (6.4.13)$$

These equations express the secretion rate of T_3 and T_4, in particular, $S_4 \text{TSH}_{\text{delay}_6}$ represents the maximum possible production of thyroxine, where the parameter S_4 identifies the amount of hormone produced per µg of stimulating TSH, while $\text{TSH}_{\text{delay}_6}$ describes the amount of TSH interacting with the thyroid where the subscript "delay" indicates the delay in the interaction of TSH with the thyroid gland imposed by the physiological barriers present and which stands at about 8 h.

RTF_{T_4} is the multiplicative parameter that modulates the hormone secretion capacity of the thyroid gland as a function of the degree of primary hypothyroidism of the patient. It can only assume positive values and, if set to zero, indicates a completely suppressed thyroid production. In contrast, a unitary value indicates a thyroid gland in perfect condition (*i.e.*, euthyroidism). Consequently, the input to the subsystem is identified in the plasma TSH value derived from the BRAIN compartment, while the output refers to the thyroid secretion values for both T_3 and T_4.

6.4.3 Input submodel

The input submodel [49] in Figure 6.5 describes the LT_4 absorption process through the main routes of administration in the body: oral, intravenous, intramuscular, and intradermal. The first absorption mode, *per os*, describes the metabolic processes of the active ingredient within the gastrointestinal tract and the subsequent release into the bloodstream [45]. Equations (6.4.14) and (6.4.15) describe the mechanism of dissolution of the drug tablet within the stomach and the subsequent absorption of the T_4 hormone at the level of the intestinal villi [57]. Similarly, Equations (6.4.16) and (6.4.17) refer to the T_3 hormone.

$$\dot{T}_4^{\text{PILL}}(t) = -k_4^{\text{dissolve}} T_4^{\text{PILL}}(t) \tag{6.4.14}$$

$$\dot{T}_4^{\text{GUT}}(t) = k_4^{\text{dissolve}} T_4^{\text{PILL}}(t) - \left(k_4^{\text{excrete}} + k_4^{\text{absorb}}\right) T_4^{\text{GUT}}(t) \tag{6.4.15}$$

$$\dot{T}_3^{\text{PILL}}(t) = -k_3^{\text{dissolve}} T_3^{\text{PILL}}(t) \tag{6.4.16}$$

$$\dot{T}_3^{\text{GUT}}(t) = k_3^{\text{dissolve}} T_3^{\text{PILL}}(t) - \left(k_3^{\text{excrete}} + k_3^{\text{absorb}}\right) T_3^{\text{GUT}}(t) \tag{6.4.17}$$

The pill dissolution terms k^{dissolve} are related to the quantities of drug administered and are preceded by a minus sign since they refer to a quantity that is exclusively consumed. The equations referring to $\dot{T}_3^{\text{PILL}}$ and $\dot{T}_4^{\text{PILL}}$ define the dynamics of pill dissolution in the stomach and thus made available for absorption in the gastrointestinal tract. Instead, $\dot{T}_3^{\text{GUT}}$ and $\dot{T}_4^{\text{GUT}}$ represent the dynamics of absorption at the intestinal level of the dissolved active ingredient. To determine this latter quantity, the difference is made between the amount of dissolved pill, and therefore available for absorption, and that both excreted and already absorbed. The terms k^{absorb} represent the absorption rate at the level of the jejunum and ileum, while the

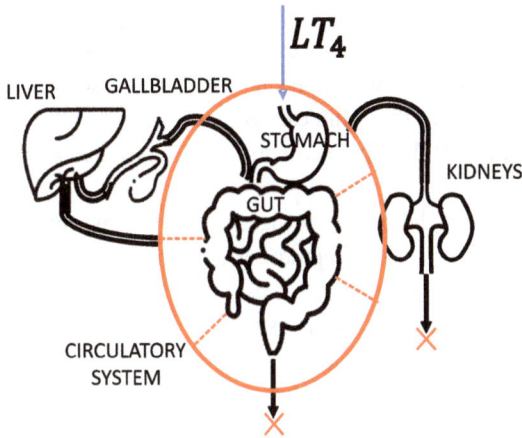

Figure 6.5: Anatomical diagram of the input/output subsystems, including drug administration and elimination.

terms k^{excrete} represent the excretion rate in urine and feces of the drug quantities introduced at the exogenous level [49].

The inactive hormones are then eliminated 20 % through the feces and the remaining 80 % through the urine, concluding the ADME pathway of LT_4 and the metabolic pathway of endogenous T_3 and T_4 [57]. In the case of intravenous administration, the drug is introduced and made immediately available in the bloodstream. The intravenous absorption term appears directly in the equations of the TH D&E subsystem in the form of the term $u(t)$, as it does not pass through the gastrointestinal compartment where it would necessarily undergo a partial degradation process.

In conclusion, the inputs to the subsystem are the quantities of drug administered, and as output, the quantity of T_4 and/or T_3 that the compartment transforms into circulating flows within the TH D&E submodel [53, 55, 58, 59].

6.5 A model-based approach to the prediction of the optimal levothyroxine dose

The *p-Thyrosim* model discussed in the previous section can simulate the HPT axis based on the patient's characteristics and, in addition, describe the possible hypothyroid condition or the dynamics of treatment based on exogenous replacement therapy. However, it should be emphasized that the model described in Section 6.4 cannot automatically calculate the optimal dose of levothyroxine nor quantify the degree of hypothyroidism of the specific patient (*i.e.*, RTF parameter). When using *p-Thyrosim*'s functionalities for treatment simulation, it is necessary to set *a priori* the value of the residual thyroid gland function (RTF) for the secretion of the respective hormones.

The present work proposes a further computational model, *PzeroT* [60], based on *p-Thyrosim*, capable of determining the optimal dosage of levothyroxine in treating patients with hypothyroidism. *PzeroT* operates in two distinct and sequential phases. The first phase involves deriving the subject's residual thyroid function (RTF). This parameter indicates the gland's remaining thyroid hormone secretion capacity in the case of primary hypothyroidism. In the second phase, the algorithm calculates the optimal dose of LT_4 for the correct application of replacement therapy based on the RTF parameter and the patient's characteristics.

To effectively understand the structure of the predictive algorithm, it is important to recall the inputs to be assigned to the model so that it reproduces the temporal trend of thyroid hormones in plasma and peripheral tissues. Initially, the user-definable parameters were limited to the patient's sex, absorption rate, and endogenous secretion rate of T_3 and T_4, along with the administrable doses of LT_3 and LT_4. Following recent developments in model individualization, it has been possible to include additional anthropometric parameters such as height and weight, which have allowed scaling the volumes of the various compartments, adapting the levothyroxine dose to each individual patient [49]. The model currently takes into account the following individual patient characteristics:
- Height [m];
- Body mass [kg];
- Patient's sex;
- Residual thyroid secretion factor for T_3 and T_4 hormones (RTF);
- Intestinal absorption factor for T_3 and T_4 hormones;
- Administered dose of LT_3 and LT_4 [µg].

The residual thyroid secretion factor (RTF) is the most critical parameter among those assignable as it is essential for defining the functional state of the thyroid (see also Section 6.4.2.1). Moreover, it can be interpreted as the residual efficiency factor of the thyroid gland in the case of primary hypothyroidism, *i.e.*, derived from pathologies directly related to gland dysfunctions. The RTF value is also correlated with plasma TSH and thyroxine (T_4) levels as described in *p-Thyrosim* (see Section 6.4). In particular, reduced T_4 levels cause the pituitary to attempt to stimulate thyroid production by raising TSH secretion to restore hormone-level homeostasis. The *in-silico* simulation of a hypothyroid subject is based on a reduced RTF value that induces a reduction in T_3 and T_4 secretion and leads to an increase in TSH characterized by supra-euthyroid values. Figure 6.6 shows the trend of the TSH circadian rhythm as a function of the RTF value for a simulated patient. A decrease in RTF leads to a general increase in TSH. It is important to emphasize that the *p-Thyrosim* model does not describe an exact inverse dependence between RTF and TSH. For example, if the RTF value is halved, a doubling of TSH levels is not obtained.

Indeed, there is an inverse log-linear dependence between the two physiological parameters fT_4 and TSH, not yet clarified at the medical level and discussed in [61]. Figure 6.7 refers to the same simulated patient of Figure 6.6, a male 1.70 m tall with a body mass of 68 kg.

The RTF parameter allows describing the thyroid state through modulation of both T_3 and T_4 secretion and, consequently, of TSH. Since it is impossible to experimentally

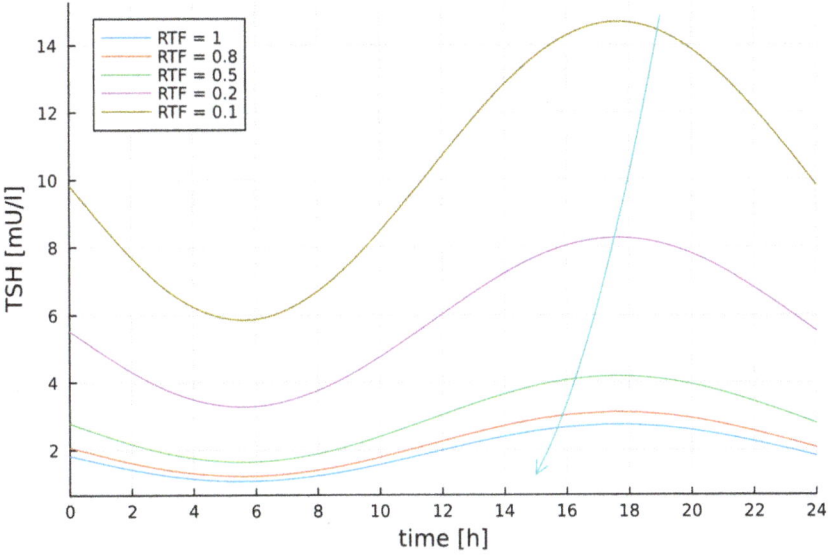

Figure 6.6: Variation of TSH trends as a function of RTF value. The arrow shows the increase in RTF values.

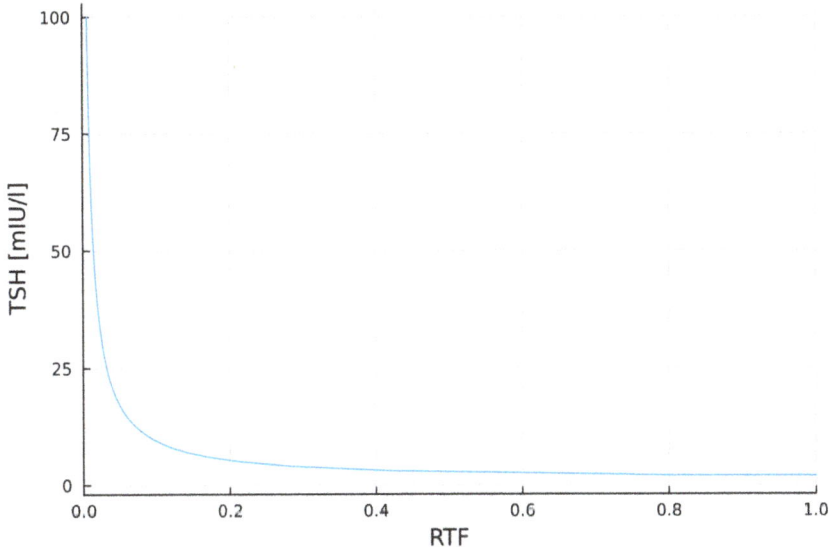

Figure 6.7: Trend of the patient's TSH as a function of RTF value.

measure the residual thyroid function (RTF) and the dependence on TSH is non-linear, the endocrinologist cannot assign an RTF value *a priori* to the patient being examined. It is therefore necessary to quantify the RTF value based on the experimental blood

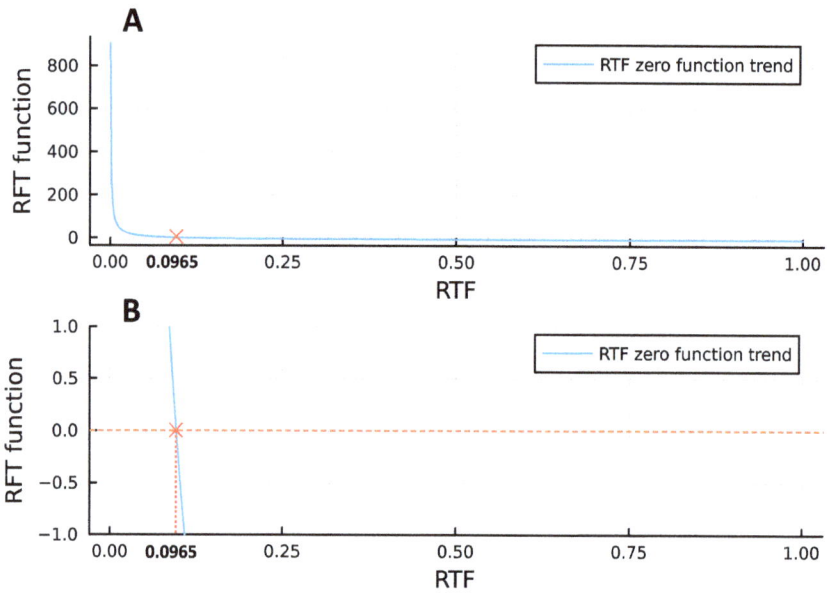

Figure 6.8: Trend of the RTF zeroing function as a function of RTF values from 0 to 1 for the patient chosen as an example. (A) Shows the complete trend, while (B) shows the restricted intersection area with the $y = 0$ axis.

measurement of TSH of the patient who needs to undergo treatment in case of hypothyroidism through a calculation procedure. The new algorithm we implemented, *PzeroT*, allows calculating through Equation (6.5.1) the specific RTF parameter of the individual patient starting from their individualized values (*i.e.*, sex, body mass, height):

$$f(\text{RTF}) = \text{TSH}_{exp} - \text{TSH}_{mod}(\text{RTF}) \tag{6.5.1}$$

TSH_{exp} and $\text{TSH}_{mod}(\text{RTF})$ represent respectively the thyrotropin value obtained from blood tests on the patient and the TSH value simulated by the model. For example, if we consider a male patient 1.70 m tall, with a body mass of 68 kg and a TSH value of 10 mIU/l, the numerical solution of Equation (6.5.1) leads to an RTF value of 0.0965. This value quantifies the degree of primary hypothyroidism of the analyzed patient. Figure 6.8 shows the functional dependence of Equation (6.5.1).

In addition, Figure 6.9 shows the temporal trend of TSH of the simulated patient, considering the individual characteristics previously mentioned. In standard medical practice, the endocrinologist, not having the dynamics shown in Figure 6.9 and not even knowing the RTF value shown in Figure 6.6, would qualitatively estimate, based on the patient's symptoms and the initial TSH value, the degree of hypothyroidism without having the quantitative value that measures the patient's residual thyroid function (RTF). What has just been described is step 1 of the algorithm, followed by step 2, namely the calculation of the optimal dose of LT_4 for the patient who needs to start treatment.

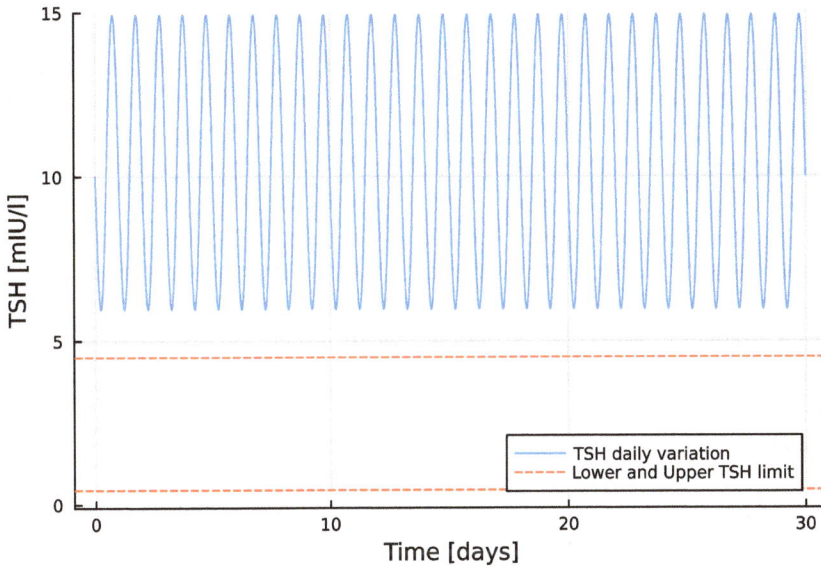

Figure 6.9: TSH trend for 30 days for the case-study patient.

The objective of the second phase of the procedure consists of the direct calculation of the optimal dose of levothyroxine according to what we define as a "one-shot" mode, *i.e.*, hopefully through the patient's first visit to the endocrinologist. The usual approach of the endocrinologist is based on correlations that return approximated dosages that are not individualized to the specific patient. Moreover, the physician's evaluation is conditioned by the limited knowledge of the subject's hypothyroid state, which cannot be objective (*i.e.*, quantitative and unbiased) but based on their own experience since measuring the RTF parameter is impossible. For these reasons, the endocrinologist proceeds with a "trial and error" approach regarding clinical treatment. In most treatments, the endocrinologist evaluates the new TSH value reached by the patient following the first LT_4 prescription and progressively adjusts the initial dose based on subsequent TSH values resulting from blood tests and the health status reported by the patient. Therefore, it is possible that during the course of treatment, the subject does not immediately take the correct dosage and continues to suffer from the symptoms caused by hypothyroidism.

On the contrary, the automated procedure we propose implements the second phase of the *PzeroT* algorithm, which aims to calculate the optimal LT_4 dose, which is hopefully correct from the first endocrinological visit, so as to lead to the euthyroid condition in the shortest possible time.

The procedure of phase 2 of *PzeroT* is numerically similar to that of phase 1 as it zeros a function of the unknown variable LT_4. To obtain this result, it is necessary to lead the TSH simulated through the model to the optimal value (aka target value) assigned by the endocrinologist based on their experience and according to the specific patient:

$$f(\text{LT}_4) = \text{TSH}_{\text{target}} - \text{TSH}_{\text{mod}}(\text{LT}_4) \qquad (6.5.2)$$

$\text{TSH}_{\text{mod}}(\text{LT}_4)$ is the thyrotropin (TSH hormone) value calculated by the model as a function of (i) the exogenous administration of T_4 due to levothyroxine (LT_4) intake and (ii) the individualized RTF parameter. The term $\text{TSH}_{\text{target}}$ is assigned by the treating physician, and the subscript "*target*" indicates the TSH value that needs to be reached for the patient to see the euthyroid state restored through exogenous administration of LT_4. Therefore, the algorithm searches for the precise amount of levothyroxine that leads the subject's TSH (simulated *in-silico*) to the desired target value. Once the individualized values of RTF and LT_4 are obtained, it is now possible to quantify the evolutionary dynamics of the (typically daily) administration of LT_4 tablets throughout the entire period of evolution of TSH levels up to the desired new target value (in clinical practice, about six weeks are necessary [60]).

Proceeding with the case study and considering the same patient described previously, we can calculate the dose necessary to restore the correct endocrine values and simulate the dynamics of the temporal trend of thyroid hormones and TSH. Figure 6.11 shows the TSH trend during the dosage of a levothyroxine quantity of 100.99 µg, a result obtained through the second step of the algorithm described previously and shown graphically in Figure 6.10.

The euthyroid reference interval is reached within 3–4 days from the first administration, while the new steady state is reached 15–20 days after the first drug intake (see

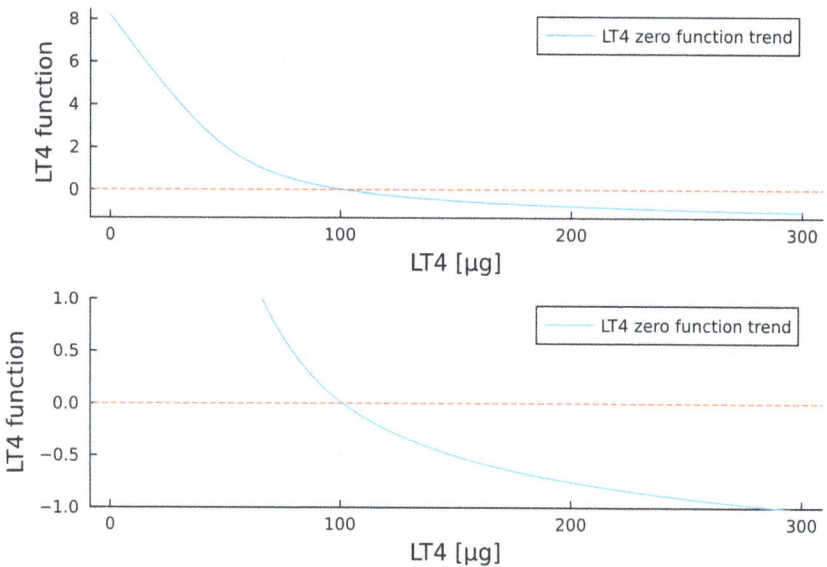

Figure 6.10: Trend of the LT_4 zeroing function as a function of LT_4 values from 12.5 µg to 300 µg for the patient chosen as an example. (A) Shows the complete trend, while (B) shows the restricted area of intersection with the $y = 0$ axis.

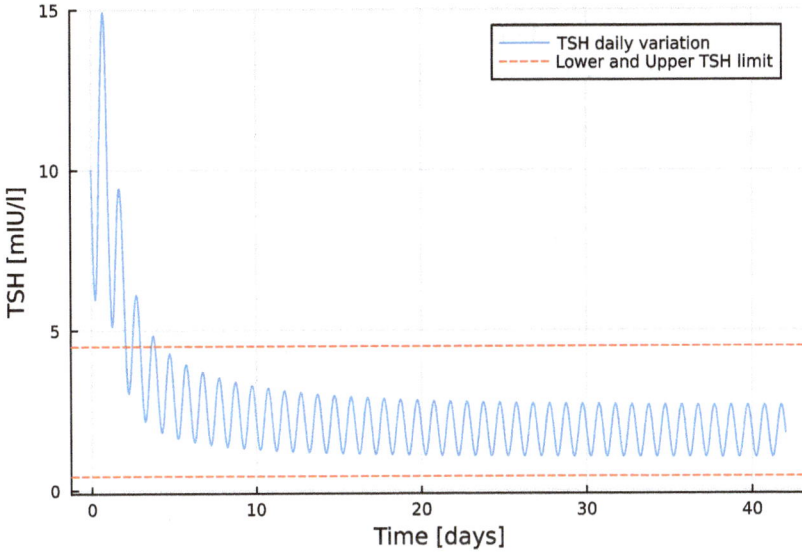

Figure 6.11: Temporal trend of TSH during LT$_4$ administration for the patient chosen as an example.

also Figure 6.12). These results were obtained by setting as the optimal target value a TSH value of 1.8 mIU/l. However, since this is a parameter imposed by the user, it can be easily modulated based on the clinical conditions of the subject and the therapy that is desired to be applied to the patient.

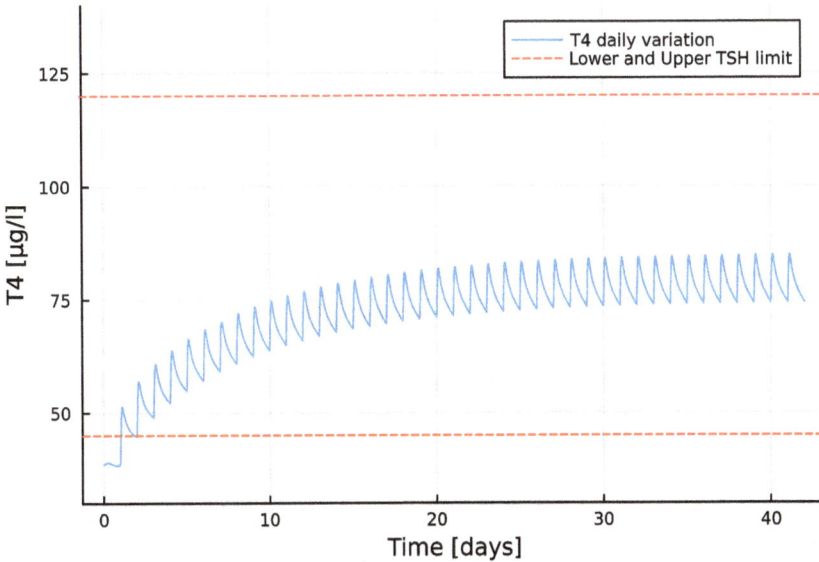

Figure 6.12: Temporal trend of T$_4$ during LT$_4$ administration for the selected patient.

The advantage of using the *p-Thyrosim* model within the *PzeroT* algorithm is the ability to account for individual information, such as the patient's sex, body mass, and height, which are fundamental for determining the individualized dose of levothyroxine. The model can scale the volumes of the involved compartments [49] according to the aforementioned individual parameters. In the case of the virtual patient, a target TSH value of 1.8 mIU/l was defined as desired by the endocrinologist without the guarantee that this is the subject's optimal value.

Section 6.3 explored the influence of age on TSH, suggesting an increase in the upper limit of the euthyroid interval with advancing age, particularly after 60 years in men and after 40 for women [41]. Indeed, there is the possibility of inducing drug overdoses for elderly patients if the limits desired for young patients are adopted. The *PzeroT* algorithm implements a functional dependence capable of modulating the optimal TSH value to be reached according to the patient's age and sex. We propose two formulas for male or female patients capable of assigning the expected optimal TSH value (attesting to euthyroid conditions) as a function of the individual's age. The study from which data were collected and processed to obtain the correlations mentioned above involved the collection of almost 300,000 TSH measurements from euthyroid subjects aged between 20 and 80 years [41]. In that study, the researchers identified an average TSH value for the lower and upper limits as a function of the individual's age (from young to elderly). Raverot and collaborators observed that the lower limit of the euthyroid interval does not change significantly. At the same time, the upper one grows considerably with age, almost reaching 6 mIU/l for females and 5 mIU/l for males.

$$\text{TSH}^{up}_{male}(\text{age}) = 4.642520589559373 - 0.02039878317500956\,x + \ldots$$

$$\ldots +0.0002614981700062368\,x^2 \tag{6.5.3}$$

$$\text{TSH}^{up}_{female}(\text{age}) = 4.1777986229928485 + 0.00463599130382207x + \ldots$$

$$\ldots +0.0001309278501772748\,x^2 \tag{6.5.4}$$

Figure 6.13 shows the trend of the variation of the upper TSH limit derived through quadratic regression from the data collected in the study:

Specifically, $\text{TSH}^{up}(\text{age})$ defines the value of the upper TSH limit while the variable x identifies the patient's age at the time of starting treatment. To avoid the risks of levothyroxine overdose, it is essential to calibrate the administration of LT_4 to TSH target levels appropriate to the patient's age, especially if the patient is elderly. The endocrinologist, using the PzeroT program, assigns the value of the parameter F (generally 2–3) to determine the target TSH value according to the patient's age and sex.

$$\text{TSH}^{target}_{age} = \frac{\text{TSH}^{up}(\text{age}) + \text{TSH}^{low}}{F} \tag{6.5.5}$$

The parameter F, assigned by the endocrinologist as input to *PzeroT*, automatically evaluates the optimal TSH value that the subject under treatment must reach to be

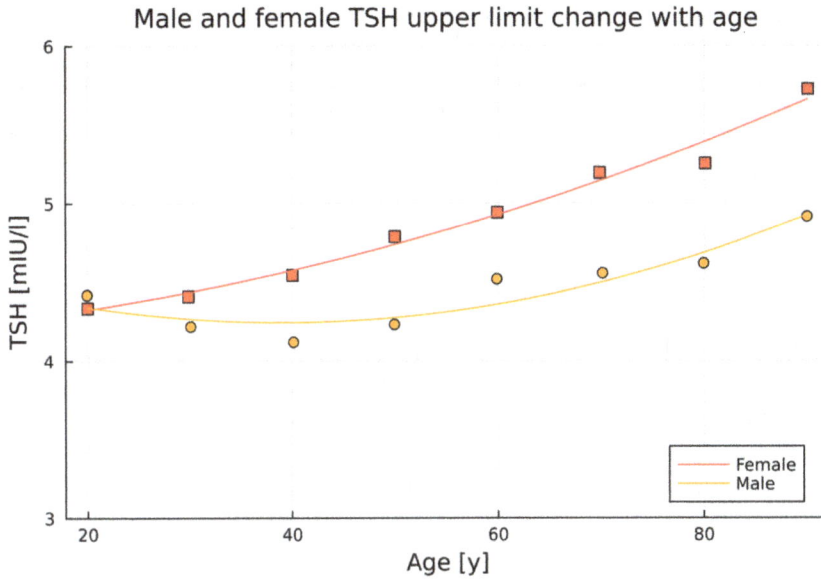

Figure 6.13: Trend of the upper TSH limit with advancing age for males (yellow) and females (red).

defined as euthyroid and to avoid possible overdoses. The execution of *PzeroT*, therefore, allows determining the optimal individualized LT_4 dose as a function of the endocrinologist's more or less aggressive approach to controlling the target TSH value.

6.5.1 Real patient case study

To demonstrate the potential of the *PzeroT* algorithm, we presented two case studies in which we want to compare the evaluation of the optimal dose to be administered by an endocrinologist with what the algorithm calculates. The algorithm (*PzeroT*) is proposed as a predictor and facilitator of correct dosage in clinical practice. It was possible to investigate the algorithm's advantages by analyzing data from hypothyroid patients, both thyroidectomized and still possessing the thyroid gland (albeit subfunctional), derived from hospital practice.

The first case we want to explore concerns the study of the therapy undertaken by a sixty-five-year-old female patient who presents at the first endocrinological visit with a suspected case of subclinical hypothyroidism. The anthropometric characteristics and the history of TSH, fT_4, and LT_4 values are reported in Table 6.2. The patient in question does not present in the outpatient reports indications of additional therapies that may interfere with the LT_4-based one, and, in addition, the reported clinical conditions exclude the presence of comorbidities with potential effects on levothyroxine absorption. Since it is not a case of overt hypothyroidism, *i.e.*, with values >10 mIU/l, the real endocrinologist decides to prescribe a dosage of 50 µg of LT_4 to be taken daily by tablet.

Table 6.2: Data of the anthropometric characteristics of patient #1 (female, 165 cm tall) and the treatment progression.

		Patient #1:		
Age [years]	Body mass [kg]	fT_4 [pmol/l]	TSH [mIU/l]	Dose [µg]
65	71	11.06821	5.74	0
66	78	13.12741	2.71	50
69	78	12.09781	2.65	50

Table 6.2 shows how the continuation of the therapy is characterized by the stabilization of TSH values within the euthyroid range and by a slight increase in the amount of free T_4 hormone in the blood. Subsequently, after the control analyses were carried out at the age of 66, the therapy was confirmed, and the patient showed correct hormonal values with the ongoing therapy even after four years from the start of the treatment.

This case study allows us to analyze the goodness of the algorithm since the necessary historical data for using the *PzeroT* algorithm are correctly reported. The dose prediction algorithm was tested with three different target values, where the first is set at 1.8 mIU/l, the second is a function of age (Equations (6.5.3) and (6.5.4)), and the last one coinciding with the final TSH value at which the patient settles (see Table 6.2). The endocrinologist is not aware of a measure of the patient's residual thyroid secretion (RTF) and, therefore, through their experience and observation of the TSH value slightly above the euthyroid range (TSH 0.45–4.5), prescribes a contained dosage of 50 µg. Conversely, the developed algorithm can quantify the patient's thyroid clinical condition by returning the RTF value as a function of her anthropometric characteristics and initial TSH, and then the optimal LT_4 dose to lead the patient to euthyroid conditions. Three distinct values of TSH_{target} are proposed to investigate three distinct operational hypotheses referring to as many objectives of the therapy to be prescribed. The first TSH target value of 1.8 mIU/l leads to a levothyroxine value corresponding to an aggressive treatment aimed at suppressing hypothyroidism symptoms. The second TSH target value is based on the specific age and sex of the patient, which results in a more moderate approach. The third TSH target value refers to the TSH condition detected in the patient after four years of therapy. It aims to reduce administration further as long as the euthyroid condition is maintained (see Table 6.3).

Table 6.3: Results of dose prediction with the *PzeroT* algorithm for patient #1 with three different TSH targets: TSH_{endo} = 1.8 mIU/l, TSH_{age} = 1.84 mIU/l, TSH_{pat} = 2.65 mIU/l. The dose prescribed by the real endocrinologist at the end of titration is equivalent to 50 µg.

TSH target		TSH targets used for dose calculation are defined in Table 6.6	
	1.8 mIU/l	1.84 mIU/l	2.65 mIU/l
Dose calculated by *PzeroT* in [µg]	94.73	92.31	53.95
Approximation to the closest commercially available dose value in [µg]	100	88	50

Once the treating physician brings the patient within the euthyroid interval, they are usually satisfied with the value obtained with the prescribed dosage and do not proceed with a fine adjustment. On the contrary, the *PzeroT* algorithm can track the patient's response over the years and dynamically adapt the dose whenever a new TSH analysis is available. Table 6.3 reports the dosage values calculated by *PzeroT* and those approximated to the closest commercially available dose (see also Table 6.7).

TSH_{pat} represents the TSH level reached by the subject under treatment at the end of the dose titration process and after four years of treatment. The different doses proposed by *PzeroT* as a function of the three target TSH values result from the other therapy objectives proposed by the algorithm based on the discretion of the endocrinologist, who can choose more drastic or mild approaches to treating hypothyroidism. The innovation of *PzeroT* consists of the possibility for the real endocrinologist to base the LT_4 dose on a therapeutic objective based on obtaining a specific target TSH value that is a function of the patient's age and sex or based on their sensitivity and experience. This procedure allows reversing the logical scheme followed by clinical practice, starting no longer from a dose calculation often based on a fixed value of micrograms per kilogram of body mass but on the evaluation of a therapy that has from the outset as an objective a target TSH value achievable with the *PzeroT* procedure through the calculation of the optimal LT_4 dose.

Figure 6.14 shows the comparison between the TSH trend with the therapy based on a target of 1.8 mIU/l compared to the treatment with the dosage obtained using the TSH_{target} equal to TSH_{pat} 2.65 mIU/l. It can be noted that obtaining a lower stationary TSH value calls for a higher dose of LT_4.

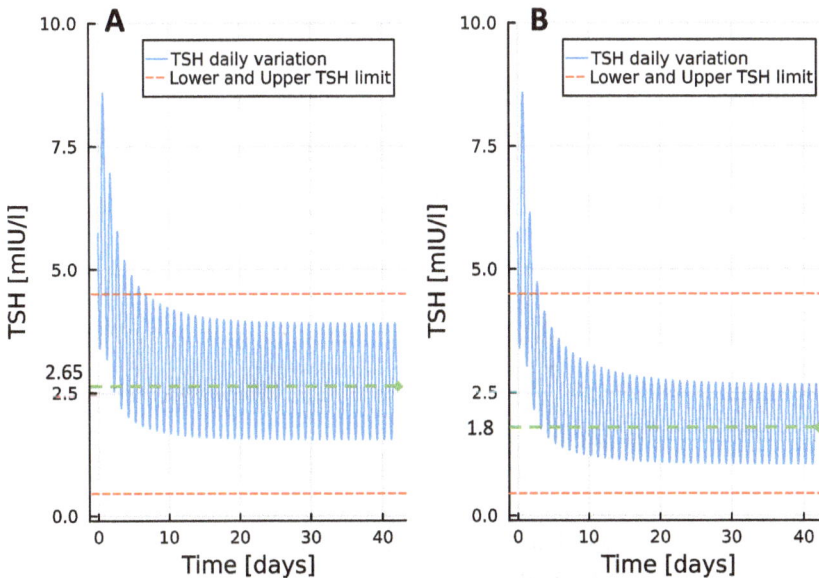

Figure 6.14: Comparison of TSH trend with two different therapies for patient #1. (A) Therapy with 50 µg with which TSH_{target} = 2.65 mIU/l is obtained. (B) Therapy with 100 µg of LT_4 with which TSH_{target} = 1.8 mIU/l is obtained.

Table 6.4: Reference intervals for the randomization of individual characteristics.

Features	Minimum value	Maximum value
Age [years]	20	90
Height [m]	1.40	2.20
Body mass [kg]	38	120
Initial TSH[mIU/l]	4.5	250

6.5.2 Robustness of the algorithm

To prove the robustness of the *PzeroT* algorithm, it was tested on tens of thousands of virtual (*i.e., in-silico*) patients belonging to a broad domain reported in Table 6.4 for both male and female individuals, using a stochastic approach for the selection of their respective physical characteristics.

6.6 Model validation

The *PzeroT* algorithm has undergone a validation process through comparison with several real case studies. This process proceeded with an analysis of data derived from comparing the algorithm's prediction with the doses proposed by endocrinologists to investigate the tool's potential and limitations.

6.6.1 Validation of clinical data from real patients

The patients' sample consists of 29 subjects with overt hypothyroidism, subclinical hypothyroidism, and thyroidectomized patients (*i.e.*, those who have had their thyroid gland removed). Based on the available historical data, the dataset consists of clinical subjects who do not present comorbidities or elements that may interfere with LT_4-based therapy. However, it is possible that some elements disturbing the treatment may not have been indicated in the clinical data or that the patients failed to present them to the treating physician during follow-up visits. The sample consists of historical information of patients under treatment, such as age, body mass, sex, height, free thyroxine (fT_4), thyrotropin (TSH), and levothyroxine dose (LT_4) (see Table 6.5). The dataset is composed of 59 % females and 41 % males. 59 % of the patients have undergone thyroidectomy, and the rest suffer from subclinical or overt hypothyroidism without having undergone thyroid gland removal.

To proceed with the algorithm validation's development, the doses necessary to restore euthyroid conditions were calculated using *PzeroT*, and three distinct prediction techniques were adopted based on three different TSH targets (Table 6.6).

Table 6.5: Description of the maximum, minimum, and average values of patients' information in the sample under analysis. The last section reports the reference values used in the *p-Thyrosim* model to scale the volumes of compartments based on the patient's body mass and height.

	Age [y]	Height [m]	Body mass [kg]	Prescribed dose [µg]
Male and female sample				
Maximum	74	1.78	95	200
Minimum	25	1.48	44	12.5
Mean	52.31	1.66	68.09	87.18
Female sample				
Maximum	73	1.67	80	150
Minimum	25	1.48	44	12.5
Mean	52.82	1.60	62.68	81.93
Male sample				
Maximum	74	1.78	95	200
Minimum	30	1.68	62	25
Mean	51.58	1.73	75.75	94.94
Reference sample defined in *p-Thyrosim*				
Male	–	1.70	65.09	–
Female	–	1.63	61.08	–

Table 6.6: Description of the different types of TSH targets chosen for dose calculation.

Type of TSH target assigned in *PzeroT*	Description of TSH target
TSH_{target} = 1.8 mIU/l	Reference value, proven to be an indicator within the model of restored thyroid functionality. Approximately coinciding with an RTF value equal to 1.
TSH_{target} = TSH_{age}	Target based on the patient's age and calculated using Equations (6.5.3) and (6.5.4).
TSH_{target} = TSH_{pat}	Value derived from the historical data of patients in the sample. The last stable TSH value from the clinical data was chosen, corresponding to a constant LT_4 dose over the time period in which the hormonal value reaches a steady state. If a TSH value within the euthyroid range is unavailable for the patient, the TSH_{pat} method for that specific subject is not used.

Having defined the TSH targets (see Table 6.6) that will be investigated in predicting the LT_4 dose for each subject in the sample under examination, it is now possible to proceed with the actual calculation of the optimized dose through the procedure shown in Section 6.5 regarding *PzeroT*. Due to how the dataset was constructed, it was possible to use the first TSH value reported in the clinical data of each patient, corresponding to the hypothyroid TSH, to perform the first phase of RTF calculation, as it exactly coincides with the value reported in the tests exhibited by the patient to the endocrinologist during the first visit. In this way, the residual thyroid function value was calculated for patients still

Table 6.7: Levothyroxine doses commercially available in the European Community.

Commercial doses [µg]
25
50
75
88
100
112
125
137
150
175
200

with the thyroid gland, while zero value was imposed for subjects who underwent thyroidectomy.

PzeroT then calculates the optimal dose value based on the target values mentioned above for the TSH. The doses calculated through the algorithm were then compared with those prescribed by the hospital endocrinologists who treated the patients of the dataset.

The dose predicted by *PzeroT* is considered correct (*i.e.*, in line with that assigned by endocrinologists) if it does not differ by more than 12.5 µg from the actual prescribed dose.

$$-12.5\,\mu g \leq LT4_{\text{prescritta}} - LT4_{\text{PzeroT}} \leq 12.5\,\mu g \tag{6.6.1}$$

The value of 12.5 µg derives from the minimum interval separating two commercially available doses (see Table 6.7).

6.6.1.1 Analysis of the overall sample

Table 6.8 refers to the doses determined by assigning a TSH target equal to 1.8 mIU/l or TSH_{age}. Regarding the method $TSH_{\text{target}} = TSH_{\text{age}}$, a correct prediction percentage by *PzeroT* of 37.9 % is evident, corresponding to 11 patients out of the total 29 present. As shown in Figure 6.15, the method using TSH_{age} as the *target* of therapy produces dosage values that are always distant and often higher than the dose prescribed.

Figure 6.15 shows that most of the arrows have the tip pointing upwards, indicating that the TSH target derived from Equation (6.5.5) often returns too-low thyrotropin (TSH) values, resulting in the prediction of excessively high LT_4 doses.

Figure 6.16 shows the results obtained by assigning a TSH target equal to 1.8 mIU/l, where a good percentage of correct doses can be observed. However, there are some significant differences between the prescribed quantity and that obtained by *PzeroT* up to values of 87.5 µg.

Table 6.8: Number and percentage of doses correctly calculated by the *PzeroT* algorithm (with method $TSH_{target} = 1.8$ mIU/l and $TSH_{target} = TSH_{age}$) and by the dose-weight correlation ($X = 1.6$ μg/kg hypothyroid patients; $X = 2.2$ μg/kg thyroidectomized subjects). Total sample size 29 patients.

	Calculated doses with TSH_{target} assigned in Table 6.6		Calculated doses with the dose-weight correlation
	1.8 mIU/l	**TSH_{age}**	**Xμg/kg**
Number of doses calculated correctly	14	11	5
Percentage of doses calculated correctly	48.3 %	37.9 %	17.2 %

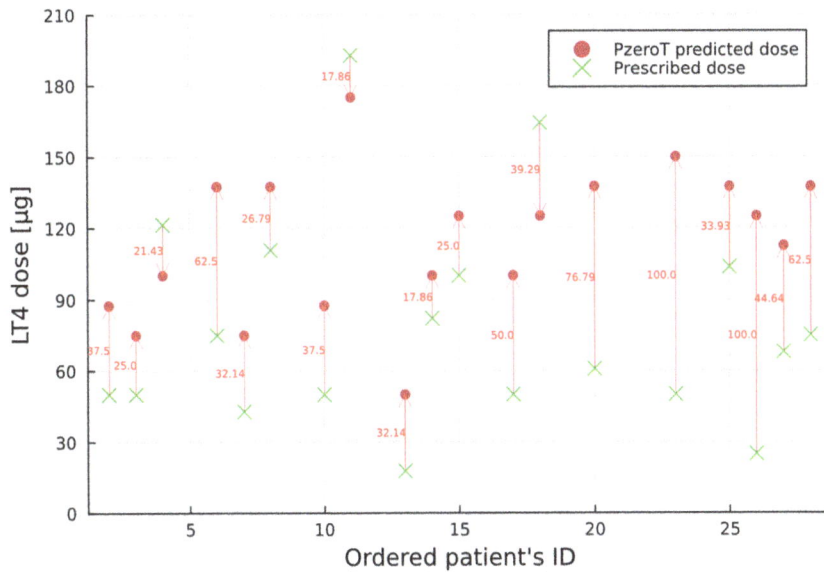

Figure 6.15: Graphical representation of the doses incorrectly calculated by the *PzeroT* algorithm using the $TSH_{target} = TSH_{age}$ method compared to those actually prescribed. The red arrows and the value placed next to them indicate the distance between the dose prescribed by the endocrinologist and that calculated by *PzeroT*.

Finally, Figure 6.17 highlights the poor accuracy of the dose-weight correlation method (2.2 μg/kg for TSH-suppressed subjects and 1.6 μg/kg for the rest). The values represented by blue squares are far from the bisector, and it is clear that this dose prediction strategy overestimates the dose actually prescribed in almost all cases since most of the values are above the blue bisector.

Table 6.9 reports the results of the *PzeroT* algorithm on the sample of 19 patients who have a final TSH within the euthyroid interval and who, therefore, have not undergone TSH-suppressive therapy. From the analysis of the algorithm's performance on the restricted

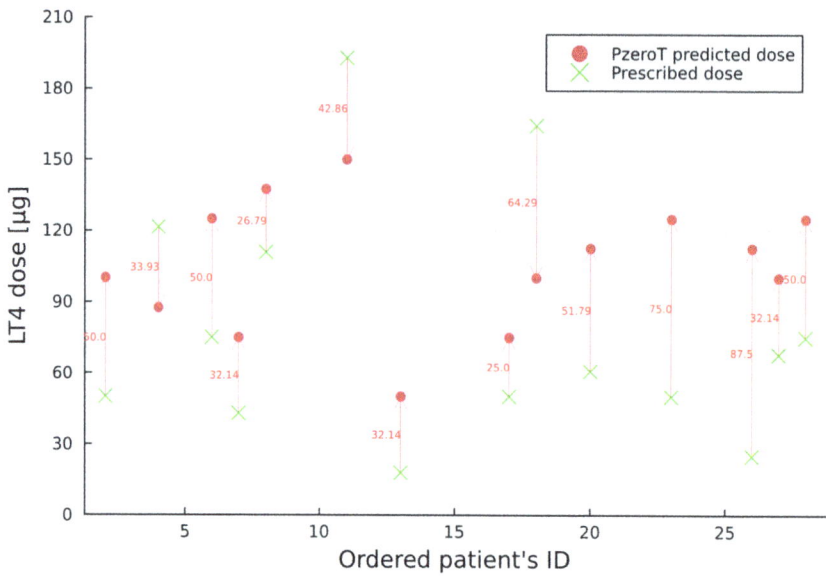

Figure 6.16: Graphical representation of the doses incorrectly calculated by *PzeroT* using the $TSH_{target} = 1.8$ mIU/l method compared to those prescribed. The red arrows and the value placed next to them indicate the distance between the dose prescribed by the endocrinologist and that calculated by *PzeroT*.

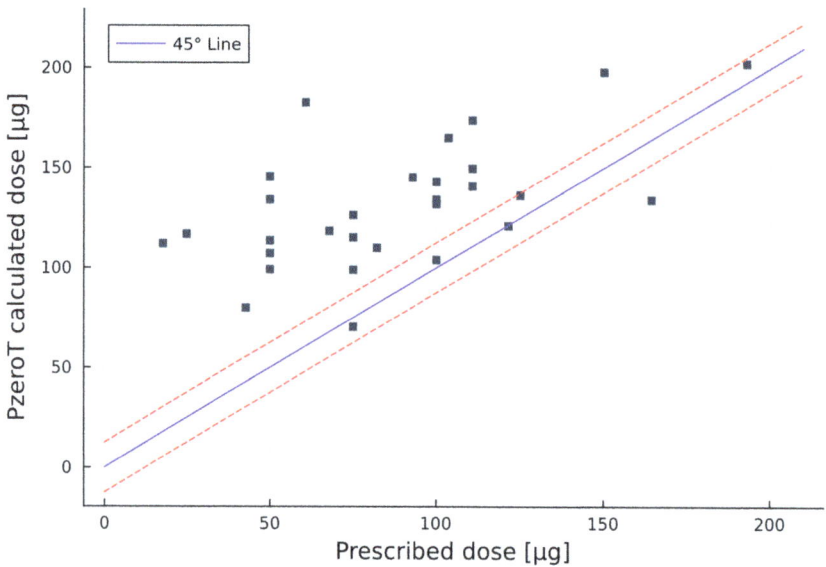

Figure 6.17: Cross-plot showing the correspondence between the prescribed dose and the dose calculated by *PzeroT* using the X µg/kg correlation. For the latter to be correct, it must lie within the range defined by the two dashed lines. If the point lies on the bisector, the correspondence is exact.

Table 6.9: Number and percentage of doses correctly calculated by *PzeroT* (with method TSH_{target} = 1.8 mIU/l, TSH_{target} = TSH_{age} and TSH_{target} = TSH_{paz}) and by the dose-weight correlation (X = 1.6 µg/kg hypothyroid patients; X = 2.2 µg/kg TSH-suppressed subjects). Total sample size 19 patients.

	Calculated doses with TSH_{target} defined in Table 6.6			Calculated doses with the dose-weight correlation
	1.8 mIU/l	TSH_{sp}(age)	TSH_{pat}	X µg/kg
Number of doses calculated correctly	6	4	10	5
Percentage of doses calculated correctly	31.58 %	21.05 %	52.63 %	26.32 %

sample of patients (Table 6.9), it can be established with certainty that *PzeroT*, having available the TSH target value to be reached equal to the patient's actual value after titration, offers better performance compared to other methods. The excellent result obtained through TSH_{pat} derives from the choice to use the real TSH value at which the patient settles following the therapy and the final dose prescribed by the endocrinologist.

We want to comment on the relative performance of the target calculation method as a function of age in both fractions of the overall sample defined previously and described in Table 6.8 and Table 6.9.

– Often, the TSH targets resulting from the equations proposed in Section 6.5 do not coincide with the values defined as euthyroid by endocrinologists, determining an error in dosage calculation. This is because the doctor does not use a precise calculation method. Still, there is a range, even quite broad, that is considered normal and for which the restoration of euthyroid conditions is determined.

– Among the overall patient sample, there is a thyroidectomized quota for which the reasoning on the variation of TSH with age is limited by the fact that these patients often undertake TSH-suppressive treatments.

Finally, we want to investigate the results achieved through the correlation based solely on the patient's body mass. In particular, it is necessary to specify how this is used by endocrinologists only as a starting point for therapy and not as an effective final dose. This is because clinical practice is based on obtaining the correct dose only after a certain time interval, which allows for establishing the patient's response in the weeks following the first or new drug intake. Moreover, it should be specified that the correlation returns values that the endocrinologist must necessarily interpret, and it is up to the doctor to decree the correct dose and modulate it according to their sensitivity based on the clinical case in front of them. Therefore, the percentage so low derives from the fact that the calculated values are compared with the final values assumed by the patient after the dose adjustment process. The calculation of the dose through correlation with body mass is not wrong. Indeed, it is used daily for the treatment of hypothyroid patients, but the issue that we want to raise concerns the patient's treatment times that could be considerably decreased if a tool like *PzeroT* were used.

6.7 Conclusions

One of the innovations offered by this work is the residual thyroid function. This characteristic parameter of the *p-Thyrosim* model [49] allows assigning a value to an elusive characteristic, such as the health status of the HPT axis, in cases of primary hypothyroidism where the pathology exclusively affects the thyroid gland. The novelty of this approach lies in the use of plasma concentrations of thyrotropin (TSH), available to the endocrinologist for determining the replacement dose of LT_4, as well as for defining the hypothyroid state of the patient based precisely on the RTF variable. From this result arises the possibility of using the algorithm in clinical practice, particularly the possibility of approaching the problem of dose calculation in an alternative, deterministic, and nonsubjective manner. The *p-Thyrosim* model is a digital twin of the patient's HPT axis and considers the subject's characteristics. The *in-silico* simulation of the subject's HPT axis allows determining, through the *PzeroT* calculation code, the optimal dose of synthetic thyroid hormone necessary to bring the subject's TSH levels back to those suitable according to medical practice. An immediate implication for patient care is a possible reduction in treatment times, while for the endocrinologist, the algorithm represents a valid support tool for calculating an individualized dose, which, through the indication of the target TSH, is also based on the actual objective of the therapy. The specialist physician's intervention remains fundamental in assigning the target value to the specific patient, but at the same time, *PzeroT* paves the way for individualized treatment of hypothyroidism.

From the data analyzed previously, the model has proven to be a reliable tool for calculating the first dose, with a percentage of predicted doses frequently above 50 %, consistently surpassing the performance of the dose-weight correlation used in clinical practice. The *p-Thyrosim* model has proven to be an excellent support for the simulation of the HPT axis and has allowed the inclusion of individual parameters such as sex, height, body mass, and age in the dose optimization.

Further developments of this work include investigating the interaction of levothyroxine with the main interfering foods (*e.g.*, coffee and foods with high fiber content) to obtain a modulating parameter of LT_4 absorption in those cases. It is also interesting to study the dependence of the LT_4 absorption rate on the main pathological conditions of the patient that tend to decrease drug absorption, such as gastritis, celiac disease, or lactose intolerance. A further sensitive parameter in the proposed model is the amount of T_3 and T_4 bound to blood transport proteins in case drugs are taken that increase or decrease that value.

A further point of in-depth study of the model relates to cases of obesity and the corresponding amount of levothyroxine to be prescribed since, in such cases, the simulation through *p-Thyrosim* is not optimal as it returns excessive LT_4 values capable of inducing overdosage. Also, the case of pregnancy in hypothyroid patients is worthy of further investigation due to the specific TSH values for the three trimesters of gestation, in the first 0.2–2.5 mIU/l and in the remaining two 0.3–3 mIU/l [62]. Finally, *p-Thyrosim* is parametrically calibrated on adult patients; therefore, extending it to pediatric patients is also interesting.

Acknowledgments: The author acknowledges the valuable contribution of Federico Appiani and Giovanni Colombo, master's degree students in Chemical Engineering at Politecnico di Milano, who worked with outstanding commitment and dedication to the discovery of thyroid pathologies and the modeling of the HPT axis, with particular attention to the condition of hypothyroidism and the identification of the optimal dose of levothyroxine.

References

1. Hall JE, Guyton AC. Guyton and Hall Textbook of medical physiology. Saunders/Elsevier; 2011. Available from: https://books.google.it/books?id=X491kgEACAAJ.
2. Singer C. A short history of anatomy from the Greeks to Harvey. Dover Publications; 1957. Available from: https://books.google.it/books?id=w7MtTIVPML0C.
3. Abbiati RA, Savoca A, Manca D. Chapter 2 – an engineering oriented approach to physiologically based pharmacokinetic and pharmacodynamic modeling. In: Manca D, editor. Computer Aided Chemical Engineering. Amsterdam, Netherlands: Elsevier; 2018, vol 42:37–63 pp.
4. Di Muria M, Lamberti G, Titomanlio G. Physiologically based pharmacokinetics: a simple, all purpose model. Ind Eng Chem Res 2010;49:2969–78.
5. Standring S, Borley NR. Gray's anatomy: the anatomical basis of clinical practice. Churchill Livingstone/Elsevier; 2008. Available from: https://books.google.it/books?id=kvhkPQAACAAJ.
6. Rivolta CM, Targovnik HM. Molecular advances in thyroglobulin disorders. Clinica Chimica Acta; J Int Fed Clin Chem 2006;374:8–24.
7. Silverthorn J, Bruce R, Ober WC, Ober CE, Impagliazzo A. Human physiology: an integrated approach, 8th ed. Indianapolis, IN: Pearson Education, Inc.; 2019.
8. Benvenga S, Robbins J. Altered thyroid hormone binding to plasma lipoproteins in hypothyroidism. Thyroid 1996;6:595–600.
9. Schussler GC. The thyroxine-binding proteins. Thyroid 2000;10:141–9.
10. Nillni EA. Regulation of the hypothalamic thyrotropin releasing hormone (TRH) neuron by neuronal and peripheral inputs. Front Neuroendocrinol 2010;31:134–56.
11. Reichlin S, Utiger RD. Regulation of the pituitary-thyroid axis in man: relationship of TSH concentration to concentration of free and total thyroxine in plasma. J Clin Endocrinol Metab 1967;27:251–5.
12. Treier M, Rosenfeld MG. The hypothalamic-pituitary axis; co-development of two organs. Curr Opin Cell Biol 1996;8:833–43.
13. Werner SC, Ingbar SH, Braverman LE, Utiger RD. Werner & Ingbar's the thyroid a fundamental and clinical text, 9th ed. Philadelphia: Lippincott Williams & Wilkins; 2005. Available from: http://lib.ugent.be/catalog/ebk01:1000000000753717.
14. Greenspan SL, Klibansk A, Schqenfeld D, Ridgway EC. Pulsatile secretion of thyrotropin in man. J Clin Endocrinol Metab 1986;63:661–8.
15. Garmendia Madariaga A, Santos Palacios S, Guillén-Grima F, Galofré JC, Ledesma F. Incidence and prevalence of thyroid dysfunction in Europe: a meta-analysis. J Clin Endocrinol Metab 2014;99:923–31.
16. Vanderpump MPJ. The epidemiology of thyroid disease. Br Med Bull 2011;99:39–51.

17. Taylor PN, Albrecht D, Scholz A, Gutierrez-Buey G, Lazarus JH, Dayan CM, et al. Global epidemiology of hyperthyroidism and hypothyroidism. Nat Rev Endocrinol 2018;14:301–16.
18. Cooper DS, Sipos J. Medical management of thyroid disease. Boca Raton: CRC Press; 2018.
19. Flynn RWV, MacDonald TM, Morris AD, Jung RT, Leese GP. The thyroid epidemiology, audit, and research study: thyroid dysfunction in the general population. J Clin Endocrinol Metab 2004;89:3879–84.
20. Vanderpump MPJ, Tunbridge WMG, French J, Appleton D, Bates D, Clark F, et al. The incidence of thyroid disorders in the community: a twenty-year follow-up of the Whickham Survey. Clin Endocrinol 1995;43: 55–68.
21. Samuels MH, Ridgway EC. Central hypothyroidism. Endocrinol Metab Clin N Am 1992;21:903–19.
22. Staub JJ, Althaus BU, Engler H, Ryff AS, Trabucco P, Marquardt K, et al. Spectrum of subclinical and overt hypothyroidism: effect on thyrotropin, prolactin, and thyroid reserve, and metabolic impact on peripheral target tissues. Am J Med 1992;92:631–42.
23. Roberts CG, Ladenson PW. Hypothyroidism. Lancet 2004;363. https://doi.org/10.1016/s0140-6736(04) 15696-1.
24. Baloch Z, Carayon P, Conte-Devolx B, Demers LM, Feldt-Rasmussen U, Henry J-F, et al. Laboratory medicine practice guidelines. Laboratory support for the diagnosis and monitoring of thyroid disease. Thyroid: Off J Am Thyroid Assoc 2003;13:3–126.
25. Means JH. Relative frequency of the several symptoms and signs of myxedema. The Thyroid and its Disease, 2nd ed. Philadelphia, PA: JB Lippencott; 1948:232–4 pp.
26. Zulewski H, Müller B, Exer P, Miserez AR, Staub J-J. Estimation of tissue hypothyroidism by a new clinical score: evaluation of patients with various grades of hypothyroidism and controls. J Clin Endocrinol Metab 1997;82:771–6.
27. Hollowell JG, Staehling NW, Flanders WD, Hannon WH, Gunter EW, Spencer CA, et al. Serum TSH, T4, and thyroid antibodies in the United States population (1988 to 1994): national health and nutrition examination Survey (NHANES III). J Clin Endocrinol Metab 2002;87:489–99.
28. Ho PY, Lisowski FP. Brief history of Chinese medicine and its influence, A. Singapore: World Scientific Publishing Company; 1997.
29. Murray GR. Note on the treatment of myxoedema by hypodermic injections of an extract of the thyroid gland of a sheep. Br Med J 1891;2:796.
30. Kendall EC. The isolation in crystalline form of the compound containing iodine which occurs in the thyroid: its chemical nature and physiological activity. Trans Assoc Am Phys 1915;30:420–49.
31. Chalmers JR, Dickson GT, Elks J, Hems BA. 715. The synthesis of thyroxine and related substances. Part V. A synthesis of L-thyroxine from L-tyrosine. J Chem Soc (Resumed) 1949:3424–33. https://doi.org/10.1039/jr9490003424.
32. Colucci P, Yue CS, Ducharme M, Benvenga S. A review of the pharmacokinetics of levothyroxine for the treatment of hypothyroidism. Eur Endocrinol 2013;9:40.
33. Izumi M, Larsen PR. Triiodothyronine, thyroxine, and iodine in purified thyroglobulin from patients with Graves' disease. J Clin Investig 1977;59:1105–12.
34. Carr D, McLeod DT, Parry G, Thornes HM. Fine adjustment of thyroxine replacement dosage: comparison of the thyrotrophin releasing hormone test using a sensitive thyrotrophin assay with measurement of free thyroid hormones and clinical assessment. Clin Endocrinol 1988;28:325–33.
35. Gottwald-Hostalek U, Razvi S. Getting the levothyroxine (LT4) dose right for adults with hypothyroidism: opportunities and challenges in the use of modern LT4 preparations. Curr Med Res Opin 2022;38:1865–70.
36. Roos A, Linn-Rasker SP, van Domburg RT, Tijssen JP, Berghout A. The starting dose of levothyroxine in primary hypothyroidism treatment: a prospective, randomized, double-blind trial. Arch Intern Med 2005; 165:1714–20.
37. Lebbink CA, Links TP, Czarniecka A, Dias RP, Elisei R, Izatt L, et al. 2022 European Thyroid Association Guidelines for the management of pediatric thyroid nodules and differentiated thyroid carcinoma. Eur Thyroid J 2022;11. https://doi.org/10.1530/etj-22-0146.

38. Burmeister LA, Goumaz MO, Mariash CN, Oppenheimer JH. Levothyroxine dose requirements for thyrotropin suppression in the treatment of differentiated thyroid cancer. J Clin Endocrinol Metab 1992;75: 344–50.
39. Santini F, Pinchera A, Marsili A, Ceccarini G, Castagna MG, Valeriano R, et al. Lean body mass is a major determinant of levothyroxine dosage in the treatment of thyroid diseases. J Clin Endocrinol Metab 2005;90: 124–7.
40. Devdhar M, Drooger R, Pehlivanova M, Singh G, Jonklaas J. Levothyroxine replacement doses are affected by gender and weight, but not age. Thyroid 2011;21:821–7.
41. Raverot V, Bonjour M, Abeillon du Payrat J, Perrin P, Roucher-Boulez F, Lasolle H, et al. Age-and sex-specific TSH upper-limit reference intervals in the general French population: there is a need to adjust our actual practices. J Clin Med 2020;9:792.
42. Rosenbaum RL, Barzel US. Levothyroxine replacement dose for primary hypothyroidism decreases with age. Ann Intern Med 1982;96:53–5.
43. Walsh JP. Thyroid function across the lifespan: do age-related changes matter? Endocrinol Metabol 2022; 37:208.
44. Eligar V, Taylor PN, Okosieme OE, Leese GP, Dayan CM. Thyroxine replacement: a clinical endocrinologist's viewpoint. Ann Clin Biochem 2016;53:421–33.
45. Hays MT. Localization of human thyroxine absorption. Thyroid 1991;1:241–8.
46. Wenzel KW, Kirschsieper HE. Aspects of the absorption of oral L-thyroxine in normal man. Metabolism 1977; 26:1–8.
47. Verhaert N, Poorten VV, Delaere P, Bex M, Debruyne F. Levothyroxine replacement therapy after thyroid surgery. B ENT 2006;3:129.
48. Mandel SJ, Brent GA, Larsen PR. Levothyroxine therapy in patients with thyroid disease. Ann Intern Med 1993;119:492–502.
49. Cruz-Loya M, Chu B, Jonklaas J, Schneider D, DiStefano JJ. Optimized replacement T4 and T4+T3 dosing in male and female hypothyroid patients with different BMIs using a personalized mechanistic model of thyroid hormone regulation dynamics. Front Endocrinol 2022;13. https://doi.org/10.3389/fendo.2022. 888429.
50. Hoermann R, Midgley JEM, Larisch R, Dietrich JWC. Advances in applied homeostatic modelling of the relationship between thyrotropin and free thyroxine. PLoS One 2017;12:e0187232.
51. DiStefano JJ, Mak PH. On model and data requirements for determining the bioavailability of oral therapeutic agents: application to gut absorption of thyroid hormones. Am J Physiol Regul Integr Comp Physiol 1979;236:R137–41.
52. DiStefano JJ. A model of the normal thyroid hormone glandular secretion mechanism. J Theor Biol 1969;22: 412–17.
53. DiStefano JJ, Jonklaas J. Predicting optimal combination LT4+ LT3 therapy for hypothyroidism based on residual thyroid function. Front Endocrinol 2019;10:746.
54. DiStefano JJ, Stear EB. Neuroendocrine control of thyroid secretion in living systems: a feedback control system model. Bull Math Biophys 1968;30:3–26.
55. Eisenberg M, Samuels M, DiStefano III JJ. L-T4 bioequivalence and hormone replacement studies via feedback control simulations. Thyroid 2006;16:1279–92.
56. Goutelle S, Maurin M, Rougier F, Barbaut X, Bourguignon L, Ducher M, et al. The Hill equation: a review of its capabilities in pharmacological modelling. Fund Clin Pharmacol 2008;22:633–48.
57. Caron P, Grunenwald S, Persani L, Borson-Chazot F, Leroy R, Duntas L. Factors influencing the levothyroxine dose in the hormone replacement therapy of primary hypothyroidism in adults. Rev Endocr Metab Disord 2021:1–21. https://doi.org/10.1007/s11154-021-09691-9.
58. Eisenberg M, Santini F, Marsili A, Pinchera A, DiStefano III JJ. TSH regulation dynamics in central and extreme primary hypothyroidism. Thyroid 2010;20:1215–28.

59. Eisenberg M, Samuels M, DiStefano III JJ. Extensions, validation, and clinical applications of a feedback control system simulator of the hypothalamo-pituitary-thyroid axis. Thyroid 2008;18:1071–85.
60. Manca D, Appiani F, Colombo G. Optimal dosing of thyroid hormones in hypothyroid patients with an individualized compartmental model. Comput Aided Chem Eng 2023;52:2643–8.
61. Van Deventer HE, Mendu DR, Remaley AT, Soldin SJ. Inverse log-linear relationship between thyroid-stimulating hormone and free thyroxine measured by direct analog immunoassay and tandem mass spectrometry. Clin Chem 2011;57:122–7.
62. McNeil AR, Stanford PE. Reporting thyroid function tests in pregnancy. Clin Biochem Rev 2015;36:109.

Carlota Guati, Lucía Gomez-Coma, Marcos Fallanza and
Inmaculada Ortiz*

7 Glucose sensors in medicine: overview

Abstract: In recent years society has seen significant progress in the development of the glucose sensing field since diabetes mellitus represents the seventh cause of death at global scale. An accurate detection method of glucose concentration can be an effective way to prevent and treat diabetes and other pathologies where glucose is an important biomarker, such as glucagonoma or acromegaly. In this way, glucose sensors play a considerable role in any healthcare system. This chapter provides a comprehensive review of numerous glucose sensors from a chemical engineering perspective. The examined sensors are based on the electrochemical detection principle due to their advantages over other detection methods. The chapter also provides important information related to design aspects and new lines of research on affordable and reliable glucose sensors.

Keywords: glucose sensors; electrochemical; chemical engineering

7.1 Glucose sensors in medicine: overview

The development of glucose sensors has heralded a revolution in medical diagnosis, particularly in the field of diabetes management. Although human health has improved, the World Health Organization (WHO) reported that, if current trends continued, chronic illnesses like cancer, diabetes, and respiratory disorders would account for 86 % of the 90 million deaths annually by approximately 2050; this represents a startling 90 % increase in absolute numbers since 2019.

This chapter provides a comprehensive review of the use of glucose sensors in medicine, emphasising their critical function in the diagnosis, management and care of type I and type II diabetes. Other pathologies are also discussed since glucose is a carbohydrate involved in most metabolic reactions of the human system.

7.1.1 Beyond diabetes: other diseases and applications

Although the management of blood sugar is still primarily focused on diabetes, maintaining optimum glycemic control is important for reasons beyond diabetes. This section

*Corresponding author: Inmaculada Ortiz, Chemical and Biomolecular Engineering Department, University of Cantabria, 39005 Santander, Spain, E-mail: ortizi@unican.es
Carlota Guati, Lucía Gomez-Coma and Marcos Fallanza, Chemical and Biomolecular Engineering Department, University of Cantabria, 39005 Santander, Spain, E-mail: carlota.guati@unican.es (C. Guati)

As per De Gruyter's policy this article has previously been published in the journal Physical Sciences Reviews. Please cite as: C. Guati, L. Gomez-Coma, M. Fallanza and I. Ortiz "Glucose sensors in medicine: overview" *Physical Sciences Reviews* [Online] 2024. DOI: 10.1515/psr-2024-0063 | https://doi.org/10.1515/9783111394558-007

examines the complex role that blood sugar regulation plays in a range of medical disorders. Several illnesses and ailments where blood sugar regulation is crucial, including hormonal disorders to rare cancers, will be considered. Understanding the effects of glycemic control in these situations is crucial to advancing the field of precision medicine, improving therapeutic approaches, and providing better patient care.

7.1.1.1 Glucagonoma

Glucagonoma is a rare tumour of the alpha cells[1] of the islets of both the body and tail of the pancreas. These cells overproduce glucagon, hormone that has the opposite effect of insulin. Patients suffering from Glucagonoma usually present hiperglycemia, glycosuria and changes in nutrient metabolism. Treatment of glucagonoma usually involves surgical removal of the tumour along with controlling symptoms and normalizing blood glucose levels.

7.1.1.2 Acromegaly

Acromegaly is an uncommon hormonal condition that is mostly brought on by a pituitary adenoma and growth hormone (GH) overproduction. This overabundance of growth hormone causes different tissues to produce more insulin-like growth factor 1 (IGF-1), which disrupts several metabolic processes, including the metabolism of glucose. Acromegaly patients commonly show insulin resistance and hyperglycemia.

Managing glucose levels in individuals with acromegaly involves addressing the underlying hormonal imbalance and implementing strategies to improve insulin sensitivity and glycemic control. Treatment options may include surgical removal, medical therapy, monitoring and testing of glucose levels.

7.1.1.3 Pheochromocytoma

A rare kind of neuroendocrine tumour called a pheochromocytoma develops from chromaffin cells found in the sympathetic ganglia or adrenal medulla. Excessive production of catecholamines by these tumours, such as norepinephrine (noradrenaline) and epinephrine (adrenaline), can cause a variety of symptoms, such as headaches, palpitations, sweating, and hypertension. Although pheochromocytoma in and of itself does not directly impact glucose metabolism, the overabundance of released catecholamines can indirectly affect glucose levels through several mechanisms: stress response, insulin resistance and release of the counter regularoty hormone.

---

1 **Alpha cells:** Endocrine cells that are found in the Islets of Langerhans in the pancreas. Alpha cells secrete the peptide hormone glucagon in order to increase glucose levels in the blood stream.

7.1.1.4 Cushing's syndrome

A rare endocrine condition known as Cushing's syndrome is caused by extended exposure to high amounts of cortisol. This may occur as a result of either prolonged administration of glucocorticoid medicines (iatrogenic Cushing's syndrome) or excessive adrenal gland production (adrenal Cushing's syndrome). A hormone called cortisol is essential for controlling glucose metabolism, and too much of it can cause a number of problems with glucose homeostasis. Cortisol is also known as the stress hormone.

All diseases in which more than 7.5 mg of corticoids per day are prescribed must include monitoring of glucose levels. Glucose measurement sensors represent a preventive tool and an early recognition system for many pathologies, their extensive implementation in health systems could reduce associated costs.

7.1.2 Diabetes mellitus: a pressing healthcare challenge

Currently, diabetes causes more than 400 million people to suffer from the disease and nearly one million deaths. Furthermore, these numbers are expected to continue to increase as a result of factors such as aging population, sedentary lifestyle, and bad eating patterns. The same trend is expected in different regions, especially in those areas called low middle-income countries, where health systems cannot afford an exhaustive control of this pathology (Figure 7.1).

Type 1 diabetes mellitus is an autoimmune condition characterized by the destruction of pancreatic beta cells,[2] resulting in an absolute deficiency of insulin production.

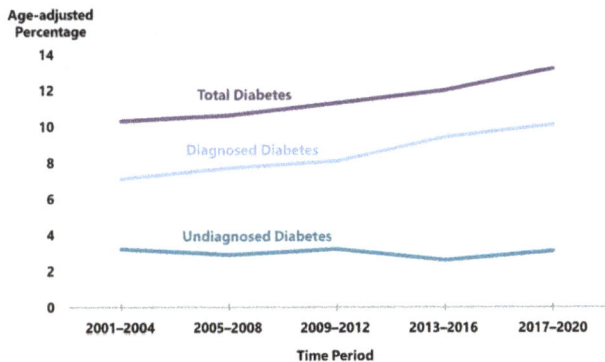

Figure 7.1: Trends in age-adjusted prevalence of diagnosed diabetes, undiagnosed diabetes, and total diabetes among adults aged 18 years or older, United States, 2001–2020 (Our World in Data, Diabetes).

---

2 **Beta cells:** Endocrine cells located within the pancreatic islets of Langerhans responsible for the production and release of insulin and amylin.

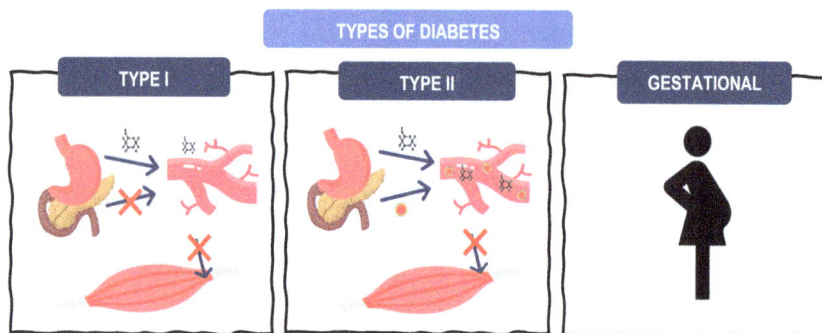

Figure 7.2: Representation of types of diabetes. Adapted from https://www.primemedic.com.au/health-library/diabetes-mellitus-type-2-32.

This chronic disease is the result of the combination of environmental and genetic factors.

Insulin is essential for the uptake and utilization of glucose by cells throughout the body, therefore, patients rely on exogenous insulin therapy to regulate blood glucose levels and prevent complications associated with hyperglycemia for the rest of their lines.

Type 2 diabetes is characterized by insulin resistance, where cells become less responsive to insulin. In most parts of the world, the prevalence of type 2 diabetes has significantly increased during the past decades. Between 1980 and 2019 (108 million people to 422 million), the prevalence of diabetes in adults nearly quadrupled globally, even after accounting for the effects of ageing population. The increase was more noticeable in men than in women, and in low- and middle-income nations (Figure 7.2).

A kind of diabetes known as gestational diabetes mellitus usually appears in the second or third trimester of pregnancy and disappears after delivery. It is characterized by elevated levels of blood glucose that are higher than normal but not high enough to meet the criteria for diabetes outside pregnancy (also called prediabetes). Insulin resistance and decreased tolerance to glucose result from gestational diabetes mellitus, which is caused by the body's inability to create enough insulin to fulfil the demands of pregnancy.

Diabetes can be effectively prevented and treated with the use of an accurate testing technology of glucose concentration. Hence, glucose sensors are crucial for controlling blood glucose levels in any type of diabetes individuals.

7.2 Glucose recognition methods

Numerous techniques for detecting glucose have been developed, including optical rotation, calorimetry, electrochemistry, conductimetry, and fluorescence spectroscopy. However, these methods often face various challenges such as laborious detection processes, interaction with coexisting cationic or anionic molecules such as ibuprofen, protracted test times, and expensive equipment [1].

Regarding lab-on-a-chip and paper-based systems, literature equally highlights both electrochemical and optical technologies. Similarly, both alternatives are extensively used in biosensors that are nowadays commercially available. Wearable biosensors, on the other hand, exhibit high preference for electrochemical sensing. The use of electrochemical techniques appears to be more straightforward, and it is especially beneficial when combined with wireless data transfer technologies [2].

Hence, most glucose sensors rely on electrochemical methods due to their portability, selectivity, and simplicity. Furthermore, they display preeminent stability, fast response time, lower cost, and low limit of detection of glucose (LOD). Typically, an electrochemical sensor works at a fixed potential applied at the working electrode where glucose is oxidized. The variation of the oxidation current is directly proportional to the concentration of glucose, identifying the detection level. Due to the recognized relevance of electrochemical methods, this section focuses on the main features of electrochemical glucose sensors.

7.2.1 Electrochemical discrete and continuous measurements

Because of their affordability, mobility, and simple testing process, blood glucose biosensor test strips have been extensively utilized for point-of-care glucose monitoring in at-home settings since the 1990s. Unfortunately, the invasive blood fingerpicks cause pain and discomfort and limit the extended use with frequent readings. As a result, these strips are unable to accurately reflect the dynamic variations in blood glucose.

Since glucose sensing has a significant scientific and clinical relevance, a significant progress has been recently made, particularly related to the development of non-invasive methods to monitor blood glucose (Figure 7.3). Non-invasive methods can be classified in

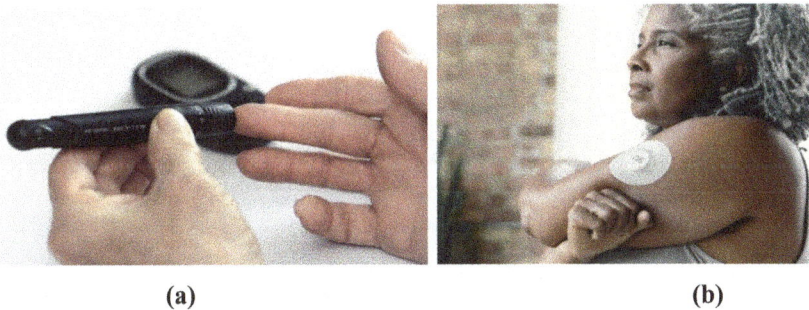

(a)   (b)

Figure 7.3: Discrete and continuous glucose measurement. (a) Finger pricking. (b) Continuous glucose monitoring device.

two major groups: minimally-invasive (MI) and fully non-invasive (NI). MI technologies are those that need to extract some form of fluid from the body (ex. tears or interstitial fluid) to measure glucose concentration. Alternatively, NI technologies rely solely on some form of detection without the need for painful access to any bodily fluid.

However, the most widely used technique for continuous glucose monitoring (CGM) employs minimally invasive methods (MI). These devices use needle-based or subcutaneous implantable sensors to measure glucose directly from the interstitial fluid and they must be replaced every two weeks. Unlike conventional glucose meters, which provide a snapshot of the blood glucose value at the time of testing, CGM sensors provide semi continuous information about glucose levels (Figure 7.4).

Importantly, CGMs allow users to make decisions regarding their day-to-day diabetes management using real-time glucose trends. Along with this information, CGM systems provide customizable hypo- and hyperglycemia alarms and display trends of the rate of change of glucose levels [3]. They have been also integrated with insulin pumps and are being used in artificial pancreas clinical trials.

Non-invasive methods, which avoid both injury to blood vessels and damage to the surface of the skin, are presumably preferred for diagnosis: such methods are painless and avoid potential infection. However, even for blood glucose the problem for its non-invasive evaluation cannot be considered as solved [4]. Although such sensors show high accuracy, they are affected by pH changes, and cannot provide rigorous continuous measurement, which gives them less advantage over subcutaneous CGM monitors based on MI systems. Some authors have studied clinical devices for glucose sensing and out of the 47 products found for non-invasive glucose monitoring, there are currently no FDA approved products on the market [5]. So far only four products have received the Conformité Européene (CE) mark of approval that meet European safety, health, and environmental standard requirements and are currently being sold in Europe.

Some attempts to introduce NI systems in clinical applications rely on iontophoresis technique. The effort to deliver interstitial fluid to the skin surface by reverse iontophoresis was unsuccessful in commercialized devices. Transdermal sensors involve

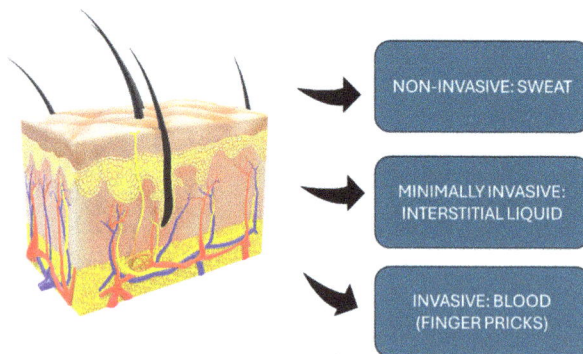

NON-INVASIVE: SWEAT

MINIMALLY INVASIVE: INTERSTITIAL LIQUID

INVASIVE: BLOOD (FINGER PRICKS)

Figure 7.4: Glucometers invasiveness.

passing a current through the skin and thereby assessing the electrical properties of the interstitial fluid. Although these sensors show very good correlations with glucose levels and have the significant benefit of being wearable, the use of electric current might irritate the skin [6]. Other attempt for non-invasive sensors is the collection of sweat: measuring its conductivity it is possible to diagnose cystic fibrosis (mucoviscidosis) [7]. It is important to note that for sweat sampling the clinically relevant procedure (sweat gland activation through pilocarpine electrophoresis) is generally accepted. The metabolite content of glucose in such samples is known to be independent of the sweating rate [8].

7.2.2 Catalytic materials: enzymes and metallic structures

As previously discussed, electrochemical sensors are the most significant type of glucose biosensors, and include both enzymatic and non-enzymatic materials. Most common enzymes to detect glucose are glucose oxidase (GOx) and glucose dehydrogenase, they offer great selectivity and sensitivity to glucose in a biological complex fluid. However, the procedures for enzyme immobilization are complex since they work under critical operational conditions and enzymatic systems usually present instability issues that shorten the sensors lifespan. Because of these reasons minimally and non-invasive enzymatic sensors become expensive. In this scenario, non-enzymatic nanostructures have gained much attention due to their outstanding properties to mimic enzyme systems.

For non-enzymatic glucose sensors, carbonaceous materials, such as graphene and its derivatives and carbon nanotubes, constitute most of the materials used in wearable electrochemical biosensors. They are usually combined with flexible noble metallic materials, such as platinum or gold, as well as metal oxides, that are widely used to improve the electrical conductivity and catalytic performance of these biosensors. Features like comfortability and high biocompatibility should be considered during their application. These sensors are still under research and have not reached the market.

7.2.2.1 Classification according to the electron transfer mechanism

Considering all possible catalytic materials, there are four primary generations of glucose biosensors, which are classified according to the electron transfer mechanism. Three generations represent the enzymatic glucose biosensor, and one generation represents the non-enzymatic glucose biosensor (Figure 7.5).

First-generation enzymatic glucose biosensors measure glucose concentration from H_2O_2 generation according to following reaction:

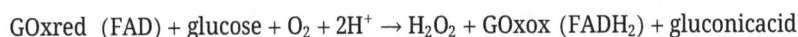

$$\text{GOxred (FAD)} + \text{glucose} + O_2 + 2H^+ \rightarrow H_2O_2 + \text{GOxox (FADH}_2) + \text{gluconicacid}$$

The immobilized enzyme uses oxygen as an electron acceptor to catalyze the oxidation of glucose ($C_6H_{10}O_6$) into gluconolactone ($C_6H_{12}O_6$), yielding H_2O_2 and water as byproducts.

First Generation

Second Generation

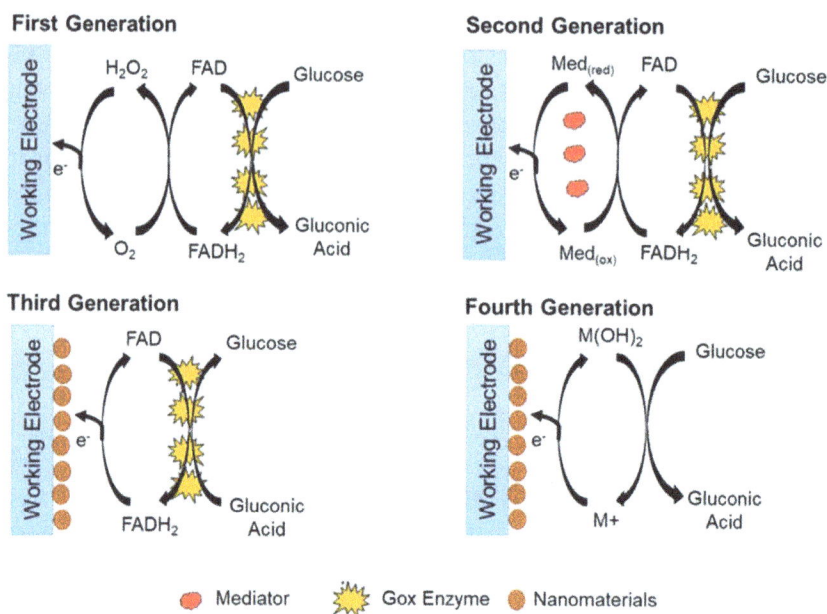

Third Generation

Fourth Generation

- 🔴 Mediator
- ✴ Gox Enzyme
- 🟠 Nanomaterials

Figure 7.5: Glucose sensors generations.

The catalyst, FAD, which is an active redox center of GOx, plays a role as the initial electron acceptor and is reduced to $FADH_2$ in the presence of glucose. The re-oxidation of $FADH_2$ with free oxygen generates the oxidized form of the enzyme FAD.

The second-generation enzymatic glucose biosensor is based on artificial redox mediators that replace the oxygen-dependency. Mediators are small, low-molecular-weight, soluble redox components that act as artificial electron transfer agents. The mediators facilitate electron transport from the FAD active redox center to the working electrode. Because of use, biosensors operate at moderate redox potentials, avoiding the oxidation of other interfering species. Some types of electron mediators that are suitable for GOx include ferrocene derivatives, ferricyanide, quinone compounds, conducting polymer salt transition metal complexes, and phenothiazine.

Third-generation enzymatic glucose sensors eliminate the need for artificial or natural mediators by introducing direct electron transfer between the enzyme and the working electrode. The FAD-active redox center of the enzyme is covalently or electro-chemically attached to the working electrode by certain nanomaterials.

Finally, the **fourth generation of glucose biosensors**, also known as non-enzymatic glucose biosensors, employs direct electron transfer through electro-oxidation of glucose to gluconic acid at the nanomaterial matrix with strong electrocatalytic activity. These sensors are discussed deeply in the next section (Table 7.1).

Table 7.1: Classification of glucose sensors.

Generation of glucose sensor	Benefits	Drawbacks
First	Simplicity	Limit to oxygen solubility
		Deactivation of enzymes
Second	No oxygen dependence	Likely reaction with interferences
	Mediator improves electron transfer	Mediator leaching
Third	Nanomaterials facilitate direct electron transfer	Need of high conductivity nanomaterials
	High selectivity and specificity	Enzyme leaching
Fourth	High stability	Low specificity
	Cost-effective	Interfering species

7.3 4th generation of glucose sensors: state of art

The relentless pursuit of non-invasive and continuous glucose monitoring (CGM) systems has led to the development of the 4th generation glucose sensors. These innovative devices hold immense promise for revolutionizing diabetes management by offering real-time glucose data without the need for finger pricking. This section delves into the state-of-art of 4th generation sensors, focusing on the advancements in catalytic materials and their impact on glucose oxidation sensitivity.

7.3.1 Beyond enzymes: a materials revolution

The transition from enzyme-based sensors to the 4th generation glucose sensors (FGGS) represents a significant leap forward. As it was previously mentioned, enzymes, while offering high selectivity, suffer from limitations like instability, high production costs, and potential immunogenic responses. FGGS leverage the unique properties of various nanomaterials as their core catalytic material, offering several advantages. These materials can be engineered to possess high surface area, exceptional electrocatalytic activity towards glucose oxidation, and improved long-term stability.

Table 7.2 summarizes the most common materials found in literature, including their strengths and limitations that could be useful to determine which catalyst material is more suitable and promising, so far, for glucose detection in minimally invasive sensors (Table 7.1). Those that best meet the ideal sensor features, will be discussed deeply at the end of this section.

Although carbon derivatives and conductive polymers do not directly catalyze glucose oxidation, they have been included in the table since they enhance the oxidation reaction by increasing conductivity. Besides, graphene and carbon nanotubes offer a large surface area to immobilize enzymes or other catalysts, promoting efficient contact

Table 7.2: Non enzymatic materials for glucose sensors.

Non enzymatic glucose sensor	Strengths	Limitations	Examples
Noble metals	Enhance electron transfer efficiency during glucose oxidation	Higher cost compared to other options Dependence of basic media	*Pt nanoparticles*
Transition metals	Price friendly High stability	Dependence of basic media	***Ni carbon doped***
Metal oxides	Price friendly Can be easily tailored	Dependence of basic media	*CuO nanoflowers*
Metallic combinations	Combine the advantages of different metals Potentially superior performance	More complex synthesis process	*Copper sulfide nanoparticles decorated with Pt nanoparticles*
Carbon derivatives	High surface area for catalyst immobilization Good electrical conductivity	Can be challenging to disperse uniformly the catalyst material Costly	*Graphene oxide-MnO$_2$ composite, Nitrogen-doped carbon nanotubes*
Conductive polymers	Enhance electron transfer between electrode and biomolecule Can be tailored for specific functionalities	May suffer from stability issues	*Polypyrrole-glucose oxidase composite, Poly(3,4-ethylenedioxythiophene) with gold nanoparticles*

with glucose molecules. However, achieving uniform dispersion of these materials can be challenging.

Conductive polymers like polypyrrole and poly(3,4-ethylenedioxythiophene) can be tailored to possess specific functionalities that enhance electron transfer between the electrode and the biomolecule, further improving sensor performance. However, their long-term stability in physiological environment remains a concern.

7.3.1.1 Copper takes center stage

Among various candidates, copper nanostructures have emerged as the frontrunners in FGGS development. Copper exhibits exceptional electrocatalytic activity for glucose oxidation, leading to enhanced sensitivity and faster response times. Additionally, copper nanostructures can be personalized to possess high surface area, further amplifying their interaction with glucose molecules, ultimately translating to more efficient signal generation.

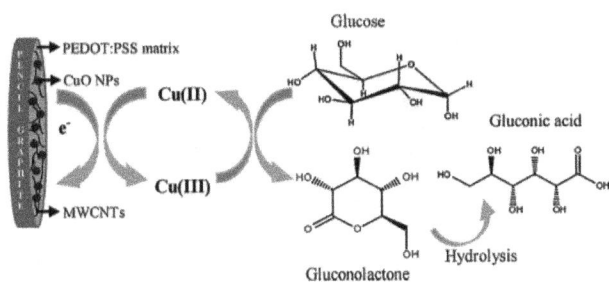

Figure 7.6: Oxidation mechanism in the electrode proposed by Amirzadeh et al. [10].

Copper nanoparticles (CuNPs): A 2020 study by Zhang et al. demonstrated the efficacy of CuNPs decorated on laser induced graphene (LIG) for glucose detection. Their sensor exhibited a high linear detection range of 0.39 μM–7 mM glucose with a high sensitivity of 495 μA mM^{-1} cm^{-2}. The synergistic effect of CuNPs and LIG provide deficient electron transfer pathways [9].

Copper oxide nanostructures (CuOx): Metal oxides offer enhanced stability compared to pure metals. In this sense, Amirzadeh et al. (2018) studied porous CuO on multi-wall carbon nanotubes using PEDOT: PSS (Poli(3,4-etilendioxitiofeno)-poli(estireno sulfonato)) as a matrix for glucose sensing. Their sensor displayed a linear detection range up to 10 mM with a sensitivity of 663.2 μA mM^{-1} cm^{-2}. Their findings describe how the porous structure maximized the surface area for glucose interaction, while the CuO facilitated electron transfer (Figure 7.6) [10].

Copper-based metal-organic frameworks (MOFs): This class of porous materials offers tunable structures with incorporated metal centers. A recent study carried out in 2022 by Anamika Ghosh et al. explored a copper-terephthalate MOF for glucose detection. Their sensor exhibited a linear detection range of 50 μM–2.0 mM with a sensitivity of 40 μA mM^{-1} cm^{-2}. The incorporation of copper within the MOF structure provided efficient catalytic sites for glucose oxidation making it possible working at physiological pH [11].

7.3.1.2 Exploring the metallic landscape

Nowadays, while copper holds a dominant position, researchers are actively exploring the potential of other metals and their alloys for FGGS.

Nickel (Ni): Nickel also emerges as a promising candidate. For example, nickel nanoparticles demonstrate good electrocatalytic activity towards glucose oxidation and offer an attractive alternative due to their lower cost compared to copper. However, nickel suffers from limitations like lower sensitivity. Here, we explore some examples from the scientific literature showcasing the potential of nickel-based materials:

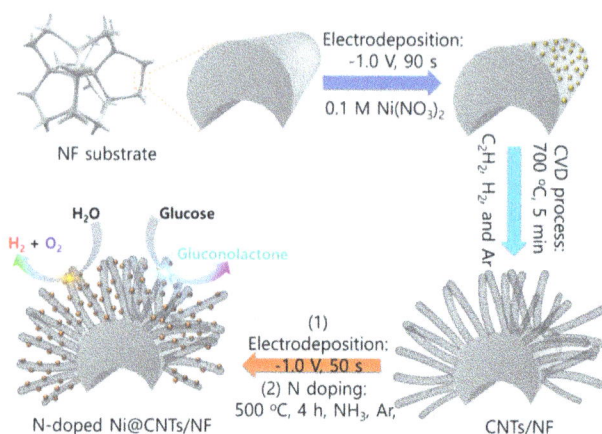

Figure 7.7: Preparation of N-doped Ni@CNTs for glucose sensing [13].

Nickel nanoparticles (NiNPs): Similar to copper, nickel nanoparticles offer a high surface area for efficient glucose interaction. A recent study investigated NiNPs decorated on reduced graphene oxide (rGO) for glucose oxidation. The sensor exhibited a linear detection range from 0.5 µM to 244 µM with a sensitivity of 185 mA mM^{-1} cm^{-2}. The combination of NiNPs and rGO provided a conductive platform with abundant catalytic sites for glucose oxidation [12].

Nickel-doped carbon nanomaterials: Doping carbon nanomaterials with nickel may incorporate catalytic centers for glucose oxidation. Recently, Jeong et al. (2023) synthetized nickel-doped carbon nanotubes (Ni-CNTs) for the effective glucose measurement. Their sensor exhibited a linear detection range from 1 µM to 3.7 mM with a sensitivity of 5.2 µA mM^{-1} cm^{-2}. The incorporation of nickel into the CNT structure provided active sites for glucose oxidation, while the CNTs facilitated efficient electron transfer [13] (Figure 7.7).

Nickel-based metal-organic frameworks (MOFs): Ren et al. (2024) studied a nickel-based metal–organic framework (Ni-MOF) on a three-dimensional (3D) conductive nickel foam (NF) for glucose detection. The fabricated Ni-MOF/NF electrode exhibits an excellent limit of detection (LOD) of 2.65 µM and an impressive sensitivity (14.31 mA cm^{-2} mM^{-1}) within the linear range 4–576 µM at neutral physiological pH. This linear range is too small compared to most biological biofluids.

Nickel-doped with oxides: Doping metal oxides with cobalt can introduce synergistic effects for glucose sensing. Babulal et al. (2021) explored nickel-cobalt oxide (NiCo$_2$O$_4$) nanosheets on graphene oxide template for glucose detection. Their sensor displayed a linear detection range from 150 nM to 8.86 mM with a sensitivity of 729 µA mM^{-1} cm^{-2}. The porous structure of the NiCo$_2$O$_4$ nanosheets maximized the surface area for glucose interaction, while the nickel and cobalt combination enhanced catalytic activity [14].

Cobalt (Co): Cobalt-based nanomaterials, particularly cobalt oxides (CoOx), exhibit good catalytic activity and can be synergistic with copper. Cobalt, with its unique electrocatalytic properties, emerges as a promising candidate alongside copper and nickel. Besides, several studies have shown that combining copper nanoparticles with Co_3O_4 enhances the overall performance by facilitating the reduction of hydrogen peroxide (H_2O_2) – a byproduct of glucose oxidation – thereby improving the signal-to-noise ratio [15].

Cobalt-doped metal oxides: Metal oxides offer stability advantages over pure metals. Chakraborty et al. (2021) synthesized porous CoO nanostructured electrodes on fluorine doped tin oxide (FTO) to detect glucose. Their sensor exhibited a linear detection range from 5 µM to 0.5 mM with a sensitivity of 887 µA mM^{-1} cm^{-2}. Salivary glucose sensing experiments were also carried out in that work and showed glucose sensitivity 854.30 µA mM^{-1} cm^{-2} [16].

Cobalt-based metal-organic frameworks (MOFs): MOFs offer tunable structures with incorporated metal centers. The work by Abrori et al. introduced a cobalt-based MOF (Co-BTC) for glucose detection. Their sensor displayed a linear detection range up to 5 mM with a sensitivity of 55 µA mM^{-1} cm^{-2}. The incorporation of cobalt within the MOF structure provided accessible catalytic sites for glucose oxidation, while the porous framework facilitated mass transport of glucose molecules [17].

Although noble metals are expensive, platinum (Pt) and palladium (Pd) are being explored for their ability to act as co-catalysts with copper. These noble metals can further enhance the electron transfer efficiency during the glucose oxidation process. Myung et al. designed a hybrid electrocatalyst consisting of copper sulfide nanoparticles decorated with Pt nanoparticles on carbon nanotubes (CNTs), achieving an impressive sensitivity of 280 µA mM^{-1} cm^{-2} at pH = 7.2 [18].

Figure 7.8 provides a visual representation of the performance of the previous discussed electrodes. Those that show response under neutral pH (physiological conditions) are shown in green. Besides, the sensitivity is included at the right of each column (units µA mM^{-1} cm^{-2}).

Nonenzymatic glucose sensor are a promising solution in the glucose detection field, however they still present some drawbacks to be solved. Most of the studies found in scientific database report sensors working at conditions distant from those of biological fluids, for example they measure glucose in electrolytes with high pH (0.1 M NaOH or 0.1 M KOH = pH 13).

The future of FGGS likely lies in exploring combinations of these materials to achieve superior performance under physiological conditions. By leveraging the strengths of each metal, researchers can create composite electrodes or bimetallic nanostructures with enhanced selectivity, sensitivity, and long-term stability. It has been reported that metal-metal (oxide) interaction helps in lowering the HOMO-LUMO energy gap [19]. In this sense, although the superior price, noble metals can be used together with transition metals to promote glucose oxidation.

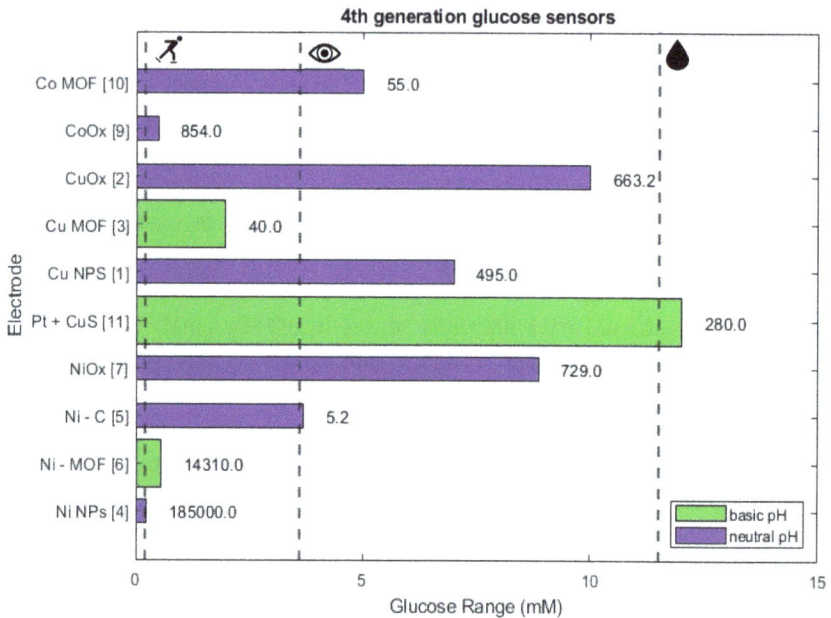

Figure 7.8: 4th generation glucose sensors (🏃 for sweat, 👁 for lacrimal biofluid and 🩸 for blood and interstitial liquid).

7.4 Challenges and considerations

7.4.1 Social considerations

The global prevalence and impact of diabetes are significant, making its control a priority area in Goal 3 of the United Nations' Sustainable Development Goals (SDGs): "Good Health and Well-Being." This objective emphasizes the value of early detection, efficient treatment, and management of chronic illnesses like diabetes mellitus. The objective is to decrease the death rate and enhance life quality of people who are affected by this condition. To achieve this goal, it is essential to implement strategies to improving healthcare access, increasing public awareness, and funding research for cutting-edge treatment alternatives.

Diabetes affected an estimated 463 million people in 2019, a number that is expected to grow to approximately 700 million by 2045. Of people with diabetes, about 90 % have type 2 diabetes and almost 80 % live in low- and middle-income countries (LMICs), where its prevalence is increasing most rapidly. This is the principal motivation to achieve reliable and cost-effective glucose sensors since health insurance is not fully covered in those areas.

7.4.2 Performance considerations

While the examples mentioned in previous section show the promising sensitivity of copper and other transition metals FGGS, several challenges remain.

– **Selectivity:** Glucose is not the only biomolecule present in physiological fluids. Interference from other substances like ascorbic acid, ibuprofen and uric acid may lead to inaccurate readings since they may also be oxidized at the applied potential. Researchers focus on the design of sensor architectures that discriminate glucose against these interferences. The selected interferences will depend on the target biofluid where glucose is measured. The different biofluids will be discussed in **linear range** discussion. Here, there are some examples with their level in blood plasma:

Ibuprofen: 20 µg/mL (in case the user has taken 400 mg of paracetamol in the past hour).

Ascorbic Acid: 0.1 mM

Uric Acid: 0.41 mM

Chlorine: 0.1 M.

Concentration was selected according to the maximum biological values in blood stream (Figure 7.9).

– **Stability**: Long-term stability in biological environments is crucial for continuous monitoring. Current commercial glucometers only last between 10 and 14 days. Copper can be susceptible to oxidation and degradation. Strategies that include surface modification and encapsulation to enhance sensor's lifespan are key to achieve a commercial product.

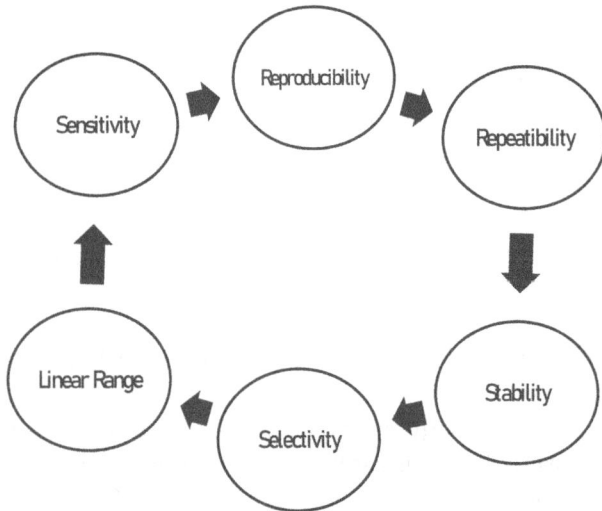

Figure 7.9: Features to consider in the development of the 4th generation glucose sensors.

- **Sensitivity:** Sensitivity is absolutely crucial when any user selects a glucose sensor. A highly sensitive sensor can detect smaller changes in blood sugar levels. This is vital for users, to make informed decisions about their insulin intake, diet, and overall diabetes management. Sensitivity allows the sensor to pick up on subtle rises or drops in blood sugar before they become severe. This can help to prevent episodes of hypoglycemia or hyperglycemia.

  With more accurate and timely blood sugar data, users can better track trends and patterns in their blood sugar levels. This empowers patients to fine tune their diabetes management strategies for optimal health.

Sensors with very high sensitivity values are a good option for applications where the target biofluid has small range of glucose concentration. These ranges are discussed below.

- **Linear range:** Glucose can be detected in many biofluids within the human body. The selected biofluid and its glucose range could be:

  Blood: 4–11 mM of glucose.

  Interstitial biofluid: 3.5–11 mM of glucose.

  Lacrimal fluid: 0–3.6 mM of glucose.

  Sweat: 0.06–0.2 mM of glucose.

  Saliva: 0.02–0.06 mM of glucose.

Depending on the target biofluid, the sensor could be designed to be minimally or a non-invasive device. For example, if glucose is to be measured in sweat, the sensor will be non-invasive. Multiple patch sensors have been tested in sweat to monitor electrolytes and other molecules such as glucose.

- **Reproducibility and repeatability:** This ensures that the sensor delivers consistent results under similar conditions, even if different people operate it or if measurements are taken at different times of the day. Consistent readings give users confidence in the sensor's accuracy and reliability.

  High repeatability that translates into the same reading for a given blood sugar level, even with multiple consecutive measurements. This consistency allows users to trust the data for making crucial diabetes management decisions.

- **Biocompatibility:** For implantable sensors, biocompatibilityy is also paramount. Careful selection of materials and surface engineering are necessary to minimize adverse tissue reactions.

More aspects to consider in the glucose sensor design stage are: the electrode surface (number of active sites where glucose is oxidized), the band gap of the bimetallic combination which represents the minimum energy that is required to excite an electron up to a state in the conduction band where it can participate in the glucose oxidation. Other features are: affordability, portability, harm to the environment, ease to use and degree of miniaturization.

7.4.3 The future challenges of FGGS

Despite these challenges, the potential of FGGS is undeniable. The continuous development of novel metal nanostructures with tailored properties offers a promising avenue for overcoming these hurdles. Future research directions include:

- Integration with microfluidic devices: Microfluidic platforms can enable miniaturized and automated continuous monitoring systems.
- Machine learning integration: Machine learning algorithms can analyze sensor data in real-time, accounting for variations and improving measurement accuracy.
- Alternative catalytic materials: While copper shows promise, research into other transition metals and their nanostructures can provide valuable insights for further development to achieve a good response under physiological conditions.

Acknowledgments: The authors would like to thank the editors David Bogle and Tomasz Sosnowski for their guidance and review of this article before its publication.

References

1. Naikoo GA, Salim H, Hassan IU, Awan T, Arshad F, Pedram MZ, et al. Recent advances in non-enzymatic glucose sensors based on metal and metal oxide nanostructures for diabetes management – a review. Front Chem 2021;9:1–20.
2. Pour SRS, Calabria D, Emamiamin A, Lazzarini E, Pace A, Guardigli M, et al. Electrochemical vs. optical biosensors for point-of-care applications: a critical review. Chemosensors 2023;11:1–29.
3. Shubrook J, Butts A, Chamberlain JJ, Johnson EL, Leal S, Rhinehart AS, et al. Standards of medical care in diabetes—2017 abridged for primary care providers. Clin Diabetes 2017;35:5–26.
4. Karpova EV, Karyakina EE, Karyakin AA. Wearable non-invasive monitors of diabetes and hypoxia through continuous analysis of sweat. Talanta 2020;215:120922.
5. Di Filippo D, Sunstrum FN, Khan JU, Welsh AW. Non-invasive glucose sensing technologies and products: a comprehensive review for researchers and clinicians. Sensors 2023;23. https://doi.org/10.3390/s23229130.
6. Davison NB, Gaffney CJ, Kerns JG, Zhuang QD. Recent progress and perspectives on non-invasive glucose sensors. Diabetology 2022;3:56–71.
7. Karpova EV, Karyakin AA. Noninvasive monitoring of diabetes and hypoxia by wearable flow-through biosensors. Curr Opin Electrochem 2020;23:16–20.
8. Nyein HYY, Bariya M, Kivimäki L, Uusitalo S, Liaw TS, Jansson E, et al. Regional and correlative sweat analysis using high-throughput microfluidic sensing patches toward decoding sweat. Sci Adv 2019;5:1–12.
9. Zhang Y, LI N, XIang Y, Wang D, Zhang P, Wang Y, et al. A flexible non-enzymatic glucose sensor based on copper nanoparticles anchored on laser-induced graphene. Carbon N Y 2020;156:506–13.
10. Amirzadeh Z, Javadpour S, Shariat MH, Knibbe R. Non-enzymatic glucose sensor based on copper oxide and multi-wall carbon nanotubes using PEDOT:PSS matrix. Synth Met 2018;245:160–6.
11. Sun Y, Li Y, Wang N, Xu QQ, Xu L, Lin M. Copper-based metal-organic framework for non-enzymatic electrochemical detection of glucose. Electroanalysis 2018;30:474–8.
12. Kurt UB, Demir Ü, Öznülüer Özer T, Öztürk Doğan H. Electrochemical fabrication of Ni nanoparticles-decorated electrochemically reduced graphene oxide composite electrode for non-enzymatic glucose detection. Thin Solid Films 2020;693. https://doi.org/10.1016/j.tsf.2019.137695.

13. Jeong H, Tran KD, Tran DT, Kim NH, Lee JH. Catalytic manipulation of Ni nanostructures-immobilized CNTs via nitrogen coupling for robust water electrolysis and effective glucose detection. Mater Today Sustain 2023;23:100413.

14. Babulal SM, Chen SM, Palani R, Venkatesh K, Haidyrah AS, Ramaraj SK, et al. Graphene oxide template based synthesis of NiCo2O4 nanosheets for high performance non-enzymatic glucose sensor. Colloids Surf A Physicochem Eng Asp 2021;621:126600.

15. Guati C, Gomez-Coma L, Fallanza M, Ortiz I. Progress on the influence of non-enzymatic electrodes characteristics on the response to glucose detection: a review (2016–2022). Rev Chem Eng 2024;40:123–48.

16. Chakraborty P, Deka N, Patra DC, Debnath K, Mondal SP. Hydrothermally grown porous cobalt oxide nanostructures for enzyme-less glucose detection. J Electron Mater 2021;50:3699–705.

17. Abrori SA, Trisno MLA, Aritonang RA, Anshori I, Nugraha S, Yuliarto B, et al. Synthesis and characterization of metal-organic framework (MOF) CoBTC as a non-enzymatic electrochemical biosensor for glucose. IOP Conf Ser Mater Sci Eng 2021;1045:012006.

18. Myung Y, Jang DM, Cho YJ, Kim HS, Park J, Kim JU, et al. Nonenzymatic amperometric glucose sensing of platinum, copper sulfide, and tin oxide nanoparticle-carbon nanotube hybrid nanostructures. J Phys Chem C 2009;113:1251–9.

19. Islam T, Hasan MM, Awal A, Nurunnabi M, Ahammad AJS. Metal nanoparticles for electrochemical sensing: progress and challenges in the clinical transition of point-of-care testing. Molecules 2020;25:8–13.

Álvaro González-Garcinuño*, Antonio Tabernero and
Eva Martín del Valle*

8 Macroscopic transport models for drugs and vehicles in cancer tissues

Abstract: Modeling drug release in solid tumors is a convergence point between chemical engineering and medicine. Consequently, many studies have been conducted to unravel the mechanisms behind drug distribution after administration. In addition, several approaches have been explored, ranging from pharmacokinetic and pharmacodynamic models to microscopic transport models through macroscopic transport models. This chapter focuses on the latter, macroscopic transport models, and discusses how these models can predict the processes involved in drug delivery, in free form or vehicle transported. We start by presenting some of the differentiating physiological parameters in cancer tissues and then the main equations used for modeling, including fluid flow, mass transport, and cell uptake. Also, the use of some dimensionless parameters explaining the processes that control transportation will be examined. Lastly, the final section will explore the process employed for building geometries to simulate solid tumors, as well as current research being conducted on patient-specific simulations made using medical images.

Keywords: drug delivery; macroscopic transport models; cancer treatment; simulation; modeling

8.1 Introduction: the importance of modeling drug transport in cancer. Types of models

Cancer is one of the major health concerns of the last century. It is estimated that by 2030, there will be around 26 million new cases of cancer and 17 million deaths per year [1]. Cancer research has, therefore, become one of the leading lines of action for improving the quality of life of an increasingly aging population [2].

---

*Corresponding authors: Álvaro González Garcinuño and Eva Martín del Valle, Department of Chemical Engineering, University of Salamanca, Salamanca, Spain; and IBSAL, Institute for Biomedical Research of Salamanca, Salamanca, Spain, E-mail: alvaro_gonzalez@usal.es (A. González-Garcinuño), emvalle@usal.es (E.M.del. Valle) (E. Martín del Valle). https://orcid.org/0000-0003-3506-2546 (E. Martín del Valle)
Antonio Tabernero, Department of Chemical Engineering, University of Salamanca, Salamanca, Spain; and IBSAL, Institute for Biomedical Research of Salamanca, Salamanca, Spain

As per De Gruyter's policy this article has previously been published in the journal Physical Sciences Reviews. Please cite as: Á. González-Garcinuño, A. Tabernero and E. Martín del Valle "Macroscopic transport models for drugs and vehicles in cancer tissues" *Physical Sciences Reviews* [Online] 2024. DOI: 10.1515/psr-2024-0059 | https://doi.org/10.1515/9783111394558-008

Cancer has been approached from various perspectives, and, as a result, extensive efforts have been made to understand the molecular mechanisms that promote cancer cell differentiation and progression [3]. In addition, intensive pharmaceutical research has promoted drug discovery, from classical cytostatic compounds to stem cells and gene therapy to immunotherapy [4]. However, the development of these techniques has not been accompanied by an in-depth study of the transport phenomena involved in cancer progression, drug distribution, and perfusion. Also, only a few mathematical studies have been carried out. Therefore, this gap presents an excellent opportunity for chemical engineers to apply the basis of transport phenomena to medicine, in particular to cancer therapy, using a promising field called Transport Oncophysics (*TOP*) [5]. Moreover, **modeling** and numerical simulations provide a powerful tool for carrying out detailed preliminary research before conducting experiments, which reduces the time required for carrying out subsequent steps in pharmaceutical development [6].

According to the classification by [7], computational models for drug delivery to solid tumors can be divided into three main categories: pharmacokinetics and pharmacodynamics-based compartmental models, microscopic transport models, and macroscopic transport models, which are the main focus of this paper.

8.1.1 Pharmacokinetics (PK)–Pharmacodynamics (PD) models

PK models explain the absorption, distribution, metabolism, and excretion of substances utilizing mass balance equations. In many cases, a biological system is divided into several compartments to represent the different organs or tissues, with connections between them and also with the circulatory and/or lymphatic system. These models can be integrated with PD models that describe the pharmacological effects of a drug within an organism. Therefore, the formulation of these models is based on ordinary differential equations (ODEs) and the principle that mass is conserved among compartments. The values of parameters for this large number of equations are sometimes experimentally determined or numerically estimated based on some measurable physiological variables [7]. In most cases, the concentration in each compartment is estimated as the area under the curve (AUC). Several PKPD models have been published for drugs with chemotherapeutic effects and many have been included in clinical trials and marketing authorization processes. [8] described that around 73 % of companies use PKPD analysis as proven data for regulatory submissions. Moreover, modern PKPD models have also included drug resistance on therapeutic efficacy, mainly mediated by P-glycoprotein, approximating more realistically the effect of drugs in tissues [9]. Figure 8.1 represents a schematic of a classical pharmacokinetic model with different compartments for each process (adsorption, distribution, metabolism, and excretion).

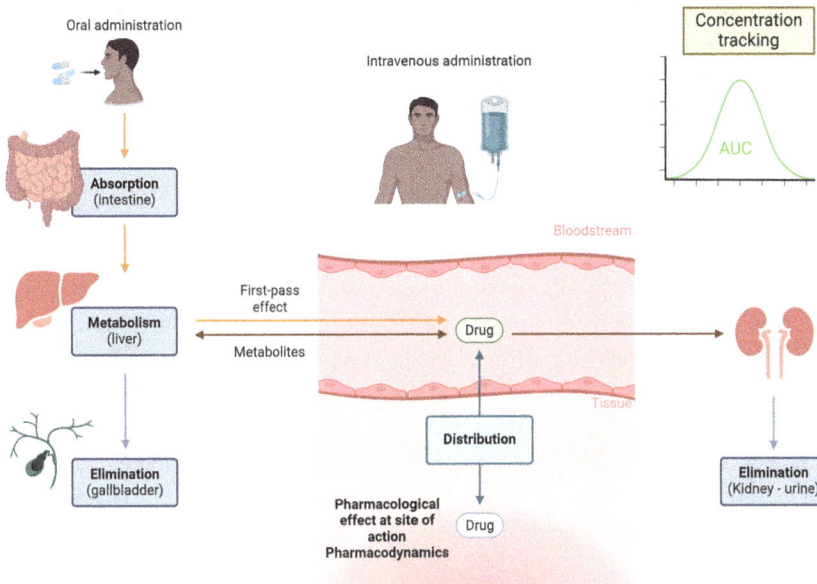

Figure 8.1: Schematic representation of pharmacokinetics models. Created using biorender.

8.1.2 Microscopic models

These models consider the true behavior of drugs in a delimited study region, and unlike PKPD models, microscopic models use partial differential equations (PDEs) and can, therefore, estimate not only progress over time but also spatial distributions in the selected geometry. Therefore, this approach provides an explicit description of both fluid flow and drug transport within a domain of interest.

Initially, these models considered the tumor as a cylinder surrounded by a closed blood circuit. These early models were known as tumor cords, which can include some internal necrotic regions with no biological activity [10].

Later on, microscopic models were developed to include tumor vasculature, creating more complex geometries that also vary over time, as tumor angiogenesis is a process coupled with tumor development and growth [11]. These models consider blood flow through vessels, diffusion of solutes and fluids, convective transport in the extracellular matrix, extravasation from blood vessels, and so on.

These approaches have been complemented using models that take into account transvascular transport in capillary vessels, controlled by interstitial fluid pressure (IFP) and vessel pore size [12] or other models that consider the heterogenicity of the interstitium [13].

Although these models offer a realistic and detailed approximation of drug transport in the tumor microenvironment, extending them to tissue-level simulations is a challenge that is solved by using macroscopic models [7].

8.1.3 Macroscopic models

Macroscopic models consider a tumor as a porous medium in which drug transport and fluid flow can be described by PDEs. Specific geometries for capillary or lymphatic vessels are not considered and are incorporated into the model as sink or source terms. This simplification is indeed necessary for maximizing computational efforts and predicting the drug concentration in the entire tumor [14]. Macroscopic models are the main focus of this chapter because of their ability to estimate drug transport in real tumor sizes and shapes. In Section 8.3, the main equations used to describe these phenomena are presented in detail, and in Section 8.4, some improvements in classical approaches using medical images to obtain more accurate models are presented [15].

8.2 Physiology of cancer and necrotic tissues

According to the World Health Organization (WHO), cancer is *"a large group of diseases that can start in almost any organ or tissue when abnormal cells grow uncontrollably, go beyond their usual boundaries to invade adjoining parts of the body and/or spread to other organs"*. Irregular growth results in changes in the affected tissue that significantly influence the potential transport of drugs within it. It is, therefore, important to know what changes are observed in cancerous and necrotic tissues because these particularities can be used as an advantage for designing new therapies or routes of administration.

First, it is important to distinguish between tumor tissue and necrotic tissue because their properties are quite different. Tissue necrosis is a response that occurs in advanced solid tumors and involves a loss of organ function due to cell death. Necrosis is independent of caspase activity (proteins responsible for apoptosis, the process of controlled cell death), and the main characteristics are cellular swelling, mitochondrial damage, and cell rupture, with the subsequent release of cell contents and considerable inflammation [16].

Solid tumors sometimes present a necrotic core surrounded by active tumor tissue, so two different compartments must be considered for modeling [17]. However, drug action must be localized to the active tumor, where its therapeutical effect is intended to reduce the viability of malignant cells.

Based on the above facts, a summary of the main physiological aspects influencing drug transport in active tumors, as well as their dissimilarities with normal tissues, is presented.

8.2.1 Pressure gradient

Tumors have a greater extracellular matrix (ECM) as compared to normal tissues, which is responsible for tumor growth and expansion. This abundant ECM increases IFP [18], which can in turn limit the penetration of macromolecules such as cancer treatment drugs [19]. Moreover, some studies have reported that greater IFP is associated with a worse prognosis [20].

The overpressure within the tumor depends on the distance to the center or edge and is highly dependent on the blood pressure of the capillaries supplying the tumor with blood. According to previous studies, overpressure ranges from 500 to 2000 Pa [21, 22]. Occasionally, the overpressure can exceed a limit that favors capillary rupture and thus the creation of a hypoxic region due to the absence of oxygen supplied by the blood [23]. This pressure gradient seems to be preserved even if the tumors are surgically removed and hydrogels are placed to fill the cavity [24].

8.2.2 Tumor vasculature. Blood irrigation

Differences in vasculature are probably the most significant between tumors and other tissues. This characteristic is often used as a target for anticancer agents also known as Tumor-Vascular Disrupting Agents (Tumor-VDAs) [25].

The architecture of normal vascular networks is hierarchically organized to ensure proper diffusion of nutrients and oxygen to cells. However, this structure shifts toward a disorganization of vessel networks in tumors due to the uncontrolled growth of neoplastic cells and overexpression of proangiogenic factors [26]. Tumor blood vessels often exhibit a high proportion of proliferating endothelial cells, aberrant basement membrane formation, and increased tortuosity [27]. This abnormal distribution promotes the creation of hypoxic regions owing to perfusion problems, which is one of the factors driving tumor metastasis and chemoresistance [28]. Figure 8.2 represents a schematic of the differences in blood vasculature in tumor and healthy tissues.

This aberrant distribution occurs through the presence of other metabolites in blood vessels that also affect the prognosis and evolution of tumor tissue. Cancer cells can adapt themselves to low O_2 stress by reprogramming their metabolism [29]. Among all the metabolites involved, nitric oxide (NO) plays the most important role in regulating responses to hypoxia and has been also studied in depth as a therapeutic strategy [30]. For this reason, in parallel, some efforts have been made to model the transport and concentration of this molecule in tumor tissues [31].

8.2.3 Lymphatic drainage

The proliferation of nonfunctional and aberrant lymphatic vessels is another physiological feature associated with the development of solid tumors. Often, the vessels are

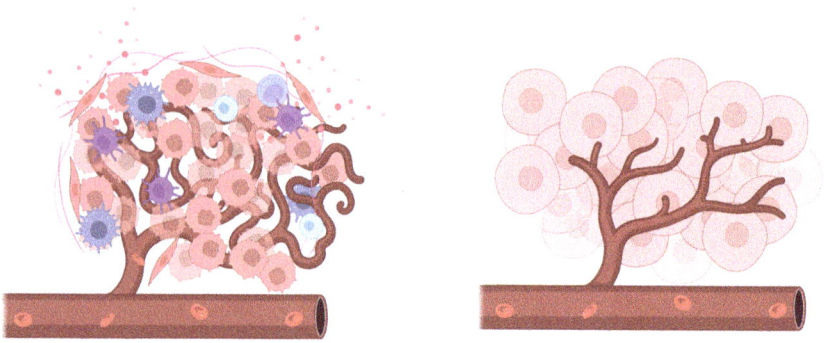

Figure 8.2: A: Blood vessels distribution in tumor tissues, B: Blood vessels distribution in normal tissues. Created using Biorender.

sacs with blind ends with odd tight junctions that modify the absorption and transport of fluids and macromolecules [32]. This modification is associated with the accumulation of inflammatory cells and promotes tumor-specific immune responses [33].

Around 80 % of solid tumors metastasize via the lymphatic system, i.e., cancer cells are internalized in lymphatic vessels and spread to other organs and tissues through this network [34]. As a result, lymphatic drainage has often been considered a target for the development of some cancer treatments [35]. Hence, it has been found that large particles (larger than 16 kDa) preferentially accumulate in lymphatic vessels to an upper limit of around 80 nm. Consequently, this drainage of therapeutic particles or substances to the lymphatic system is a key factor to be considered when studying transport within tumors from a macroscopic perspective [36, 37]. In addition, particles smaller than 10 nm are easily cleared because they can pass through the tight junctions of blood vessels [38]. For these reasons, classical transport equations for describing the behavior of drugs in tissues should be modified to account for the important role of lymphatic drainage in tumors.

8.3 Classical transport equations and phenomena

As described in Section 8.1, macroscopic transport models consider the tumor as a porous system but do not consider specific geometries for blood or lymphatic vessels. This issue will be addressed in Section 8.4, as an improvement to the classical approach.

At this point, the conservation of mass and momentum (equations (8.1) and (8.2)), according to the Navier–Stokes equation, are the governing equations for determining pressure and, consequently, velocity [7].

$$\rho \nabla \cdot \vec{u} = 0 \tag{8.1}$$

$$\rho\frac{\partial\vec{u}}{\partial t} + \rho\left(\vec{u}\cdot\nabla\right)\vec{u} = \nabla\cdot\left(-p\vec{I}+\vec{\tau}\right) + \rho\vec{g} + \vec{F} \qquad (8.2)$$

Where ρ is the density, $\vec{u}$ is the velocity vector, p is the pressure, $\vec{I}$ is the inertial term, $\vec{\tau}$ is the shear stress, $\vec{g}$ is the gravity, and $\vec{F}$ is the vector for the external forces applied. The shear stress can be calculated according to equation (8.3):

$$\vec{\tau} = \mu\left(\nabla\vec{u} + \nabla\vec{u}^T\right) \qquad (8.3)$$

Equation (8.1) is specifically modified for this case, in order to consider fluid exchange to the surrounding vessels, and can be reformulated using equation (8.4):

$$\nabla\vec{u} = F_{BV} + F_{LV} \qquad (8.4)$$

Where F_{BV} is the interstitial fluid exchange rate between tissue and circulatory system and F_{LV} is the fluid adsorption rate by the lymphatic system. Both rates are governed by **Starling's law** [39] and can be expressed as follows (equations (8.5) and (8.6)):

$$F_{BV} = K_{BV}\frac{S_{BV}}{V_{TU}}\left[p_{IVS} - p_{ECS} - \sigma_T\left(\pi_{IVS} - \pi_{ECS}\right)\right] \qquad (8.5)$$

$$F_{LV} = K_{LV}\frac{S_{BV}}{V_{TU}}\left(p_{ECS} - p_{LV}\right) \qquad (8.6)$$

Where K is the hydraulic conductivity of vasculature, the quotient S/V represents the relation between vessel surface area per tissue volume, π is the osmotic pressure, and σ_T is the averaged osmotic reflection coefficient (a value that depends on each protein or substance to be transported). The subindexes refer to IVS (intravascular space), ECS (extracellular space), LV (lymphatic vessels), or BV (blood vessels). Table 8.1 represents the values (or the range of values) for some of the previous parameters according to published literature.

Table 8.1: Value of parameters for Starling's equations in tumor tissue.

Parameter	Value	Units	Reference
Hydraulic conductivity blood vessels (K_{BV})	$2.1\cdot10^{-7}$	m/Pa·s	[40]
Hydraulic conductivity lymphatic vessels (K_{LV})	$2.1\cdot10^{-7}$	m/Pa·s	[40]
Surface area of blood vessels per unit tissue volume (S_{BV}/V_{TU})	From 7 to 45	mm^{-1}	[41]
Surface area of lymphatic vessels per unit tissue volume (S_{LV}/V_{TU})	16.5	mm^{-1}	[42]
Pressure at intravascular space (p_{IVS})	19.5	mmHg	[43]
Pressure at extracellular space (p_{ECS})	From 7.5 to 30	mmHg	[44]
Pressure in lymphatic vessels (p_{LV})	−15.6	mmHg	[45]
Osmotic pressure intravascular space (π_{IVS})	From 15 to 20	mmHg	[45]
Osmotic pressure extracellular space (π_{ECS})	From −0.75 to −2	mmHg	[44]

Equation (8.2) can also be simplified into equation (8.7), according to **Darcy's law**, which governs transport in porous media:

$$\vec{u} = -\frac{k}{\mu}\left(\nabla p - \rho\vec{g}\right)$$

(8.7)

Where k is the permeability of the tissue (m^2) and μ is the dynamic viscosity of the interstitial fluid. Gravity ($\vec{g}$) is often discarded and not considered for modeling in many works. However, the relative position of the tumor may force the consideration of gravity as an important vector, especially in those organs that are externally located (breast, testicles, etc.).

Permeability is defined as the capacity of the medium to transport fluid and is strongly related to porosity (φ) and tortuosity (T), as well as the diameter of the cells involved in this porous medium [46]. These three magnitudes are associated through Kozeny-Carman's law, which is formulated in equation (8.8), [47]:

$$k = \frac{\varphi^3}{cT^2S^2}$$

(8.8)

Where c is the shape factor (equal to 1 for spheres) and S is the specific surface area of pores (where particle diameter is considered). For spherical cells, the previous equation can be reformulated in equation (8.9), which is the one most considered for many works [48]:

$$k = \frac{d_p^2 \cdot \varphi}{180\left(1 - \varphi\right)^2}$$

(8.9)

Where d_p is the diameter of the particles (cells in this case). Cell diameter is often obtained after microscopic visualization of the tissue, or from isolated cells obtained from it. However, tissue porosity is more difficult to determine, and, in some cases, it is easier to determine the permeability instead of porosity, using uniaxial compression tests [49]. Table 8.2 shows the permeability values of different tumor tissues according to the results of published studies:

Table 8.2: Permeability values of different types of tumor tissue.

Tissue	Permeability (m^2)	Reference
Breast cancer	$7.6 \cdot 10^{-13}$	[50]
Colorectal cancer	$2.55 \cdot 10^{-17}$	[51]
Ovarian cancer	$2.14 \cdot 10^{-17}$	[51]
Pancreatic cancer	$1.44 \cdot 10^{-17}$	[51]
Brain cancer	$1 \cdot 10^{-15}$	[52]
Cervix cancer	$1.81 \cdot 10^{-15}$	[53]

Therefore, according to Table 8.2, tissue permeability ranges from 10^{-13} to 10^{-17} m^2, and it is considered that there is an increase in tumor tissue permeability compared to healthy tissue (one or two orders of magnitude), promoted by the well-known enhanced permeation and retention effect (EPR) [53].

For model simulation, some boundary conditions are required. Often, the zero-flux boundary condition is imposed at the boundaries of the simulation domain. Also, some values of pressure must be provided on different surfaces in 3D models. According to [21], the overpressure inside the tumor (at the center) can be estimated between 1,000 and 1,600 Pa, and these values can be provided as boundary conditions.

Once the fluid velocity has been determined, it is necessary to define the transport of substances in the tissue, based on the hydraulic parameters calculated from Navier–Stokes-derived equations. The global mass balance can be written as equation (8.10) for a substance (i):

$$\frac{d(\varphi \cdot C_i)}{dt} + \nabla \cdot \vec{J_i} + \vec{u_i} \cdot \nabla C_i = R_i \tag{8.10}$$

Thus, equation (8.10) considers a term for accumulation (the first), a term for diffusive flux (the second), and another term for convective flux (the third), as well as a reaction term (R_i), which is the way to simplify drug exchange from/to lymphatic or blood vessels or how the drug is internalized by cells in the tissue. The diffusive flux term is calculated by equation (8.11) according to Fick's law:

$$\vec{J_i} = -\left(D_{D_i} + D_{ef_i}\right)\nabla C_i \tag{8.11}$$

Where the effective diffusion (D_{ef}) is calculated from free diffusion (D_D) by considering the porosity and tortuosity (equation (8.12)):

$$D_{ef_i} = \frac{\varphi}{T}D_{D_i} \tag{8.12}$$

The reaction term can be calculated as the contribution of many terms, as indicated in equation (8.13):

$$R_i = R_{BV} + R_{LV} + R_{cell} \tag{8.13}$$

The reaction term, therefore, includes first, the drug exchange with the blood (R_{BV}); second, the lymphatic drainage (R_{LV}); and finally, the cell uptake rate (R_{cell}). Equation (8.13) can be extended to include other less frequent phenomena, such as protein binding or physical degradation, which can affect the local concentration of the drug in the tissue. Drug exchange with the blood and lymphatic system is formulated in equations (8.14) and (8.15), respectively, taking into account the fluid exchange rate, calculated using Starling's law (equations (8.5) and (8.6)) [7]:

$$R_{BV} = F_{BV}(1 - \sigma_T)C_{i,BV} + P_{BV}\frac{S_{BV}}{V_{TU}}(C_{i,BV} - C_{i,Ts})\frac{Pe_{BV}}{\exp(Pe_{BV}) - 1} \tag{8.14}$$

$$R_{LV} = F_{LV} \cdot C_{i,Ts} \tag{8.15}$$

Therefore, the exchange with blood capillaries depends on the difference in drug concentration between both compartments: blood vessels (*BV*) and tissue (*Ts*). Nevertheless, lymphatic drainage follows a first-order kinetic and only depends on the drug concentration within the tissue.

Cell uptake is often receptor-mediated. Therefore, it can be formulated according to Scatchard's model (equation (8.16)), where the internalization rate is corrected by the concentration of the drug in the tissue [54].

$$R_{cell} = k_{int}\frac{C_{i,Ts}}{k_a + C_{i,Ts}} \tag{8.16}$$

The internalization rate (k_{int}) is often calculated from translational times, which depend on the substance and takes values from 0.5 to 2 h, depending on the size [55]. Along the domain boundaries, the zero-flux boundary condition is often imposed, i.e., $-n \cdot (\vec{J_i} + \vec{u} \cdot C_i) = 0)$

Figure 8.3 represents all of the transport phenomena involved in drug or vehicle transport in cancer tissues, where the different colored arrows represent phenomena that have already been described using their equations.

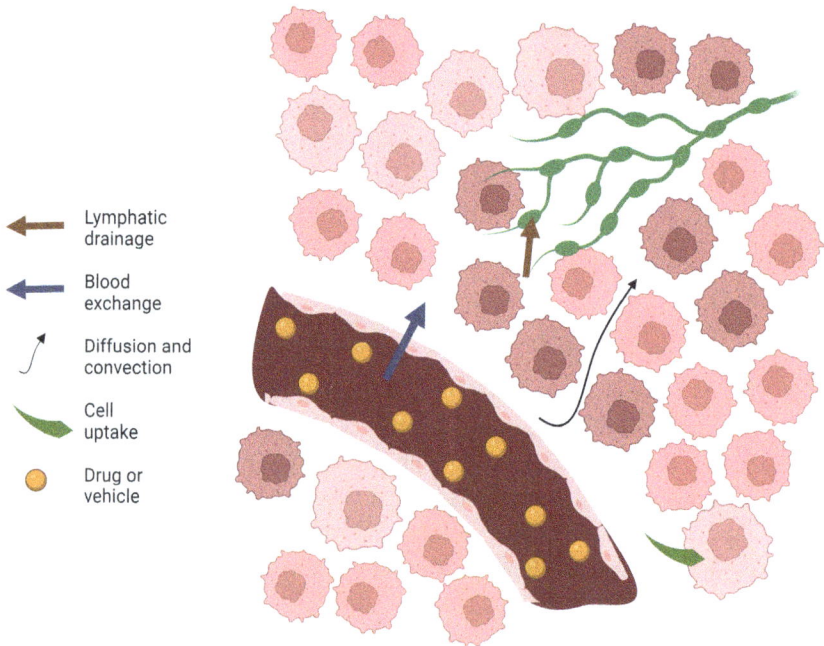

Figure 8.3: Schematic representation of the transport phenomena of a drug or vehicle in cancer tissue. Created using biorender.

Finally, in this section, some **frequently used Dimensionless parameters** are presented. These numbers are useful for assessing the importance of different factors in total drug transport [56].

First, the ratio of interstitial to vascular resistance to fluid flow, also known as Rt, was proposed by [57] **to determine the importance of tumor morphology in drug transport. These authors concluded that the optimal** volumetric flow rate was proportional to Rt^2 for a spherical tumor. They also studied the effect of shape with prolate and oblate spheroids as tumor geometries. Equation (8.17) is used to calculate this parameter:

$$R_t = R_{TU}\sqrt{\frac{\mu\left(K_{BV}\cdot S_{BV} + K_{LV}\cdot S_{LV}\right)}{\kappa\cdot V_{TU}}} \tag{8.17}$$

Where R_{TU} is defined as the equivalent radius of tumor/normal tissue with the same volume and κ is the permeability of the interstitial space.

The Peclet number is often used because it expresses the relative importance of drug diffusion and drug convection. The **Peclet number (Pe)** can be formulated for transport in the extracellular space (Pe_{ECS}) and transvascular transport (Pe_{BV}). Both parameters are defined in Equations (8.18) and (8.1), respectively:

$$Pe_{ECS} = \frac{v_{ECS}}{D_{ef}}R_{TU} \tag{8.18}$$

$$Pe_{BV} = \frac{F_{BV}\left(1-\sigma\right)}{P_{BV}\frac{S_{BV}}{V_{TU}}} \tag{8.19}$$

The velocity (v_{ECS}) in equation (8.18) is calculated from Darcy's law, and the effective diffusion is estimated according to equation (8.12).

The relationship between drug reaction (uptake or elimination) and drug diffusion is expressed as **Thiele modulus (φ)** [58], and its mathematical formulation is presented in equation (8.20).

$$\phi = R_{TU}\sqrt{\frac{k_{elim}}{D_{ef}}} \tag{8.20}$$

Where k_{elim} is the drug elimination rate and may include all of the possible phenomena involved (protein binding, cell uptake, etc.).

Lastly, the **Karlovitz number (Ka)** expresses the relationship between convective transport and drug reaction (or elimination), and it is expressed in equation (8.21), [59]

$$Ka = \frac{v_{ECS}}{R_{TU}\cdot k_{elim}} \tag{8.21}$$

However, more recently, [59] have proposed a new dimensionless parameter, called KT<!–index: KT–>, which can include both transport phenomena (convection and diffusion) and the reaction process. This dimensionless number can be defined as the ratio between the time scale of the reaction rate and the cumulative time scale of convective

Table 8.3: Main models for describing drug release from vehicles.

Model name	Specification or consideration	Equation	Ref.
Higuchi	Matrix solution is negligible Diffusion coefficient unidirectional	$\frac{M(t)}{M_\infty} = k_H \sqrt{t}$	[61]
Peppas	N for the mechanism that controls release and K depends on the carrier	$\frac{M(t)}{M_\infty} = K \cdot t^n$	[62]
Peppas–Sahlin	Considers diffusion (K_1) and polymer chain relaxation (K_2)	$\frac{M(t)}{M_\infty} = K_1 \cdot t^n + K_2 \cdot t^n$	[63]
Peppas with a lag phase	Includes barriers before release	$\frac{M(t)}{M_\infty} = K(t - t_l)^n$	[64]
Peppas with an initial burst	b As quick release at initial stages (burst)	$\frac{M(t)}{M_\infty} = K \cdot t^n + b$	[64]
Corrigan	Three phenomena coupled: burst, lag phase, and polymer losses	$\frac{M(t)}{M_\infty} = F_{BIN}(1 - exp(-k_b \cdot t))$ $+(1 - F_{BIN}) \cdot \left(\frac{exp(k(t-t_{max}))}{1+exp(k(t-t_{max}))} \right)$	[65]
Hopfenberg	Includes polymer degradation during release	$\frac{M(t)}{M_\infty} = 1 - \left(1 - \frac{K_{hp} \cdot t}{C_0 a_0} \right)^n$	[66]

and diffusive transport. It is defined by the Karlovitz number and by the Thiele modulus, according to equation (8.22).

$$KT = \frac{Ka}{\phi^2}. \tag{8.22}$$

The above equations have been presented for a drug that is administrated in a free form. All of them can also be used for drug-carrying vehicles such as liposomes, polymeric micelles, organic and inorganic nanoparticles, etc.

In these cases, other equations should be considered to study drug release during the transportation process, as well as possible phenomena of erosion and particle degradation that modify the amount of drug available in the tissue or blood vessels.

Many authors have proposed different mathematical models to study drug release phenomena from vehicles [60], and the most commonly used models with their specifications and equations can be found in Table 8.3. Generally, these equations are formulated as a quotient between the mass of the drug released in the external medium ($M(t)$) and the maximum mass to be released (M_∞).

8.4 Improving models using realistic geometries

Initially, macroscopic models have worked using quite simple geometries known as *"Tumor cord models*<!–index: Tumor cord models–>*"* (Figure 8.4). These models consider the tumor as the association of several tumor cords, which are two concentrical

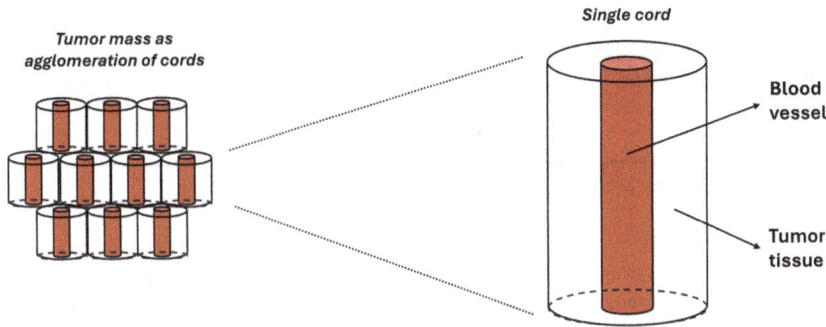

Figure 8.4: Schematic representation of tumor cord models. Adapted from [67].

cylinders: the smallest one located in the center, defined as the blood vessel, and the other one surrounding it, defined as the tumor tissue [67]. A representation of these structures can be seen in Figure 8.4.

However, this is a simplification that provides results that always depend on the radial position (drug concentration, cell survival, etc.).

Other authors have considered even more simple geometries to study drug transport in tumors. As an example, [68] studied the transport and adsorption of lipid nanoparticles injected intramuscularly, but considered the geometry of a cube (1 cm side). Similarly, [69] used a cube (10 cm) to study the delivery of monoclonal antibodies after subcutaneous injection.

Another approach often adopted is the use of simple geometric figures. However, two compartments are differentiated: an inner compartment, which simulates the necrotic core, surrounded by non-necrotic cancerous tissue. This strategy has been used in studies such as those by [17, 70].

Based on the previously mentioned facts, more complex geometries are needed to explain different phenomena that often take place in patients [71]. Consequently, several studies have recently been carried out regarding realistic geometries. For this purpose, medical images are essential for providing the information for reconstructing 3D geometry. Recently, [72] compared drug release from thermo-sensitive liposomes using an imaged-based vascularized tumor and a volume-averaged porous media model and concluded that volume averaging is a suitable approach for making fast calculations. Nevertheless, imaged-based models provide more accurate predictions and information. These strategies, based on images, can lead to patient-specific simulations aimed at improving treatments or doses [73].

The use of magnetic resonance images (MRI) to construct geometries for Multiphysics simulations began by studying the progress and evolution of brain tumors (glioblastoma); first, in 2D [74] and, later on, in 3D [75]. Several studies have considered this alternative over the last few years. Table 8.4 summarizes Multiphysics simulations using macroscopic transport models that have used 3D real geometries taken from

Table 8.4: Multiphysics 3D simulations based on MRI images of patients.

Cancer type	Drug	Number of patients studied	Mesh elements	Reference
Glioblastoma (brain tumor)	Not provided	1	8 million	[75]
Brain tumor	Tracer (model)	1	0.010 million	[76]
Brain tumor	Methotrexate, cisplatin, doxorubicin	4	0.52 million	[77]
Liver tumor	Doxorubicin (free and inside liposomes)	1	0.088 million	[78]
Breast ductal tumor	Doxorubicin	10	Not provided	[79]
Brain tumor	Bevacizumab and temozolomide	2	0.082	[80]
Brain tumor	Not provided	1	3.5 million	[81]
Hypopharyngeal cancer	Nanoparticles (model)	1	0.015 million	[82]
Breast cancer	Liposomes loaded with MZ1	6	0.34 million	[50]

human patients for cancer drug delivery. Other studies and simulations have been performed in murine models, a summary of which can be found in [71].

However, as shown in Table 8.4, it can be seen that most of the studies have been carried out using brain tissues. This is the case because MRI is widely used in this area, and more research is needed using other types of tissues.

Other studies have examined these phenomena in 2D, and have also generated virtual tissues (varying some properties), as a means to understand the significance of anisotropy in tissues for modeling and patient-specific simulations [83].

8.5 Conclusions and perspectives

Developing models to study and understand how a vehicle "travels" through tissues (specifically cancerous ones) is one way to improve a potential medical treatment. In this context, chemical engineering and the basis of transport phenomena may be essential for acquiring a deeper understanding.

This chapter summarizes the usefulness of macroscopic models and Multiphysics for understanding the physiology of necrotic tissues, by taking into account specific parameters such as pressure gradient, blood irrigation, and lymphatic drainage.

In this regard, MRI is a tool that can provide more accurate 3D geometries. However, MRI imaging has mainly been used to study brain tissues and should be tested using other tissue types. In addition, despite the growing body of research that has been carried out in recent years, more experiments employing more precise techniques to determine tissue properties, such as intravascular or extravascular pressures, and surface areas among others, are needed to improve the accuracy and prediction of pharmacodynamics and pharmacokinetics using knowledge on transport phenomena and chemical engineering.

Acknowledgment: Authors want to acknowledge the funding support from spanish ministry of Science, PID2022-1405990B-I00. Authors also want to acknowledge professors David Bogle and Tomas Sosnowski for the reviewing process.

References

1. Thun MJ, DeLancey JO, Center MM, Jemal A, Ward EM. The global burden of cancer: priorities for prevention. Carcinogenesis 2010;31:100–10.
2. McAleer S. A history of cancer and its treatment. A history of cancer and its treatment. Ulster Med J 2022;91: 124–9.
3. Motofei IG. Biology of cancer, from cellular and molecular mehcanisms to developmental processes and adaptation. Semin Cancer Biol 2022;86:600–15.
4. He W, Li Q, Lu Y, Ju D, Gu Y, Zhao K, et al. Cancer treatment evolution from traditional methods to stem cells and gene therapy. Curr Gene Ther 2022;22:368–85.
5. Nizzero S, Ziemys A, Ferrari M. Transport barriers and Oncophysics in cancer treatment. Trends Cancer 2018;4:277–80.
6. Kenjeres S. On recent progress in modelling and simulations of multi-scale transfer of mass, momentum and particles in biomedical applications. Flow, Turbul Combust 2016;96:837–60.
7. Zhan W, Alamer M, Xu XY. Computational modelling of drug delivery to solid tumour: understanding the interplay between chemotherapeutics and biological system for optimized delivery systems. Adv Drug Del Rev 2018;132:81–103.
8. Schuck E, Bohnert T, Chakravarty A, Damian-Iordache V, Gibson C, Hsu CP, et al. Preclinical pharmacokinetic/pharmacodynamic modeling and simulation in the pharmaceutical industry: an IQ consortium survey examining the current landscape. AAPS J 2015;17:462–73.
9. Eigenmann MJ, Frances N, Lavé T, Walz AC. PKPD modeling of acquired resistance to anti-cancer drug treatment. J Pharmacokinet Pharmacodyn 2017;44:617–30.
10. Bertuzzi A, Gandolfi A. Cell kinetics in a tumour cord. J Theor Biol 2000;204:587–99.
11. Sefidgar M, Soltani M, Raahemifar K, Sadeghi M, Bazmara H, Bazargan M, et al. Numerical modeling of drug delivery in a dynamic solid tumor microvasculature. Microvasc Res 2015;99:43–56.
12. Chauhan VP, Stylianopoulos T, Martin JD, Popovic Z, Chen O, Kamoun WS, et al. Normalization of tumour blood vessels improves the delivery of nanomedicines in a size-dependent manner. Nat Nanotech 2012;7: 383–8.
13. Rejniak KA, Estrella V, Chen T, Cohen AS, Lloyd M, Morse DL. The role of tumor tissue architecture in treatment penetration and efficacy: an integrative study. Front Oncol 2013;3:111–23.
14. Penta R, Ambrosi D, Quarteroni A. Multiscale homogenization for fluid and drug transport in vascularized malignant tissues. Math Model Methods Appl Sci 2015;25:79–108.
15. Kashkooli FM, Soltani M, Momeni MM. Computational modeling of drug delivery to solid tumors: a pilot study based on a real image. J Drug Deliv Sci Technol 2021;62:102347.
16. Liu ZG, Jiao D. Necroptosis, tumor necrosis and tumorigenesis. Cell Stress 2020;4:1–8.
17. Kashkooli FM, Soltani M, Hamedi MH. Drug delivery to solid tumors with heterogeneous microvascular networks: novel insights from image-based numerical modeling. Eur J Pharm Sci 2020;151. https://doi.org/10.1016/j.ejps.2020.105399.

18. Kim HG, Yu AR, Lee JJ, Lee YJ, Lim SM, Kim JS. Measurement of tumor pressure and strategies of imaging tumor pressure for radioimmunotherapy. Nucl Med Mol Imag 2019;53:235–41.
19. Heldin CH, Rubin K, Pietras K, Ostman A. High interstitial fluid pressure - an obstacle in cancer therapy. Nat Rev Cancer 2004;4:806–13.
20. Milosevic M, Fyles A, Hedley D, Pintilie M, Levin W, Manchul L, et al. Interstitial fluid pressure predicts survival in patients with cervix cancer independent of clinical prognostic factors and tumor oxygen measurements. Cancer Res 2001;61:6400–5.
21. Liu LJ, Brown SL, Ewing JR, Ala BD, Scheneider KM, Schlesinger M. Estimation of tumor insterstitial fluid pressure (TIFP) noninvasively. PLoS One 2016;11:e0140892.
22. Netti PA, Baxter LT, Boucher Y, Jain RK, Skalak R. Time-dependent behavior of interstitial fluid pressure in solid tumors: implications for drug delivery. Cancer Res 1995;20:20.
23. Milosevic MF, Fyles AW, Hill RP. The relationship between elevated interstitial fluid pressure and blood flow in tumors: a bioengineering analysis. Int J Rad Oncol Biol Phys 1999;43:1111–23.
24. Lee GH, Huang SA, Aw WY, Rathod ML, Cho C, Ligler FS, et al. Multilayer microfluidic platform for the study of luminal, transmural, and interstitial flow. Biofabrication 2022;14:025007.
25. Siemann DW. The unique characteristics of tumor vasculature and preclinical evidence for its selective disruption by tumor-vascular disrupting agents. Cancer Treat Rev 2011;37:63–74.
26. Konerding MA, Fait E, Gaumann A. A 3D microvascular architecture of pre-cancerous lesions and invasive carcinomas of the colon. Br J Cancer 2001;84:1354–62.
27. Brigger I, Dubernet C, Couvreur P. Nanoparticles in cancer therapy and diagnosis. Adv Drug Deliv Rev 2002; 54:631–51.
28. Baik AH. Hypoxia signaling and oxygen metabolism in cardio-oncology. J Mol Cell Cardiol 2022;165:64–75.
29. Al Tameemi W, Dale TP, Kh Al-Jumaily RM, Forsyth NR. Hypoxia-modified cancer cell metabolism. Front Cell Dev Biol 2019;7:4.
30. Tu J, Tu K, Xu H, Wang L, Yuan X, Qin X, et al. Improving tumor hypoxia and radiotherapy resistance via in situ nitric oxide release strategy. Eur J Pharm Biopharm 2020;150:96–107.
31. Chen YH, Peng CC, Cheng YJ, Wu JG, Tung YC. Generation of nitric oxide gradients in microfluidic devices for cell culture using spatially controlled chemical reactions. Biomicrofluidics 2013;7:064104.
32. Padera T, Stoll B, Tooredman J. Cancer cells compress intratumour vessels. Nature 2004;427:695.
33. Kataru RP, Ly CL, Shin J, Park HJ, Baik JE, Rehal S, et al. Tumor lymphatic function regulates tumor inflammatory and immunosuppressive microenvironments. Cancer Immunol Res 2019;7:1345–58.
34. Alitalo A, Detmar M. Interaction of tumor cells and lymphatic vessels in cancer progression. Oncogene 2012;31:4499–508.
35. Cote B, Rao D, Alany RG, Kwon GS, Alani AWG. Lymphatic changes in cancer and drug delivery to the lymphatics in solid tumors. Adv Drug Deliv Rev 2019;144:16–34.
36. Bagby TR, Cai S, Duan S, Thahi S, Aires DJ, Forrest L. Impact of molecular weight on lymphatic drainage of a biopolymer-based imaging agent. Pharmaceutics 2012;4:276–95.
37. Oussoren C, Zuidema J, Crommelin DJA, Storm G. Lymphatic uptake and biodistribution of liposomes after subcutaneous injection. Biochim Biophys Acta Biomembr 1997;1328:261–72.
38. Xie Y, Bagby TR, Cohen MS, Forrest ML. Drug delivery to the lymphatic system: importance in future cancer diagnosis and therapies. Expet Opin Drug Deliv 2009;6:785–92.
39. Soltani M, Chen P. Numerical modeling of fluid flow in solid tumors. PLoS One 2011;6:e20344.
40. Baxter LT, Jain RK. Transport of fluid and macromolecules in tumors I. Role of interstitial pressure and convection. Microvasc Res 1989;37:77–104.
41. Forster JC, Harriss-Phillips WM, Douglass MJJ, Bezak E. A review of the development of tumor vasculature and its effects on the tumor microenvironment. Hypoxia (Auckl) 2017;5:21–32.
42. Jafarnejad M, Ismail AZ, Duarte D, Vyas C, Ghahramani A, Zawieja DC, et al. Quantification of the whole lymph node vasculature based on tomography of the vessel corrosion casts. Sci Rep 2019;9:13380.
43. Shore AG. Capillaroscopy and the measurement of capillary pressure. Br J Clin Pharmacol 2000;50:501–13.

44. Voutouri C, Stylianopoulos T. Evolution of osmotic pressure in solid tumors. J Biomech 2014;47:3441–7.
45. Rasouli SS, Jolma IW, Friis HA. Impact of spatially varying hydraulic conductivities on tumor interstitial fluid pressure distribution. Inform Med Unlock 2019;16. https://doi.org/10.1016/j.imu.2019.100175.
46. Graczyk KM, Matyka M. Predicting porosity, permeability, and tortuosity of porous media from images by deep learning. Sci Rep 2020;10:21488.
47. Koponen A, Kataja M, Timonen J. Permeability and effective porosity of porous media. Phys Rev E 1997;56. https://doi.org/10.1103/physreve.56.3319.
48. Majumder S, Islam MR, Righetti R. Non-invasive imaging of interstitial fluid transport parameters in solid tumors in vivo. Sci Rep 2023;13:7132.
49. Ramazanilar M, Mojra A. Characterization of breast tissue permeability for detection of vascular breast tumors: an in vitro study. Mat Sci Eng C 2020;107. https://doi.org/10.1016/j.msec.2019.110222.
50. González-Garcinuño A, Tabernero A, Nieto C, Martín del Valle E, Kenjeres S. Mutiphysics simulation of liposome release from hydrogels for cavity filling following patient-specific breast tumor surgery. Eur J Pharm Sci 2025;204. https://doi.org/10.1016/j.ejps.2024.106966.
51. Salavati H, Pullens P, Debbaut C, Ceelen W. Hydraulic conductivity of human cancer tissue: a hybrid study. Bioeng Trans Med 2023;9:e10617.
52. Yang Y, Zhan W. Role of tissue hydraulic permeability in convection-enhanced delivery of nanoparticle-encapsulated chemotherapy drugs to brain tumour. Pharm Res (N Y) 2022;39:877–92.
53. Stapleton S, Milosevic M, Allen C, Zheng J, Dunne M, Yeung I, et al. A mathematical model for enhanced permeability retention effect for liposome transport in solid tumors. PLoS One 2013;8:e81157.
54. Duzgunes N, Nir S. Mechanisms and kinetics of liposome-cell interactions. Adv Drug Del Rev 1999;40:3–18.
55. Vainsht I, Roskos LK, Cheng J, Sleeman MA, Wang B, Liang M. Quantitative measurement of the target-mediated internalization kinetics of biopharmaceuticals. Pharm Res (N Y) 2015;32:286–99.
56. Zhan W, Wang CH. Convection enhanced delivery of chemotherapeutic drugs into brain tumour. J Contr Release 2018;271:74–87.
57. Soltani M, Chen P. Effect of tumor shape and size on drug delivery to solid tumors. J Biol Eng 2012;6:4.
58. de Monte F, Pontrelli G, Becker S. Chapter 3: drug release in biological tissues. Transport in Biological Media 2013:59–118.
59. Yadav KS, Dalal DC. Penetration and distribution efficacy of chemotherapeutic drugs in biological tissues: a computational investigation. Mathem Comp Simul 2023;214:152–71.
60. Trucillo P. Drug carriers: a review on the most used mathematical models for drug release. Processes 2022; 10:1094.
61. Paul DR. Elaborations on the Higuchi model for drug delivery. Int. J. Pharm. 2011;418:13–17.
62. Peppas NA. A model of dissolution-controlled solute release from porous drug delivery polymeric systems. J Biomed Mater Res 1983;17:1079–87.
63. Peppas NA, Sahlin JJ. A simple equation for the description of solute release. III. Coupling of diffusion and relaxation. Int. J. Pharm. 1989;57:169–72.
64. Costa P, Sousa Lobo JM. Modeling and comparison of dissolution profiles. Eur J Pharm Sci 2001;13:123–33.
65. Corrigan OI, Li X. Quantifying drug release from PLGA nanoparticulates. Eur. J. Pharm. Sci. 2009;37:477–85.
66. Hopfenberg HB. Membranes. In: Polymers in Medicine and Surgery. Boston, MA, USA: Springer; 1975: 99–107 pp.
67. Eikenberry S. A tumor cord model for Doxorubicin delivery and dose optimization in solid tumors. Theor Biol Med Model 2009;6:16.
68. Di J, Hou P, Corpstein CD, Wu K, Xu Y, Li T. Multiphysics modelling and simulation of local transport and absorption kinetics of intramuscularly injected lipid nanoparticles. J Contr Release 2023;359:234–43.
69. Zheng F, Hou P, Corpstein CD, Xing L, Li T. Multiphysics modeling and simulation of subcutaneous injection and absorption of biotherapeutics: model development. Pharm Res (N Y) 2021;38:607–24.

70. Steuperaert M, D'Urso Labate GF, Debbaut C, De Wever O, Vanhove C, Ceelen W, et al. Mathematical modelling of intraperitoneal drug delivery: simulation of drug distribution in a single tumor nodule. Drug Deliv 2017;24:491–501.

71. Bhandari A, Gu B, Kashkooli FM, Zhan W. Image-based predictive modelling frameworks for personalized drug delivery in cancer therapy. J Contr Release 2024;370:721–46.

72. Adabbo G, Andreozzi A, Iasiello M, Vanoli GP. Numerical evaluation of heat-triggered drug release via thermos-sensitive liposomes: a comparison between image-based vascularized tumor and volume-averaged porous media models. Int J Heat Mass Transfer 2024;220. https://doi.org/10.1016/j.ijheatmasstransfer.2023.124942.

73. Jarrett AM, Hormuth DA, Wu C, Kazerouni AS, Erkut DA, Virostko J, et al. Evaluating patient-specific neoadjuvant regimens for breast cancer via mathematical model constrained by quantitative magnetic resonance imaging data. Neoplasia 2020;22:820–30.

74. Linninger AA, Somayaji MR, Mekarski M, Zhang L. Prediction of convection-enhanced drug delivery to the human brain. J Theor Biol 2008;250:125–38.

75. May CP, Kolokotroni E, Stamatakos GS, Büchler P. Coupling biomechanics to a cellular level model: an approach to patient-specific image driven multi-scale and Multiphysics tumor simulation. Prog Biophys Mol Biol 2011;107:193–9.

76. Bhandari A, Bansal A, Singh A, Sinha N. Perfusion kinetics in human brain tumor with DCE-MRI derived model and CFD analysis. J Biomech 2017;59:80–9.

77. Bhandari A, Bansal A, Singh A, Gupta RK, Sinha N. Comparison of transport of chemotherapeutic drug in voxelized heterogeneous model of human brain tumor. Microvasc Res 2019;124:76–90.

78. Zhan W, Gedroyc W, Xu XY. Effect of heterogeneous microvasculature distribution on drug delivery to solid tumour. J Phys D Appl Phys 2014;47. https://doi.org/10.1088/0022-3727/47/47/475401.

79. Wu C, Hormuth DA, Lorenzo G, Jarrett AM, Pineda F, Howard FM, et al. Towards patient-specific optimization of neoadjuvant treatment protocols for breast cancer based on image-guided fluid dynamics. IEEE Trans Biomed Eng 2022;69:3334–44.

80. Bhandari A, Jaiswal K, Singh A, Zhan W. Convection-enhanced delivery of antiangiogenic drugs and liposomal cytotoxic drugs to heterogeneous brain tumor for combination therapy. Cancers 2022;14:4177.

81. Vidotto M, Pederzani M, Castellano A, Pieri V, Falini A, Dini D, et al. Integrating diffusion tensor imaging and neurite orientation dispersion and density imaging to improve the predictive capabilities of CED models. Ann Biomed Eng 2021;49:689–702.

82. Caddy G, Stebbing J, Wakefield G, Adair M, Xu XY. Multiscale modelling of nanoparticle distribution in a realistic tumour geometry following local injection. Cancers 2022;14:5729.

83. Zhan W, Rodriguez y Baena F, Dini D. Effect of tissue permeability and drug diffusion anisotropy on convection-enhanced delivery. Drug Deliv 2019;26:773–81.

Nunzio Cancilla*, Luigi Gurreri, Michele Ciofalo, Andrea Cipollina,
Alessandro Tamburini and Giorgio Micale

9 Mathematical modelling of hollow-fiber haemodialysis modules

Abstract: This chapter provides an overview of the principles and modelling of membrane-based modules for haemodialysis, the most common renal replacement therapy. Following an introduction on the structure, function and diseases of the kidney, the technological evolution of membranes for blood purification is outlined and the main transport mechanisms involved are described, making a distinction between pure haemodialysis, haemodiafiltration and haemofiltration. The main performance figures of a hollow-fiber module are introduced and their dependence on the parameters that characterize the device is illustrated. A multi-scale modelling approach is then presented, in which preliminary single-fiber CFD simulations are used to derive the hydraulic permeability of a fiber bundle and the relevant mass transfer coefficients as functions of the local velocities. The predicted correlations are then fed to a module-scale model, in which blood and dialysate compartments are simulated as interpenetrated porous media while appropriate source terms account for the exchange of solutes and water between the two fluids. The model predictions are three-dimensional flow and concentration distributions, from which, in particular, performance figures such as clearance and ultrafiltration flow rate can be extracted as functions of the module geometrical and physical characteristics. Validation tests are also presented and the results of a parametrical sensitivity assessment are discussed.

Keywords: renal replacement treatment; haemodialysis; porous media; mass transfer; computational fluid dynamics; hollow-fiber membrane

9.1 Introduction

Although this chapter is dedicated to the mathematical modelling of renal replacement devices (notably haemodialysis modules), a brief introduction on the healthy kidney and

*Corresponding author: Nunzio Cancilla, Dipartimento di Ingegneria, Università Degli Studi di Palermo, Viale Delle Scienze Ed. 6, 90128 Palermo, Italy, E-mail: nunzio.cancilla@unipa.it. https://orcid.org/0000-0003-3065-3291
Luigi Gurreri, Dipartimento di Ingegneria Elettrica, Elettronica e Informatica, Università di Catania, Viale Andrea Doria 6 Ed. 3, 95125 Catania, Italy, E-mail: luigi.gurreri@unict.it
Michele Ciofalo, Andrea Cipollina, Alessandro Tamburini and Giorgio Micale, Dipartimento di Ingegneria, Università Degli Studi di Palermo, Viale Delle Scienze Ed. 6, 90128 Palermo, Italy,
E-mail: michele.ciofalo@unipa.it (M. Ciofalo), andrea.cipollina@unipa.it (A. Cipollina),
alessandro.tamburini@unipa.it (A. Tamburini), giorgiod.maria.micale@unipa.it (G. Micale)

As per De Gruyter's policy this article has previously been published in the journal Physical Sciences Reviews. Please cite as: N. Cancilla, L. Gurreri, M. Ciofalo, A. Cipollina, A. Tamburini and G. Micale "Mathematical modelling of hollow-fiber haemodialysis modules" *Physical Sciences Reviews* [Online] 2024. DOI: 10.1515/psr-2024-0062 | https://doi.org/10.1515/9783111394558-009

its pathologies can be useful to identify the functions that a replacement treatment must reproduce and the main causes that may make it necessary.

9.1.1 Structure and function of the kidney

The function of the kidney is to filter the blood, allowing free flux of water and small solutes (salts and potentially toxic molecules such as urea), but sieving macromolecules and retaining large plasma proteins (e.g. albumin) and all the cellular components of blood.

Most of these functions are accomplished in the kidney glomerulus [1]. As illustrated in Figure 9.1, it is a tuft of anastomosing capillaries surrounded by a spheroidal enclosure (Bowman's capsule). The blood enters the glomerulus through an afferent arteriole, which branches into the capillary tuft. The glomerular filtrate is forced out of the capillaries by the hydrostatic pressure of the blood, is collected in Bowman's capsule and is then funnelled into the renal tubule (whose proximal portion is visible in the bottom part of Figure 9.1), where re-absorption of most of the fluid and small ionic solutes (salts) occurs.

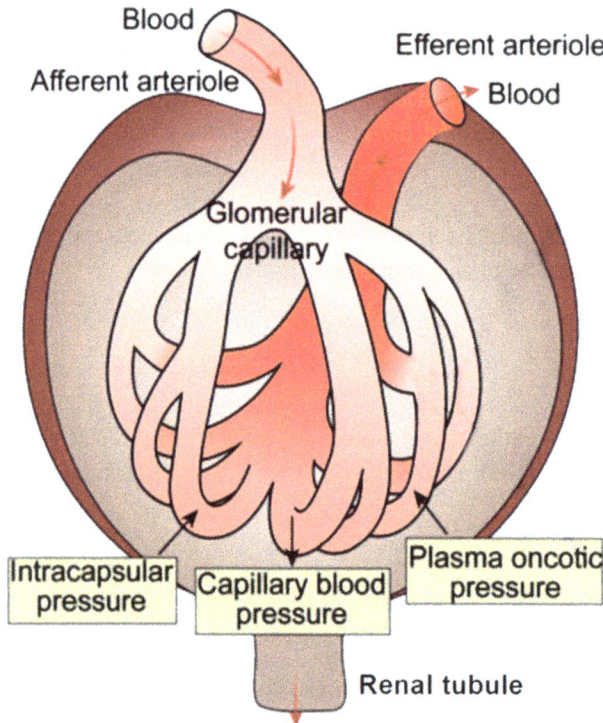

Figure 9.1: The kidney glomerulus. Reproduced (adapted) from Huang et al. [2].

The typical (relative) hydrostatic pressure in Bowman's capsule is ~20 mmHg, while that inside the glomerular capillaries is ~50 mmHg [3]; taking the adverse osmotic pressure gradient into account, the driving pressure difference (ultrafiltration pressure) is of the order of 10 mmHg, or ~1,330 Pa [4].

A section of the glomerular capillary wall (GCW) is shown schematically in Figure 9.2. It includes, from top to bottom (luminal to capsule sides):

- The endothelial layer, widely and irregularly fenestrated. **Fenestrae** have diameters of 50–100 nm and, unlike in other fenestrated capillaries, are not closed by true diaphragms;
- The glomerular basement membrane (GBM), or basal lamina;
- The foot processes (podocytes) of the epithelial cells, which face the urinary spaces (Bowman capsule) and are separated by gaps of ~25 nm (epithelial slits).

The GBM [5, 6] is the main structure where renal filtration takes place. It is composed of three layers, from luminal to capsule side: a **lamina rara interna** (LRI); a **lamina densa** (LD); and a **lamina rara externa** (LRE). In most mammals, the **lamina densa** is ~80–100 nm thick, while the **laminae rarae** are thinner (20–40 nm). The three **laminae** are all of fibrous nature, but differ in ultrastructure and chemical composition:

- The **laminae rarae** are networks of heparan sulphate proteoglycans and attachment glycoproteins including entactin, laminin and fibronectin, which anchor the endothelial or epithelial cells to the GBM and are continuous with their glycocalyx [7, 8];
- The **lamina densa** is a more compact fibrillar meshwork layer mainly containing type IV collagen and sialic acid; individual **fibrillae** are ~3 nm thick.

Several reviews of glomerular filtration and its molecular, structural and functional determinants have been presented [9, 10]. Generally speaking, the GBM has size–, shape–and charge–selective properties.

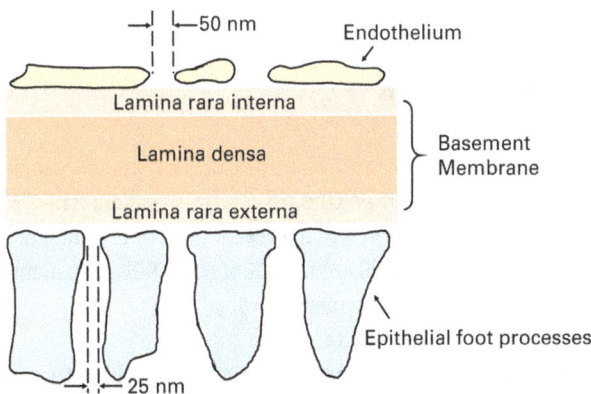

Figure 9.2: Cross section of the glomerular capillary wall (GCW).

- In regard to size selectivity, it has been known for a long time that large macromolecules do not have access to the urine [11]. Chang et al. [12], using dextran, showed that neutral molecules with diameters less or equal to that of inulin (2.8 nm) have a fractional clearance of 1; as size increases, the fractional clearance decreases following a sigmoidal curve and is ~0.1 for albumin (~7 nm diameter). The clearance for neutral molecules is practically zero for diameters above 8–9 nm in all animal species.
- In regard to charge selectivity, it is well known that the glomerular barrier is more permeable to cationic macromolecules, as a consequence of possessing fixed anionic charges [13–15].
- Also the shape and flexibility of molecular species can influence their transmission through the glomerular barrier [16]. For example, for the same molecular diameter, Ficoll – an uncharged, highly coiled polymer – is arrested in the glomerular capillary wall to a greater extent than the less coiled neutral dextran.

Bohrer et al. [17] compared clearance curves obtained in normal rats for neutral dextran, anionic dextran sulfate and cationic DEAE (Diethylaminoethyl) dextran, and showed that clearance was highest for the cationic species, lowest for the anionic one and intermediate for neutral dextran.

The main size–and charge–selective "sieve" in the GBM is the network of proteoglycans, particularly in the **lamina rara interna**. The GAG moieties of heparan sulphate proteoglycans are among the most highly negative (anionic) biomolecules, and their presence in the **laminae rarae**, where they are arranged in lattice-like regular arrays, is crucial to the size- and charge-selectivity of the glomerular capillary wall.

An additional function of the sulphated proteoglycans is to protect the glomerular capillary wall from being "clogged" by plasma macromolecules [18]. Work with synthetic membranes constructed from similar sulphated polymers [19] has shown that the sulphate groups are highly hydrophilic and thus do not form hydrogen bonds with the molecules present in the solution to be filtered; a similar mechanism may be operating in natural, biological membranes.

9.1.2 Kidney diseases and malfunction

Kidney diseases affect today over 850 million people in the world [20]. Two million people worldwide suffer from end-stage renal disease (ESRD), and the growth rate of patients is 5–7 % per year [21]. These figures are expected to increase due to the recent COVID–19 pandemic: according to the US National Institutes of Health, in 2020 around 5 % of the COVID–19 patients were having acute kidney injury requiring renal replacement therapy [22].

Renal diseases can be divided into two main groups:
- Acute kidney injury (AKI) refers to a kidney malfunction characterized by a rapid deterioration of its functions. AKI is usually reversible but an incomplete recovery can lead to progress to the later stages of the disease.

- Chronic kidney disease (CKD) refers to a sustained kidney damage indicated by the presence of structural or functional abnormalities. There are five levels of CKD, the last of which requires treatments such as dialysis or kidney transplantation as the only option.

Renal pathophysiology in general is treated, for example, by Leaf et al. [23]. Proteinuria, the anomalous increase of the excretion of proteins and other macromolecules in the urine, occurs whenever a pathologic or toxic condition alters the permselectivity of the renal glomerulus [24].

In the same paper cited shortly above [17], Bohrer et al. showed that the charge selectivity exhibited by clearance curves for normal rats was lost when rats affected by nephrotoxic serum nephritis (NSN) were tested. Similar results are obtained for other kidney diseases such as aminonucleoside nephrosis, or ANN [25, 26].

Puromycin, the drug used to induce ANN, causes changes in the structure of the glomerular wall similar to those seen clinically in patients with the so called minimal change nephrotic syndrome, or MCNS [27]. These effects are also similar to those produced by neuraminidase [18] and can be attributed to a partial disruption of the glycoprotein matrix in the epithelial glycocalix and in the **lamina rara externa** of the glomerular basement membrane. Robson et al. [28] and Bohrer et al. [29] observed that ANN or the related MCNS cause a reduced clearance of neutral molecules, but increase the clearance of anionic species (e.g. albumin). This is the effect expected if a partial disruption of anionic sites leads to macromolecular "clogging" of the GBM, thus reducing charge selectivity but possibly increasing the resistance to uncharged, large macromolecules.

Charge selectivity remains basically unchanged in other syndromes, e.g. autologus immune complex nephritis and adriamycin-induced proteinuria [30].

Barnes and Venkatachalam [31] studied the influence of polyanion neutralisation by the synthetic polycation polyethyleneimine (PEI) or by platelet factor 4 (PF4), which also behaves as a cationic macromolecule, on the glomerular permeability to native (anionic) and cationised ferritin in the rat. Neutralisation resulted in the increase (by a factor of 100 or more) of the clearance of native (anionic) ferritin, but affected to a much lesser extent that of cationised ferritin, confirming the electrostatic nature of the main glomerular resistance to anionic molecules. However, the residual influence of neutralisation on the penetration of cationic ferritin was interpreted as a sign that PEI somehow perturbed also the structural integrity (size selectivity) of the barrier; the simple neutralisation of polyanionic sites, with no change in the architecture of the glomerular basement membrane and its annexes, should lead to a reduction of the clearance of cationic probes, not to its (however moderate) increase. Platelet factor 4 was shown to bind avidly to glomerular polyanions, suggesting that endogenous cationic molecules released from platelets during immune glomerular disease may alter glomerular permeability and favour the precipitation of immune complexes.

Seiler et al. [32] observed that perfusion of rat kidneys with the polycation protamine sulphate produced a fusion of foot processes of the epithelium of glomerular capillaries similar to that observed in experimental nephrotic syndromes induced by puromycin or neurominidase (see above), but reversible by perfusion with the strong polyanion heparin. This suggests that neutralisation, and not removal, of glomerular polyanions is implied here. It also suggests that one of the consequences of nephrotic diseases and of polycation administration may be the loss of the repulsive forces between epithelial foot processes which maintain their normal architecture, thus leading to their disorganisation and fusion.

In regard to the influence of pressure and flow on the permeability of glomerular capillaries, Barnes and Venkatachalam [31] reported that changes in the kidney perfusion pressure had no effect on the permeability to ferritin. However, data from Chang et al. [12, 33] indicate a significant influence of glomerular capillary pressure and trans-capillary flow on dextran clearance profiles.

The effect of angiotensin has been studied, for example, by Eisenbach et al. [34], while the effect of vasodilators was investigated by Baylis et al. [35]. As expected, renal vasoconstriction reduces renal perfusion and glomerular filtration rate, whereas vasodilators like calcium antagonists reverse renal vasoconstriction and improve renal perfusion.

9.2 Membrane–based renal replacement treatments (RRT)

Most renal replacement treatments (RRT) are extracorporeal blood filtering procedures which typically make use of hollow fiber membrane modules. An alternative is peritoneal dialysis, a treatment which uses the body's own peritoneal membrane, lining the abdominal cavity and highly vascularized, to assist or replace the kidneys' functions. Waste solutes and excess water move through diffusion and ultrafiltration from the blood vessels into a fluid (dialysate) filling the peritoneal cavity. After a set amount of time, the dialysate with the filtered waste is let to flow out of the abdomen and is disposed of.

9.2.1 Technological evolution of membrane modules for haemodialysis

The basic functions of a haemodialysis membrane are the following:
- Separating waste solutes and excess fluid from the patient's blood;
- Restoring the electrolyte balance in the body;
- Achieving the lowest possible activation of blood components at the membrane surface (haemocompatibility);
- Possessing adequate thermal, mechanical and chemical stability (properties must remain unaltered during the manufacturing steps and the sterilization).

To this purpose, some characteristics are required. First, a thin and hydrophilic sepa-ration layer is necessary to provide high transmembrane flux in conjunction with low protein absorption. Second, the membrane should have a narrow pore size distribution to attain the right selectivity; the maximum pore size should be such that the loss of albumin is prevented. Third, a high overall porosity of the membrane wall is desired to achieve high hydraulic permeability. Finally, also the choice of the material is important for the characterization of the separation properties and the biocompatibility of the membrane.

Haemodialysis membranes have historically been classified into three categories according to the material composition of the polymers: unmodified cellulosic membranes, modified cellulosic membranes, and synthetic membranes [36–40].

Cellulosic membranes are highly hydrophilic due to the presence of hydroxyl groups, and form a hydrogel when absorbing water. Intensively used in the past, they have now been dismissed for two main reasons. One is their high permeability to water, which induces the swelling phenomenon enhancing water flow but reducing selectivity and, thus, compromising the patient's health. Another reason is that the hydroxyl groups cause biocompatibility problems [41–43]. Modified cellulose derivatives such as cellulose diacetate, cellulose triacetate, and diethylaminoethyl–substituted cellulose were devel-oped with the aim of improving biocompatibility. Most cellulose membranes (modified or not) have a thickness of 5–11 μm and a surface of 0.8–2.5 m².

Synthetic membranes are now those most used for dialysis treatments. Their thick-ness is 20–50 μm, larger than in cellulosic membranes [44]. They include sulphonated polyacrylonitrile and polymethylmethacrylate membranes [45], which are structur-ally symmetric (like the cellulosic membranes) and possess a uniform homogenous structure throughout the entire membrane wall. However, most synthetic membranes (i.e., polysulfone, polyethersulfone, polyamide, polyacrylonitrile polyvinylchloride copolymer) are asymmetric [36]. They are characterized by a thin selective skin layer of ~1 μm at the membrane–blood interface, where the actual separation process takes place, and by a thick spongy bulk providing mechanical strength. For high-flux syn-thetic membranes, the average pore size of the skin layer is usually in the range of 3–5 nm, while the pore size in the spongy layer can be greater than 10 nm. For low-flux synthetic membranes, the inner skin layer mean pore size is ~1 nm [46]. Polyethersulfone (PES) membranes are typically additivated using polyvinylpyrrolidone (PVP) to make the final hollow fibers sufficiently hydrophilic. PVP increases the viscosity of the polymer solution and improves the hollow fiber properties during manufacturing [47]. This blend is higher in porosity, with well-interconnected pores and a very small macrovoid formation. PVP is mainly located at the surface of the pores in the skin thanks to its hydrophilicity [48].

Another criterion often used to categorize dialysis membranes is their hydraulic permeability. The clinical parameter used is the ultrafiltration coefficient, K_{UF}, typically expressed in mL/(m² h mmHg) (multiply K_{UF} by ~$2 \cdot 10^{-12}$ to express it in SI units, i.e. m/(s Pa)). K_{UF} is empirically measured from *in vitro* experiments by membrane manufac-turers as the ratio between the ultrafiltration flow rate (Q_{UF}) and the transmembrane pressure. Membranes having K_{UF} lower than 10 mL/(m² h mmHg) are classified as low–

flux ones, those with K_{UF} higher than 25 mL/(m^2 h mmHg) as high–flux ones and those with $10 \leq K_{UF} \leq 25$ mL/(m^2 h mmHg) as medium-flux ones [44, 49].

9.2.2 Transport mechanisms of solute removal: haemodialysis, haemofiltration, haemodiafiltration

Haemodialysis is a membrane-based technique where solute removal primarily occurs through diffusion across the membrane [50]. It involves two fluids: the blood, containing toxic substances, and a rinsing solution called dialysate, separated by the membrane. The dialysate is prepared by diluting a concentrated aqueous solution of electrolytes and sometimes glucose with ultrapure water. It contains sodium, chloride and magnesium ions at concentrations equivalent to those found in normal plasma. To preserve the pH balance of the solution, bicarbonate or acetate may also be added [51, 52].

The core of the process is the semi-permeable membrane [44]. A membrane is characterized by its cutoff, defined as the lowest molecular weight of a solute 90 % of which is retained by the membrane. In haemodialysis, the cutoff can vary from one membrane to another but, usually, it is less than 50,000 Da. This value is slightly lower than the molecular weight of albumin (~69,000 Da), an important blood protein that, as already mentioned, must not be removed during the haemodialysis process as it regulates some biological functions such as the maintenance of osmotic pressure and the transport of various hormones.

Most devices used in haemodialysis therapies (haemodialyzers) are cylindrical modules, typically 2–5 cm in diameter and 15–25 cm in length. The housing is typically made from a transparent polymeric material, such as polycarbonate or polypropylene, and encompasses a bundle of several thousand (approximately 8,000–16,000) hollow fibers. The bundle has defined characteristics, including the fiber spatial arrangement and packing density. The module (Figure 9.3) is also equipped with inlet and outlet ports for the two fluids [53, 54].

Within the hollow fibers, blood flows through the lumen, while the dialysate flows outside the fiber bundle in a counter-current arrangement. The main driving force for

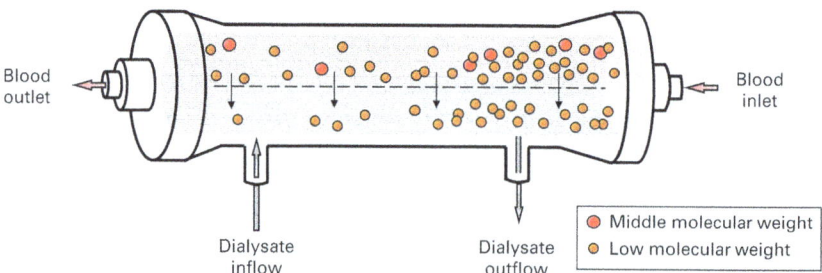

Figure 9.3: Schematic of the diffusion mechanism in a haemodialysis module.

solute mass transfer is the concentration gradient between the two compartments. Solutes are transferred from the blood to the dialysate through the membrane wall via diffusive–convective mass transfer, driven by both concentration gradients and pressure differences between the blood and dialysate [54].

In principle, haemodialysis can be divided into **standard** haemodialysis and **high-flux** haemodialysis, according to whether low-flux or high-flux membranes are employed. In modules using low-flux membranes, the contribution of ultrafiltration is negligible, while it is significant in high-flux modules, since they use membranes of higher hydraulic permeability.

Diffusive mass transfer mainly occurs according to the molecular weight of the solute to be removed. Solutes in the blood can be classified into three main categories, according to their molecular weight (Table 9.1), as defined by the European Uremic Toxin Work (EUTox).

Molecules with a molecular weight less than 500 Da (e.g. urea or creatinine) are referred to as low-molecular weight solutes [55, 56]; they are removed from the blood mainly by diffusion. In particular, urea is often used as the main marker for the success and control of the dialytic treatments. Medium-molecular weight solutes are in the range between 500 Da and 15,000 Da; they include various proteins (e.g., Beta–2 microglobulin). Solutes of this category are mainly removed by convective mass transport and the influence of convection on total removal rises with rising molecular size [57]. Molecules with molecular weight higher than 15,000 Da (e.g. Myoglobin and EPO) are considered high-molecular weight solutes.

Table 9.1: Molecular weight of the main solutes in human blood.

Solute	Molecular weight (Da)
Albumin	69,000
Erythropoietin (EPO)	34,000
Myoglobin	17,000
Beta–2 microglobulin	11,800
Endotoxin fragments	1,000–15,000
Inulin	5,200
Vancomycin	1,448
B_{12}Vitamin	1,355
Aluminum/Desferoaxamine complex	700
Glucose	180
Uric acid	168
Creatinine	113
Phosphate	80
Urea	60
Potassium	35
Phosphorus	31
Sodium	23

Significant diffusive removal can only occur if the membrane cut–off is greater than the size of the solute. In **standard haemodialysis** this threshold is very low, so that medium and high molecular weight solutes are not removed; in **high-flux** haemodialysis, the internal ultrafiltration caused by a transmembrane pressure gradient is not negligible [58, 59], so that convective mass transfer gives an important contribution, although it is smaller than in haemofiltration or haemodiafiltration.

In regard to flow rates, typical operating conditions are in the range 200–500 mL/min for the blood and 500–800 mL/min for the dialysate. The blood flow rate is limited by the vascular entry; regarding dialysate, the flow rate can potentially be enhanced, but clinical practice has shown that the upper limit is ~twice the blood flow rate. This condition is preferred in order to maximize the diffusive transport. If the blood flow rate is to be increased, also the dialysate one must be enhanced in order to keep this ratio constant.

Haemofiltration is a blood treatment in which a large amount of ultrafiltration is realized, through a high hydraulic pressure applied on the membrane, characterized by a high hydraulic permeability, without the use of a dialysis bath (Figure 9.4). Solute removal occurs only by convection, up to the membrane cutoff. This technique removes solutes with a molecular weight higher than those of the toxins rejected by **standard** haemodialysis treatments.

In haemofiltration, the plasmatic water subtracted by ultrafiltration is replaced by reinfusion. It is carried out with sterile and non-pyrogenic liquids with a controlled composition that allows the reconstitution of the blood volume. Reinfusion can take place before or after the blood purification in the module (**pre–** or **post–dilution**). Pre–dilution allows to operate in better blood rheological conditions, improving the performance of the module in the long term. In fact, the reinfusion leads to decreased values of haematocrit and viscosity: possible problems, such as **clotting** or coagulation inside the membranes, are thus limited. The disadvantage is that, by increasing the volume of the plasma before the treatment, the clearance of each solute is obviously lower. Conversely, post–dilution increases the risk of incurring in blood **clotting**, but allows for higher clearance values to be achieved. With haemofiltration, it is very difficult to obtain clearances for low molecular weight solutes (e.g., urea and creatinine) comparable to those achieved by haemodialysis. Therefore, on one

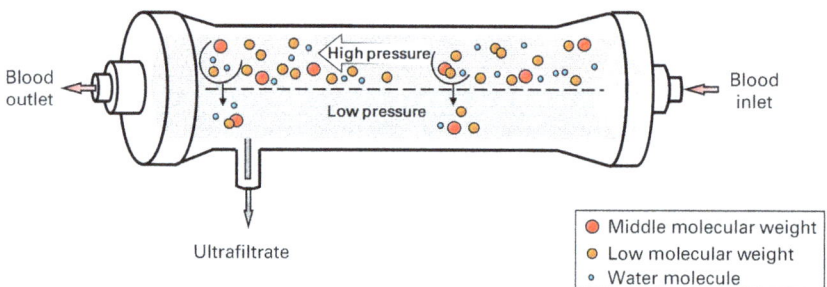

Figure 9.4: Schematic of the ultrafiltration mechanism in a haemofiltration module.

hand, haemofiltration guarantees better performance regarding medium–high molecular weight solutes while, on the other hand, it is characterized by a slower removal of the smaller solutes, actually reversing the problem of standard haemodialysis.

Haemodiafiltration is a diffusive and convective treatment which combines the advantages of haemofiltration with a good purification of small molecules allowed by the dialysate flow rate. Many researchers have studied the simultaneous effect of diffusion and convection on mass transfer [60–66]. The process consists of obtaining a certain amount of ultrafiltration, one part of which is reintegrated by infusion of suitable liquid (haemofiltration), and the other part is simultaneously passed through the module (haemodialysis). Also for haemodiafiltration, reinfusion can take place both before and after the module, although **post–dilution** is more common. The pros and cons of **pre–** and **post–dilution** are the same discussed above for haemofiltration. The two approaches are schematically illustrated in Figure 9.5.

There is a negative interference between diffusion and convection, so that, as the ultrafiltration flow rate increases, the convective effect also increases to the detriment of the diffusive one [67]. Thus, the removal of different molecular weight solutes can be selectively tuned, favouring diffusion or convection, by modifying Q_{UF}. A fairly common ultrafiltration flow rate for haemodiafiltration is Q_{UF} = 90 mL/min.

The introduction of the convective transport mechanism results in the appearance of **backfiltration**. It occurs when the transmembrane pressure gradient at some location in the module becomes negative: the dialysate pressure, together with the oncotic pressure, exceeds the pressure of the blood compartment. This allows the passage of water and solutes from dialysate to blood [68]. Rangel et al. [69] extensively reviewed various aspects of backfiltration, in particular the effect of increasing or diminishing this phenomenon in the different haemodialysis techniques, investigating the possibility of exploiting backfiltration to enhance the convective clearance of middle and large solutes.

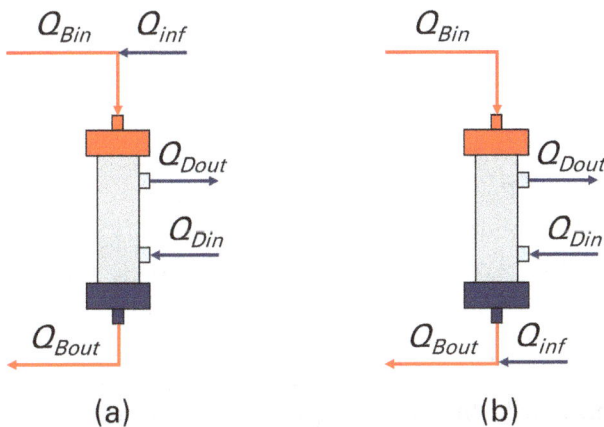

Figure 9.5: Schematic representation of modules for haemodiafiltration treatment: (a) reinfusion in pre–dilution and (b) reinfusion in post–dilution.

Table 9.2: Extracorporeal blood treatment for end–stage renal disease.

Treatment	Diffusive solute transport	Convective solute transport
Standard haemodialysis	High	Minimal
High flux haemodialysis	High	Medium
Haemodiafiltration	High	High–very high
Haemofiltration	None	Very high

Extracorporeal blood treatments for end–stage renal disease are summarized in Table 9.2, divided according to the transport phenomena involved.

9.3 Performance figures and quantities affecting them

For any given solute to be removed from the blood, the main performance figure characterizing a haemodiafiltration module is the clearance CL, commonly defined as the ratio of solute mass removal rate and solute concentration in the inflowing blood:

$$CL = \frac{Q_{Bin}C_{Bin} - Q_{Bout}C_{Bout}}{C_{Bin}} \tag{9.1}$$

where Q_{Bin} and Q_{Bout} are the blood flow rates at the module inlet and outlet, respectively, while C_{Bin} and C_{Bout} are the inlet and outlet bulk solute concentrations in the blood. Clearance can be interpreted as the blood volume which should be completely purified in the time unit to yield a given solute removal rate. For urea (MW = 60 Da), typical clearance values range from 80 % to 90 % of the inlet blood flow rate Q_{Bin} (e.g. from 240 to 270 mL/min for Q_{Bin} = 300 mL/min). Clearance values are markedly lower for larger solutes, e.g. from 50 % to 60 % of Q_{Bin} for B12 vitamin (MW = 1,355 Da).

A performance figure which characterizes the nature of the haemodiafiltration process occurring in the module is the ultrafiltration flow rate $Q_{UF} = Q_{Bin}-Q_{Bout}$, which is nil in pure haemodialysis and increases as the relative importance of ultrafiltration increases.

Eq. (9.1) can be re-formulated so as to evidence the contribution of Q_{UF}:

$$CL = \frac{C_{Bin} - C_{Bout}}{C_{Bin}}Q_{Bin} + \frac{C_{Bout}}{C_{Bin}}Q_{UF} \tag{9.2}$$

Performance figures depend on the physical, geometric and operating parameters characterizing the module, and the main object of a parametrical study aimed at improving or optimizing the module performance will be their prediction as functions of said parameters.

Assuming that the cylindrical, counter-flow configuration has been adopted, a possible set of such parameters includes the following 11 independent quantities:
- Fiber inner diameter, d_i
- Fiber outer diameter, d

- Blood inlet flow rate, Q_{Bin}
- Dialysate inlet flow rate, Q_{Din}
- Relative blood outlet pressure, p_{Bout}
- Module aspect ratio (active length to inner diameter), L/D
- Bundle porosity, ε
- Membrane surface area, S
- Membrane diffusive permeability, k_M
- Membrane hydraulic permeability, L_p
- Solute rejection coefficient σ

Also the geometry of the headers may play some role, by affecting to some extent the flow distribution in the module. Note that k_M and σ are solute-dependent, while all other parameters are the same for all solutes. Note also that, if blood and dialysate are regarded as incompressible fluids, their absolute pressure is irrelevant and thus the outlet pressure of the dialysate can be arbitrarily assumed as zero (i.e., all pressures will be interpreted as relative to it).

Other quantities characterizing the module can be derived from the above ones. For example, the following relations exist between bundle porosity ε, number of fibers N, fiber outer diameter d, and module inner diameter D and active length L:

$$1 - \varepsilon = \frac{N\pi d^2/4}{\pi D^2/4} \tag{9.3}$$

$$S = N\pi dL \tag{9.4}$$

(assuming the fibers to be straight and parallel), from which explicit expressions are obtained for the module inner diameter D and length L:

$$D = \left[\frac{Sd}{\pi(1-\varepsilon)(L/D)}\right]^{1/3} \tag{9.5}$$

$$L = \left[\frac{Sd}{\pi(1-\varepsilon)}\right]^{1/3}(L/D)^{2/3} \tag{9.6}$$

9.4 Small–scale (unit cell) modelling of the haemodialysis process

9.4.1 Regular lattices: single–fiber models

While the modelling of the lumen side flow is quite simple, the study of the shell side flow is more complex. A simplified way of modelling these devices is to consider a regular (square or hexagonal) uniform fiber lattice. A set of simplifying assumptions can be made:

- The flow is steady, fully developed and laminar.
- The fibers are cylindrical, straight and oriented parallel to the longitudinal z axis.
- All fibers have the same diameter.
- The flow and concentration structures strictly follow the spatial periodicity of the fiber arrangement.
- The fluid's physical properties, including density, dynamic viscosity and scalar diffusivity, are constant.
- Gravity is neglected, as its only effect in a constant-density fluid is to induce vertical static pressure stratification, which does not impact the flow field.

The first four assumptions allow the adoption of the unit cell approach [70]: the computational domain is two-dimensional and consists of a repetitive periodic unit of the bundle, including a single fiber.

The following sections mainly cover the case of fibers bundle arranged in a regular hexagonal lattice, since it represents the most realistic case with respect to a real bundle. Similar modelling strategies are adopted by several researchers [71–74] by assuming the fibers arranged in a square lattice. The different CFD modelling tools have been developed by finite-volume (FV) or finite-element (FE) methods. Several studies adopted commercial software, for example, Ansys CFX® [75] or Fluent® [76] (FV codes), or COMSOL Multiphysics® [77, 78] (FE code). The open-source FV OpenFOAM code [79] is another option.

9.4.1.1 Definitions for flow and mass transfer characterization

The bundle porosity ε was defined as:

$$\varepsilon = \frac{A}{A_{tot}} \tag{9.7}$$

in which A_{tot} is the total area while A is the fluid area in a generic cross section.

The definition of Reynolds number along a generic direction s of unit vector $\vec{\sigma}$ is:

$$\mathrm{Re}_s = \frac{\rho \langle u_s \rangle d_h}{\mu} \tag{9.8}$$

where ρ is density, μ is dynamic viscosity, $\langle u_s \rangle$ is the average of the superficial velocity component $u_s = \vec{u} \bullet \vec{\sigma} \varepsilon$ along the same direction and $d_h = 4\,V/S$ is the hydraulic diameter, V being the volume of fluid and S the wet surface in the computational domain (in a 2-D domain, d_h can be expressed as $4A/(\pi d)$). The Darcy friction coefficient f_s relative to the generic direction s is defined:

$$f_s = \frac{|dp/ds|2d_h}{\rho(u_s)^2} \qquad (9.9)$$

in which p is pressure. The Darcy permeability K_s relative to the generic direction s is:

$$K_s = \frac{\mu(u_s)}{|dp/ds|} \qquad (9.10)$$

In the literature, the permeability is often expressed in dimensionless form, e.g. as K_s/d^2 (d being the outer fiber diameter) or by introducing the so called Kozeny "constant" k_K:

$$k_K = \frac{\varepsilon^3}{(1-\varepsilon)^2} \frac{1}{\Sigma^2 K_s} \qquad (9.11)$$

where Σ is the specific surface of the medium particles (for cylinders, $\Sigma = 4/d$). Eq. (9.11) is usually adopted under the assumption of an isotropic permeability, so that the direction subscript "s" can be omitted from K.

In regard to mass transfer, the average shell-side mass transport coefficient k_D is:

$$k_D = \frac{\bar{J}}{\bar{C}_w - C_b} \qquad (9.12)$$

in which $\bar{J}$ is the wall–averaged molar flux at the wall, $\bar{C}_w$ is the wall–averaged solute concentration at the wall and C_b is the bulk concentration, defined as the mass flow–weighted average of the solute concentration on an arbitrary cross section.

Consistently, the average shell-side Sherwood number is calculated as:

$$\text{Sh} = k_D \frac{d_h}{D} \qquad (9.13)$$

where D is the diffusion coefficient of the solute.

9.4.1.2 Governing equations and physical properties

For a Newtonian incompressible fluid, the steady-state continuity and momentum equations are:

$$\nabla \cdot \mathbf{u} = 0 \qquad (9.14)$$
$$\rho \mathbf{u} \cdot \nabla \mathbf{u} = -\nabla p + \mu \nabla^2 \mathbf{u} \qquad (9.15)$$

in which $\mathbf{u}$ is the local velocity vector and p is pressure.

The convection–diffusion transport equation governing the concentration field is:

$$\mathbf{u} \cdot \nabla C = D\nabla^2 C \qquad (9.16)$$

C being the solute concentration and D its diffusion coefficient in the fluid.

The fluid was representative of the dialysate in a haemodialysis module. The solution properties were set to $\rho = 1{,}000 \text{ kg/m}^3$, $\mu = 7.62 \cdot 10^{-4}$ Pa s. For urea, the diffusivity D of the solute in the solution was set to $1.8 \cdot 10^{-9}$ m^2/s, so that the Schmidt number, $\mu/(\rho D)$, was 423. For B12-vitamin, D was set to $5 \cdot 10^{-10}$ m^2/s so that the Schmidt number was 1,524.

9.4.1.3 Treatment of periodicity for unit cell simulations

In the unit cell approach, in a spatially periodic computational domain, translational periodicity boundary conditions are imposed to all variables on the couples of opposite boundaries under the hypothesis of fully developed flow and concentration fields. However, it is necessary to allow for a streamwise variation of pressure, due to the hydraulic resistance of the medium, and of the bulk concentration, due to solute inflow or outflow through the membrane fiber wall. To this purpose, Eqs. (9.15) and (9.16) are treated as follows.

In the fully-developed region of a bundle, the static pressure $p(x, y, z)$ and the concentration $C(x, y, z)$ are decomposed into spatially periodic components $\tilde{p}(x, y, z)$ and $\tilde{C}(x, y, z)$, respectively, whose spatial distribution repeats itself identically in each unit cell, and large-scale components ($-G_p s$ and $G_c s$, respectively) linearly varying with a coordinate s:

$$p(x, y, z) = \tilde{p}(x, y, z) - G_p s \tag{9.17}$$

$$C(x, y, z) = \tilde{C}(x, y, z) + G_c s \tag{9.18}$$

By substituting p and C as expressed by Eqs. (9.17) and (9.18), respectively, in the momentum (Eq. (9.15)) and convection–diffusion (Eq. (9.16)) equations, they become:

$$\rho \mathbf{u} \cdot \nabla \mathbf{u} = -\nabla \tilde{p} + \mu \nabla^2 \mathbf{u} + \mathbf{f} \tag{9.19}$$

$$\mathbf{u} \cdot \nabla \tilde{C} = D \nabla^2 \tilde{C} + S_C \tag{9.20}$$

where $\mathbf{f} = G_p \vec{\sigma}$ is a forcing term along the arbitrary direction of unit vector $\vec{\sigma}$, accounting for the non-periodic component of the pressure gradient and compensating for large-scale pressure loss, and $S_C = -G_c u_s$ is a source term compensating the large-scale concentration gradient. From a global balance of solute in the computational domain, G_c can be written as:

$$G_c = \frac{\bar{J} S}{V} \frac{1}{\langle u_s \rangle} \tag{9.21}$$

in which the quantity $\bar{J} \, S/V$ is the average value of the source term and $\langle u_s \rangle$ is the volume-averaged velocity component along the s direction.

Apart from numerical approximations, this approach guarantees solute mass conservation: the mean value of the bulk concentration adopted as the initial guess is conserved through the simulation.

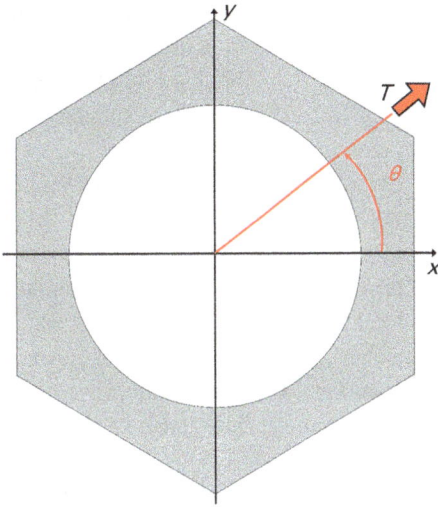

Figure 9.6: 2-D cross section of a regular hexagonal lattice with ε = 0.5. The cross flow attack angle θ and the mean cross flow direction T in the xy plane are indicated.

9.4.1.4 Computational domain and boundary conditions

Figure 9.6 shows the 2-D computational domain (unit cell) for a regular hexagonal lattice with bundle porosity ε = 0.5, a typical value for commercial haemodialyzers.

As shown in Figure 9.6, the cross-flow attack angle θ is the angle formed in the xy plane by the mean flow direction T with the x-axis. In addition to the longitudinal Reynolds number Re_z, which is calculated using the mean superficial velocity $\langle u_z \rangle$ along the axial direction z, a cross flow Reynolds number Re_T can also be determined. It is defined using the mean superficial velocity $\langle u_T \rangle$, resultant from the mean superficial velocities $\langle u_x \rangle$, $\langle u_y \rangle$

$$\langle u_T \rangle = \langle u_x \rangle \cos\theta + \langle u_y \rangle \sin\theta \qquad (9.22)$$

In regard to hydrodynamics, the cylindrical surfaces representing mass exchange walls were considered as no slip walls.

In regard to mass transfer, a Neumann boundary condition was typically applied, with an arbitrarily assigned value for the mass flux (Sherwood numbers remain unaffected by this choice). The motivation behind this is that the mass flux J crossing the membrane can be described as $\Delta C/(r_l + r_m + r_s)$, in which ΔC is the bulk concentration difference between the lumen and the shell sides, and r_l, r_m and r_s represent the areal resistances of lumen-, membrane- and shell-side, respectively. In haemodialysis, the resistance associated with the membrane is usually the largest between the three resistances in series. Both r_l and r_m can be considered uniform around the circumference of a fiber. On the other hand, the only component showing significant circumferential variations is $r_s = k_D^{-1}$, see Eq. (9.12), which is only a minor component of the overall resistance. Consequently, J is expected to be almost uniform around a fiber, making Neumann boundary conditions the most representative of the real-world scenarios.

In some simulations, Dirichlet boundary conditions were also evaluated, with the wall concentration set to an arbitrary uniform value (which does not impact k_D). For both boundary conditions, another arbitrary value was assigned to the bulk concentration of the dialysate. As explained in Section 9.4.1.3, periodicity conditions were applied to all variables at the opposite boundaries of the computational domain.

All runs were conducted in double precision and were stopped once the dimensionless residuals of all variables reduced below 10^{-12}, indicating a very stringent convergence criterion.

A careful grid-independence analysis on the present geometry [75] revealed that both triangular and quadrilateral meshes converge to the same results for increasing number of cells. Convergence is achieved earlier (i.e., for a smaller number of cells) for quadrilateral meshes. ~16,000 cells in the domain's cross sectional plane are sufficient to achieve practically grid-independent results (discrepancy < 1 % with respect to the finest grids tested, which included ~128,000 cells in the same plane).

By applying the methodology described in the previous sections, Cancilla et al. [75] developed a single-fiber (unit-cell scale) model. Numerous simulations were carried out, allowing the longitudinal Reynolds number, Re_z, the cross flow Reynolds number, Re_T, and the cross flow attack angle, θ, to vary. For each set of input parameter, the main computational results included the axial and cross-flow Darcy friction coefficients (or Darcy permeabilities) and the average Sherwood number.

9.4.1.5 Results for axial flow

In axial flow, a pressure gradient was imposed only along the z direction. The Darcy friction coefficient f_z closely follows a Re_z^{-1} behavior, indicating that the permeability K_z, is independent of Re_z. The values of the product $f_z Re_z$, K_z, Kozeny's "constant" and average Sherwood numbers are reported in Table 9.3. For comparison purposes, results for the square lattice are also given.

For $\varepsilon = 0.5$, the two lattices provided quite different friction coefficients, with the hexagonal lattice exhibiting a ~23 % higher value. A comparison of the CFD predictions in [75] with other results from the literature can be performed using the Kozeny "constant"

Table 9.3: Values of $f_z \cdot Re_z$, permeability K_z, Kozeny's k_K and average Sherwood numbers predicted for regular lattices in axial flow at $\varepsilon = 0.5$. From results in [75].

Geometry	Hexagonal	Square
$f_z \cdot Re_z$ [–]	226	180
$K_z \cdot 10^{10}$ [m^2]	7.60	9.54
Kozeny's k_K [–]	3.57	2.88
Sh, uniform wall mass flux [–]	9.86	5.15
$Sh^{(CW)}$, uniform wall concentration [–]	9.90	5.82

k_K as defined by Eq. (9.11), which remains unaffected by the fiber diameter. The results in [75] yielded $k_K \approx 3.57$ and $k_K \approx 2.88$ for the hexagonal and the square lattice, respectively, which are in good agreement with the literature. Happel [72] formulated a simplified analytical model that does not depend on the fiber array. For flow parallel to cylinders at $\varepsilon = 0.5$, the calculated k_K value was 3.67. Sparrow and Loeffler [73] derived analytical solutions for longitudinal laminar flow between cylinders in hexagonal or in square lattices. Their prediction indicated k_K values of ~3.5 and ~2.9, respectively. Skartsis et al. [80] presented both experimental and theoretical results from various authors for axial flow through straight cylinder configurations. This includes the numerical solution by Larson and Higdon's [81] for square lattices, which estimates k_K to be approximately 2.75 at $\varepsilon = 0.5$.

In regard to mass transfer, the predicted Sherwood number remains unchanged as the longitudinal Reynolds number rises. Table 9.3 provides the Sherwood numbers Sh calculated for uniform wall mass flux boundary conditions, as well as the $Sh^{(CW)}$ values calculated for uniform wall concentration boundary conditions. For the hexagonal lattice, the Sherwood number is significantly higher compared to the square one. The Sherwood number values predicted under different boundary conditions are much closer to each other in the case of the hexagonal lattice compared to the square lattice.

Experimental measurements of the shell-side mass transfer coefficient in fiber bundles are influenced by entry effects as well as irregularities within the bundle that induce cross flow. As a result, experiments often deviate from the assumption of fully developed, purely axial flow and typically reveal a certain degree of Reynolds number dependence in the Sherwood number [82].

9.4.1.6 Results for cross flow

In cross flow, a driving pressure gradient was applied only within the cross-sectional plane, involving both x and y components. Both the Darcy permeability K_T and the Sherwood number Sh are expected to vary with changes in the cross flow Reynolds number Re_T and the cross flow attack angle θ. The simulation results reported in [75] predicted a complex behavior.

In the hexagonal lattice, the angular dependence of any quantity follows a 60° periodicity. However, it is sufficient to study θ only between 0 and 30°, as the range from 30° to 60° can be obtained through reflection about the 30° direction.

The dependence of the permeability on the flow attack angle is shown in Figure 9.7(a), which reports the polar chart of the Darcy permeability K_T for different values of the cross flow Reynolds number Re_T (10, 30, 50, 100). Up to $Re_T \approx 10$ there is practically no influence of θ: the fiber lattice is hydraulically isotropic and the flow is self-similar. At higher Re_T, as inertial effects become significant, also anisotropy does: K_T departs from the uniform trend and starts to depend on θ. K_T develops an absolute maximum for $\theta = 0°$ (or 60°) and a minimum for $\theta = 30°$, which are the directions of symmetry of the hexagonal

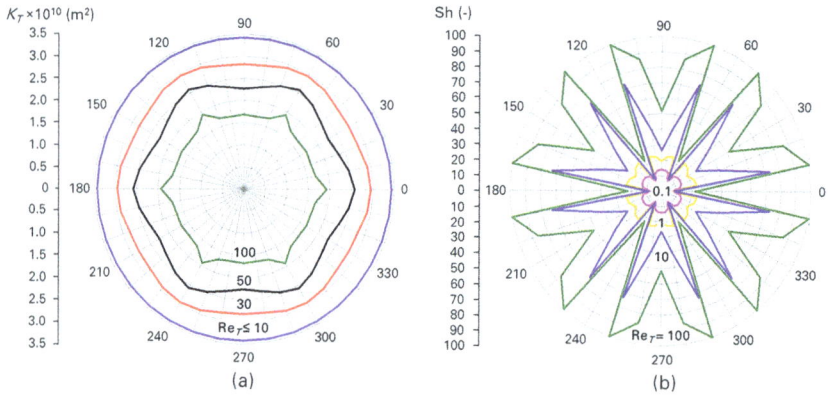

Figure 9.7: Polar chart of the Darcy permeability K_T (a) and of the Sherwood number (b) for cross flow in a hexagonal lattice with $\varepsilon = 0.5$ at different values of the Reynolds number Re_T. Data from [75].

lattice. As Re_T increases further ($Re_T > 50$), the maximum at 0°–60° persists but a secondary maximum develops for $\theta = 30°$, while two minima appear for $\theta° \approx 15°$ and 45°.

The simultaneous dependence of mass transfer on Re_T and θ is evidenced in Figure 9.7(b), which reports the polar chart of the uniform wall mass flux Sherwood number, Sh, for four values of Re_T (0.1, 1, 10 and 100). Only at very low Reynolds numbers ($Re_T = 0.1$) Sh is about uniform with θ whereas, already at $Re_T = 1$, it develops maxima at $\theta \approx 10$ and 50° ($+k \cdot 60°$) and two minima at $\theta = 0°$ and 30° ($+k \cdot 60°$) (symmetry directions).

The comparison of graphs (a) and (b) of Figure 9.7 reveals that the hexagonal lattice remains hydraulically almost isotropic up to $Re_T \approx 10$ but, in regard to mass transfer, exhibits anisotropy at significantly lower Re_T values (0.1–1).

Figure 9.8 reports maps of the normalized velocity u^* and of the dimensionless concentration C^* (for urea) in the unit cell of a regular hexagonal lattice with $\varepsilon = 0.5$. The angle is $\theta = 30°$ and two different values of Re_T (0.001 and 0.01, respectively) are considered. These two quantities are defined here as:

$$u^* = \frac{u}{\langle u_T \rangle} \tag{9.23}$$

$$C^* = \frac{\tilde{C} - C_b}{C_w - C_b} \tag{9.24}$$

(refer to Section 9.4.1.1 for the various definitions).

Although maps (a) and (b) of u^* in Figure 9.8 show that the flow is self-similar, the comparison of maps (c) and (d) for C^* shows how the fluid flow, even at low Re_T values, has a considerable impact on the scalar distribution. The thick line in the C^* maps represents the iso-concentration curve $C^* = 0$, i.e. $\tilde{C} = C_b$.

At $Re_T = 0.01$, map (d), the concentration at the wall consistently exceeds C_b. Otherwise, at very low $Re_T = 0.001$, map (c), the iso-line $\tilde{C} = C_b$ intersects the wall, resulting in some

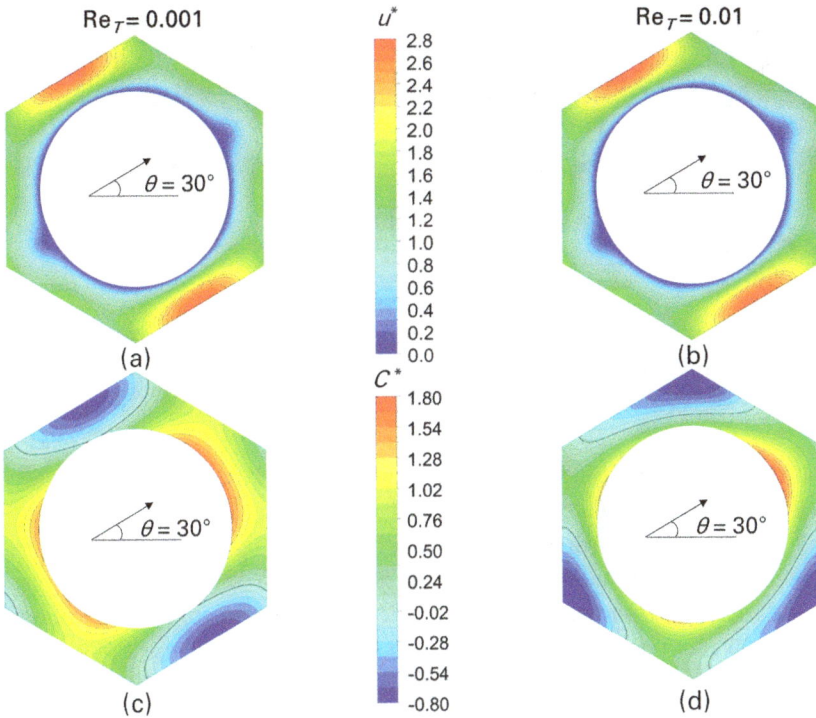

Figure 9.8: Normalized velocity (a, b) and dimensionless concentration (c, d) in the unit cell of a hexagonal lattice with $\varepsilon = 0.5$ for $\theta = 30°$: (a, c) $Re_T = 0.001$; (b, d) $Re_T = 0.01$. Reproduced (adapted) from [75], with permission from Elsevier (2021).

regions where $C_w > C_b$, others where $C_w < C_b$, and some points where $C_w = C_b$. In this case, the concentration distribution is nearly symmetrical between the upstream and downstream regions of the wall. However, at $Re_T = 0.01$, advection disrupts this symmetry, resulting in a distinctly asymmetric scalar distribution. This is attributable to the high Schmidt number (423): the transverse Péclet number, $Re_T Sc$, is 0.423 in case (c) and 4.23 in case (d). Although these values are low, they are not insignificant. Even as the cross flow Reynolds number approaches zero, the concentration distribution does not align with the centro-symmetric configuration expected in pure diffusion or purely axial flow. On the contrary, the scalar distributions along the flow direction and its perpendicular direction remain distinctly different. The intricate manner in which the cross flow distorts the iso-concentration curves accounts for the complex and non-monotonic relationship between the Sherwood number and Re_T, as illustrated in Figure 9.7(b).

The efficiency of solute transfer from the lumen-side compartment to the dialysate, and thus the magnitude of the Sherwood number, is closely tied to the shape of the iso-concentration profiles for various cross flow attack angles. For example, Figure 9.9 shows simplified concentration maps for three angles (0°, 15° and 30°) at $Re_T = 1$. For clarity, a

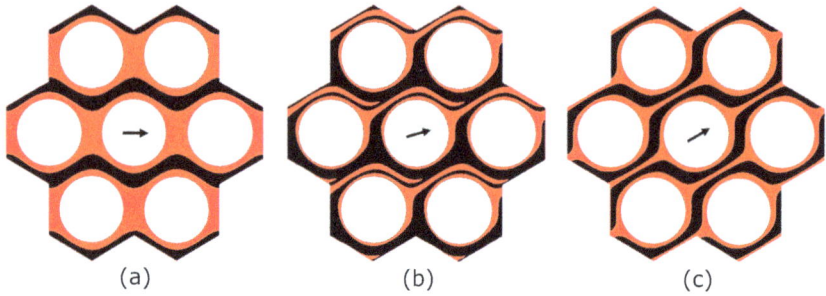

Figure 9.9: Simplified concentration maps in a hexagonal lattice at $Re_T = 1$, uniform wall mass flux and three different flow attack angles: (a) $\theta = 0°$; (b) $\theta = 15°$; (c) $\theta = 30°$. Red regions: $C > C_b$; black regions: $C < C_b$. The arrows denote the mean cross flow direction. Reproduced (adapted) from [75], with permission from Elsevier (2021).

section of the lattice comprising seven periodic unit cells is illustrated. Regions where $C < C_b$ are shown in black, while regions in which $C > C_b$ are in red.

At $\theta = 0°$, the wake with high concentration formed downstream of each fiber merges directly with the wake of the following fiber, resulting in a wide area of high concentration that impairs mass transfer. A comparable effect is observed, albeit to a lesser extent, at $\theta = 30°$. Conversely, at $\theta = 15°$, a direction that does not align with the lattice symmetry, the high concentration wake meanders around the fibers before eventually merging with the bulk flow. This significantly thins the concentration boundary layer and lowers the mean concentration at the fiber wall, leading to an improvement in mass transfer efficiency.

9.4.2 Non-ideal phenomena: effects of non-uniform and random fiber distributions

A common issue of haemodialyzers and, more in general, of hollow-fiber membrane contactors, is the management of shell-side non-ideal flow phenomena originating from the non-uniform fibers distribution. The most common one, usually named in the literature as **channelling** [83, 84], occurs when the dialysate flows mainly through preferential passages of the bundle while in some regions the fluid is essentially stagnant. As reported, among others, by Bao and Lipscomb [85, 86], this phenomenon is observed in axial, cross- and mixed flow across non-uniform bundle distributions. Recently, several researchers have dealt with this topic. Sun et al. [87] investigated the influence on the performance of an axial-flow hollow fiber contactor presenting a radially non-uniform porosity between the core and peripheral regions of the bundle. Also Cancilla et al. numerically studied the effects of a non-uniform porosity on shell-side flow and mass transfer in both axial-flow [88] and cross-flow [89] conditions. The most noteworthy conclusion is that, in axial flow, non-uniformity produces a significant rise of the Darcy

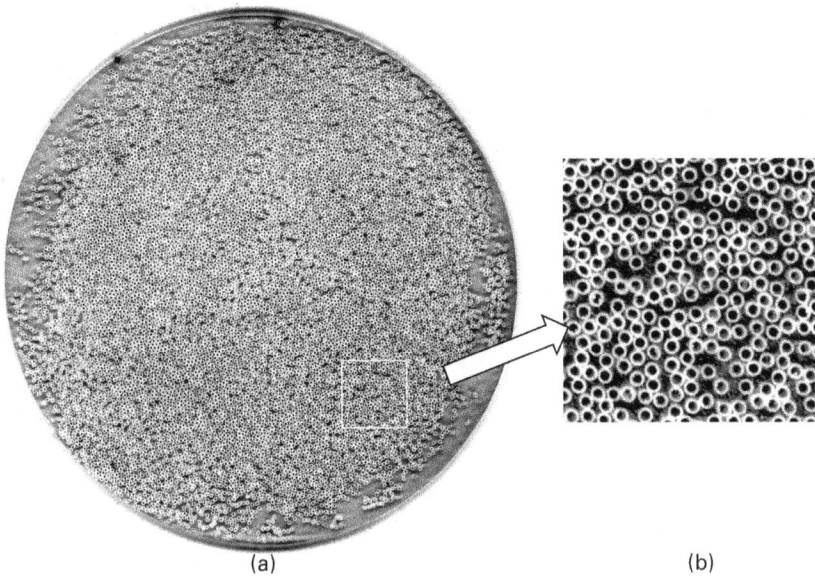

Figure 9.10: Scanned images of a cross section of a real hollow fiber bundle used in a commercial haemodialyzer (Clearum™ HS Series high flux dialyzer, manufacturer: Medtronic®): (a) entire bundle (diameter ~40 mm, ~10,000 fibers, mean porosity ~0.5); (b) detail of a 5 × 5 mm square portion, exhibiting the non-uniform fiber distribution.

permeability and an even larger drop of the mass transfer coefficient. In cross-flow the behaviour is more complex, being observed a more important dependence both on the cross-flow attack angle and on the Reynolds number considered.

Figure 9.10 shows a cross-sectional view of a hollow fiber bundle for haemodialysis.

The peripheral regions, close to the cylindrical housing of the contactor, exhibit an appreciably lower packing density compared to the central one. Even within the central regions, although this displays a more uniform distribution, scattered gaps intermingled with clusters of densely packed fibers can be observed, see magnification in Figure 9.10(b). Similar insights were also reported by Frank et al. [90].

In axial flow, simulations for random clusters of fibers predicted values of f_z which follow almost exactly a Re_z^{-1} trend, as already observed for the regular lattices in Section 9.4.1.5. The Darcy permeability K_z increases by 1.85 times with respect to the hexagonal lattice and 1.47 times with respect to the square lattice at the same porosity. In regard to mass transfer, the value of the Sherwood number is constant as Re_z increases, as expected in axial flow. Notably, as pointed out by Bao and Libscomb [86], results for random fiber arrangements show that mass transfer coefficients decrease dramatically in the fully developed region: values of Sh predicted for random distributions are only 5–10 % of those predicted for regular lattices. This large drop is due to high flows through regions of the bundle characterized by high local porosity (channelling). Similar conclusion was also obtained by the present authors [88], who studied the channelling phenomenon using a simplified approach.

In cross flow conditions, random clusters of fibers behave as an orthotropic medium at low Reynolds numbers and their permeability polar chart changes little in amplitude, shape and orientation at higher Reynolds numbers. The amount of anisotropy of random distributions is very large only for small clusters (~16 fibers) and decreases with the number of fibers, until it becomes negligible for clusters embedding more than 100 fibers [113]. This scale-dependence of the anisotropy should be kept in mind when choosing a finite cluster of random fibers as computationally representative of a much larger set. Of course, ensemble averaging over a sufficient number of realizations destroys anisotropy. Ensemble averaged values of the Darcy permeability exhibited a significant decrease with respect to the values computed for both square and hexagonal regular lattices: notably, the lower the porosity, the highest the decrease. On the other hand, at $\varepsilon = 0.8$–0.9, permeabilities computed for random clusters start to coincide with those for regular arrays [91–95]. In regard to mass transfer, random realizations of 81 fibers exhibited a quite isotropic polar chart of the average shell-side Sherwood number. At $\varepsilon = 0.5$ (a typical value for most commercial haemodialyzers), Sh varies in a narrow range of values, exhibiting a reduction of ~ 20–50 % with respect to the angle-averaged value predicted for regular lattices. As noted for hydrodynamics, ensemble averaging over an adequate number of realizations destroys such anisotropy.

9.5 Module-scale 3–D porous media models

The most effective method for modelling haemodialyzers is likely the porous media approach. This method involves treating one or both fluids as moving through aniso-tropic porous media, as described by Darcy's law. Hydraulic permeabilities and mass transfer coefficients are obtained either through numerical simulations of a single fiber or based on experimental data. For example, Lemanski and Lipscomb [96] used literature values for the Darcy permeability [97, 98] in regular fibers arrays. They performed a theoretical 2-D analysis of shell-side flow and its influence on mass transfer neglecting ultrafiltration. Liao et al. [99] addressed this limitation, by incorporating both convection and diffusion into their 2-D model. The shell-side was treated as a porous medium with Darcy permeabilities derived from experiments as well as membrane properties. Eloot et al. [100] implemented a CFD model of a haemodialyzer, defining the blood and dialysate compartments as two porous media with uniform axial and radial permeabilities. Other 2-D models using the concept of interpenetrating porous media include those developed by Łabęcki et al. [101], Lemanski and Lipscomb [102] and Ding et al. [103]. Ding et al. [104] developed a 3-D model of a haemodialyzer to more accurately capture the effects of inlet and outlet headers and the interaction between blood and dialysate flows. Darcy per-meabilities were sourced from existing literature; the authors used a global mass transfer coefficient obtained from experimental data in the literature.

In this section, starting from the concept of two interpenetrating porous media, the model of fluid flow and mass transfer in hollow fiber modules for haemodialysis proposed by Cancilla et al. [105] is reported. The model is based on two-scale approach. Predictions from single-fiber models at a small-scale level (refer to Section 9.4) were translated into equivalent properties for a porous medium. Simulations at the module-scale were then carried out to predict the three-dimensional flow fields and solute concentrations in both the blood and dialysate compartments of a haemodialyzer.

9.5.1 Small-scale CFD correlations

The main results that can be carried over from the unit cell-scale model discussed in Section 9.4 to the porous media model of the whole haemodialyzer are the shell-side axial and cross flow Darcy permeabilities and the shell-side Sherwood number.

In regard to Darcy permeabilities K_z and K_T, suitable two-parameters correlations derived by fitting in the range $0.2 < \varepsilon < 0.8$ the CFD results reported in [106] are:

$$K_z = \left(10^{-4} d^2\right) \cdot \exp\left(9.2\varepsilon\right) \tag{9.25}$$

$$K_T = \left(1.66 \cdot 10^{-1} d^2\right) \cdot \varepsilon^5 \tag{9.26}$$

For the shell-side Sherwood number, a correlation of the CFD results reported in Section 9.4 for regular hexagonal lattices with $\varepsilon = 0.5$ is:

$$Sh = a\left(1 + b \cdot Re_T^c\right) \tag{9.27}$$

For $a = 9.85$, $b = 1.41$ and $c = 0.38$, Eq. (9.27) align well with the CFD results of the single-fiber model within the Reynolds number range $Re_T = 0.005$–50. The coefficient a is chosen to ensure that, at $Re_T = 0$, the correlation yields the value of Sh for purely axial flow. The Sherwood number estimated by Eq. (9.27) represents an average value across all possible cross-flow directions relative to a hexagonal lattice. The results reported in Section 9.4 showed that at the low Reynolds numbers (approximately 0.1–1) typical of a real haemodialyzer, the orientation of the cross flow has limited effects on the Sherwood number.

For the lumen side Sherwood number, a value of 4 was adopted as a compromise between the exact values for uniform wall concentration and uniform wall mass flux in circular pipes, which are 3.66 and 4.36, respectively [107].

9.5.2 Porous media approach

The fluid on each side (whether blood or dialysate) was modelled as flowing through its own distinct equivalent porous medium. Each porous medium was characterized by its bundle porosity ε and the addition of the following momentum source terms to the right-hand side of the momentum (Navier–Stokes) equations:

$$S_{M,T} = -\frac{\mu}{K_T}\langle u_T \rangle \tag{9.28}$$

$$S_{M,z} = -\frac{\mu}{K_z}\langle u_z \rangle \tag{9.29}$$

in which $\langle u_T \rangle$ and $\langle u_z \rangle$ are the superficial velocities along the T and z directions, respectively. For the Darcy permeabilities K_z and K_T, equations (9.25) and (9.26) were adopted.

To account for ultrafiltration effects, the mass source term S_M (kg m^{-3} s^{-1}) was added to the right-hand side of the continuity equation:

$$S_M = \pm\frac{A_{ext}}{V_{tot}}\rho L_p \left(p_B - p_D - p_{onc}\right) \tag{9.30}$$

where the "plus" sign is used for dialysate and the "minus" sign for blood; A_{ext} is the total external surface area of the hollow fibers, V_{tot} is the total volume of the module, L_p is the hydraulic permeability of the membrane, p_B and p_D are the pressures in the blood and dialysate compartments, respectively, and p_{onc} is the oncotic pressure of the blood proteins. Likewise, to account for solute mass flux, the source term S_C (in mol m^{-3} s^{-1}) was added to the right-hand side of the scalar transport equation for the solute:

$$S_C = \pm\frac{A_{ext}}{V_{tot}}j \tag{9.31}$$

with, again, the "plus" sign applying to dialysate and the "minus" sign to blood. The total molar flux of solute per unit membrane area, j, expressed (in mol m^{-2} s^{-1}), is:

$$j = L_p \cdot \left(p_B - p_D - p_{onc}\right) \cdot (1 - \sigma) \cdot C_M + U \cdot (C_B - C_D) \tag{9.32}$$

The first term of Eq. (9.32) accounts for the convective contribution to mass transport due to ultrafiltration. Here, σ is Staverman's reflection coefficient and C_M represents the concentration of the solute in the fluid passing through the membrane. Notably, C_M can be expressed as the arithmetic mean $(C_B + C_D)/2$ [99] or the logarithmic mean $(C_B-C_D)/\ln(C_B/C_D)$[104] of the lumen- and shell-side bulk concentrations C_B, C_D. An additional approach could be to equate C_M with the upstream bulk concentration, specifically C_B if the ultrafiltration flux is from blood to dialysate, or C_D if it is the reverse. Comparing these alternatives revealed no substantial differences in the results.

The second term of Eq. (9.32) accounts for diffusive mass transfer, driven by the concentration gradient. U denotes the overall mass transfer coefficient, defined as:

$$U = \frac{1}{\frac{1}{k_B} + \frac{1}{k_M} + \frac{1}{k_D}} \tag{9.33}$$

in which k_B, k_M and k_D represent the mass transport coefficients for blood, membrane and dialysate, respectively. Rigorously, Eq. (9.33) is applicable to a planar membrane configuration. However, it is widely used in the literature for cylindrical fiber geometries as well, with the coefficients k_B and k_M incorporating the necessary geometric adjustments.

The mass transfer coefficient on the blood-side, k_B, can be computed using the following formula:

$$k_B = Sh_B \frac{D_B}{d_i} \tag{9.34}$$

where D_B is the diffusivity of the solute in the blood, d_i is the internal fiber diameter and Sh_B is the Sherwood number on the blood-side.

The mass transfer coefficient on the dialysate-side, k_D, was calculated as:

$$k_D = Sh_D \frac{D_D}{d_h} \tag{9.35}$$

in which d_h is the fiber bundle hydraulic diameter, D_D is the diffusivity of the solute in the dialysate and Sh_D is Sherwood number on the dialysate-side. For Sh_D, Eq. (9.27) was used, expressing it as a function of the shell-side cross-flow Reynolds number Re_T and averaging over all possible cross flow directions.

The term k_M in Eq. (9.33) denotes the membrane's diffusive permeability for the specified solute. This parameter depends on the membrane structure, composition and thickness.

9.5.3 Estimation of mass transport resistances

In Eq. (9.33) the three components (blood, dialysate and membrane) are treated as in a resistance in series model. Identifying the "controlling" step, i.e., the one that most significantly contributes to the overall resistance to mass transfer, is crucial for understanding and optimizing solute removal. To perform a preliminary estimation of the mass transport resistances, values of k_M for commercial polyphenylene membranes relative to two solutes (urea and B12 vitamin) are considered. Such data are reported, together with the hydraulic permeability L_p, in Table 9.4; for the physical fluids and solutes properties, data are reported in Table 9.5.

Estimates are conducted for membranes having internal and external fiber diameters $d_i = 200$ μm and $d = 260$ μm, respectively, and a bundle porosity $\varepsilon = 0.5$. Sherwood numbers of 4 for the blood-side and 9.85 for the dialysate-side, corresponding to axial flow, are considered. Results of such estimates are given in Figure 9.11. According to the literature [44, 54], the membrane accounts for more than half of the resistance to mass

Table 9.4: Membrane properties used in the simulations by Cancilla et al. [105].

Membrane property	Urea	B12 vitamin
k_M (m s^{-1})	$(1.1 \pm 0.2) \times 10^{-5}$	$(3.1 \pm 0.2) \times 10^{-6}$
L_p (m s^{-1} Pa^{-1})	$(6.6 \pm 0.4) \times 10^{-11}$	

Table 9.5: Fluids and solutes properties used in the simulations by Cancilla et al. [105].

Fluid	Density, ρ (approx, kg m^{-3})	Viscosity, μ (Pa s)	Diffusivity, D (m^2 s^{-1})	Schmidt number, Sc (–)	Inlet concentration, C_i (mol m^{-3})	Inlet volume flow rate, Q (mL min^{-1})
Blood	1,000	3.5×10^{-3}	7.4×10^{-10} (urea) 4.0×10^{-10} (B12)	4,730 8,750	20 (urea) 3×10^{-2} (B12)	300
Dialysate	1,000	7.62×10^{-4}	1.8×10^{-9} (urea) 5.0×10^{-10} (B12)	423 1,524	0	500

transport in current high-flux modules. This is particularly evident for high–molecular–weight solutes like B12 vitamin (MW = 1,355 Da [108]), where membrane resistance is the predominant one. For smaller solutes such as urea (MW = 60 Da [108]), the resistance within the blood compartment becomes more significant.

9.5.4 Computational domain and simulation strategy

Figure 9.12 reports the cylindrical geometry simulated by Cancilla et al. [105]. The computational domain, representative of a commercial haemodialysis module, includes eight inlets and eight outlets for dialysate flow, simulating the presence of a fluid distributor. Arrows indicate the flow direction, with red representing blood and blue denoting dialysate.

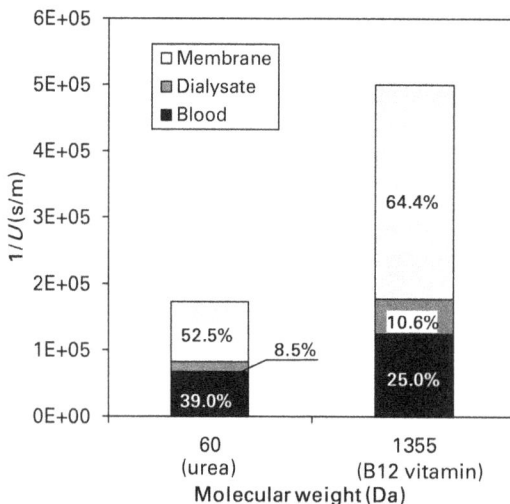

Figure 9.11: Component of the total mass transfer resistance (in s/m) for urea and B12 vitamin. Reproduced (adapted) from [105], with permission from Elsevier (^{2}022).

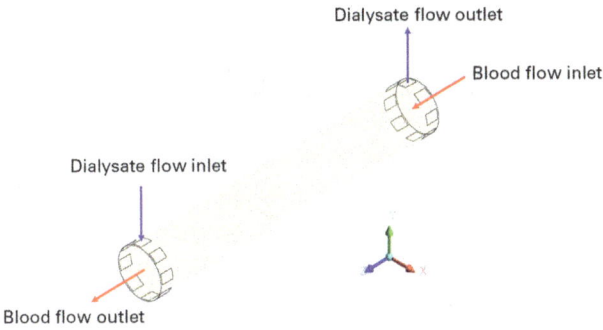

Figure 9.12: Geometry of the 3-D computational domain for the simulated module. Reproduced (adapted) from [105], with permission from Elsevier (2022).

The model was implemented using the finite volume code Ansys-CFX 18® [109]. Blood and dialysate were simulated as separate fluids flowing through two different porous media that occupy the entire internal volume of the module. The two fluids interact by transferring both the solution and solutes between them. This required an iterative approach: flow rates and solute concentrations on both the blood and the dialysate sides were interconnected through proper sink/source terms that represent solute exchange. These values were recalculated alternately until the results converged.

Figure 9.13 illustrates the flow chart of the computational procedure. Here and below, the subscripts "B" and "D" are for blood and dialysate, respectively.

The two fluid were described by the relevant physical properties (ρ, μ, D), the inlet volume flow rate (Q) and the inlet concentration (C_i), as shown in Table 9.5, along with their specific inlet and outlet configurations. It was assumed that each fluid flowed through a porous medium characterized by porosity (ε), longitudinal permeability (K_z) and cross flow permeability (K_T), as defined by Eqs. (9.25) and (9.26). The Sherwood number on dialysate-side was calculated using Eq. (9.27).

The solute markers were urea and B12 vitamin, with Staverman's reflection coefficients σ set at 0 and 0.15, respectively. The membrane's hydraulic permeability L_p and the diffusive permeabilities k_M for these solutes were as in Table 9.4.

In regard to boundary conditions, a no–slip wall condition with zero mass flux was applied to the internal cylindrical shell surface. Outlet conditions for both blood and dialysate were set by pressure, while inlets were defined by flow rates. Outlet pressure of the dialysate was set to zero (relative) while, for the blood, it was adjusted to achieve a 10 mL/min ultrafiltration flow rate. Both fluids used the same computational grid.

The procedure begins with the first iteration for the blood-side (BLOOD 1). In this step, in the mass transfer source term S_C for blood (using a negative sign in Eq. (9.31)) assumes zero dialysate-side pressure p_D and concentration C_D. After completing this iteration, the predicted blood-side pressure p_B and concentration C_B distributions are saved in the blood-side data file "BSDF[1]".

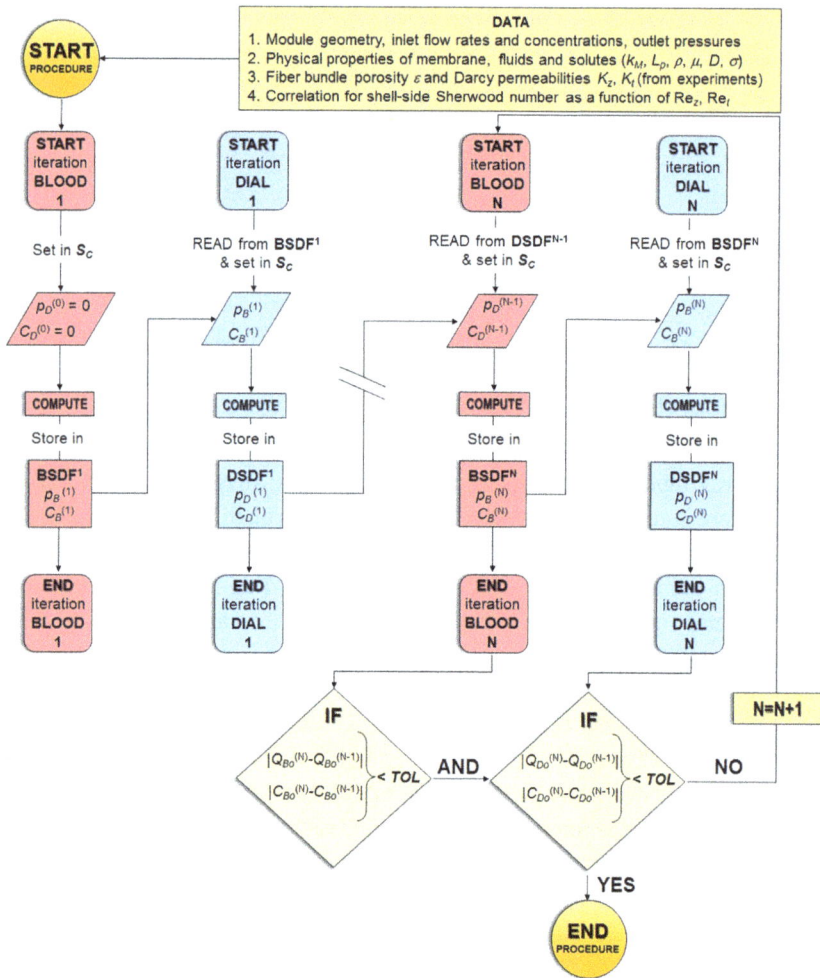

Figure 9.13: Flow chart illustrating the computational procedure for the porous media model. Reproduced from [105], with permission from Elsevier (2022).

The next step of the simulation procedure (DIAL 1) focuses on the dialysate side. In this iteration, the mass transfer source term S_C for the dialysate (using a positive sign in Eq. (9.31)) uses the blood-side pressure p_B and concentration C_B retrieved from the previously saved blood-side data file. Once this iteration is complete, the resulting dialysate-side pressure p_D and concentration C_D distributions are saved in the dialysate-side data file "DSDF[1]".

In the following iterations (BLOOD N – DIAL N), each side retrieves the most recent concentration and pressure fields for the opposite side from the corresponding saved file. After updating its own pressure and concentration fields, each side records these results in its respective data file.

Convergence is reached when the differences in outlet flow rate and solute concentration between successive iterations for both blood and dialysate drop below a specified tolerance (*TOL*). Typically, convergence to within 0.5 % was attained within 6–9 couples of iterations.

9.5.5 Model validation

To validate the model, the predicted clearance values for urea and B12 vitamin were compared with experimental clearances measured in commercial modules. Experiments referred to PHYLTHER® HF SD15 (membrane area 1.5 m²) and SD17 (membrane area 1.7 m²) modules commercialized by Medtronic® using a saline solution instead of blood. Hence, simulations were performed by substituting the blood in the lumen with a fluid matching the physical properties of the saline solution used in the experiments and setting the corresponding oncotic pressure to zero. The dialysate flow rate was set at 500 mL/min and simulations were conducted with lumen-side flow rates of 200, 300 and 400 mL/min. As in the experiments, the ultrafiltration flow rate was held constant at 10 mL/min. The data for membrane diffusive permeability and hydraulic permeability was those reported in Table 9.4.

Figure 9.14 presents a comparison between the solute clearances predicted by the model and the corresponding experimental data.

Clearance rises with the blood flow rate and with the module size. Model predictions consistently fall within the range of the experimental data. For all modules and solutes, the closest match to experimental results is observed at the lowest blood flow rate of 200 mL/min. The greatest deviation occurs for B12 vitamin with the 1.5 m² module at a blood flow rate of 400 mL/min.

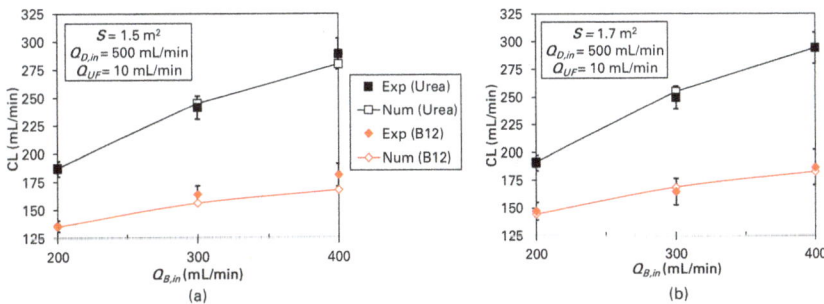

Figure 9.14: Clearance of urea (black) and B12 vitamin (red) as functions of the inlet blood flow rate for the 1.5 m² (a) and the 1.7 m² (b) modules. Model predictions (solid lines and hollow symbols) are compared with experimental results (solid symbols) provided with dispersion bars. Reproduced (adapted) from [105], with permission from Elsevier (2022).

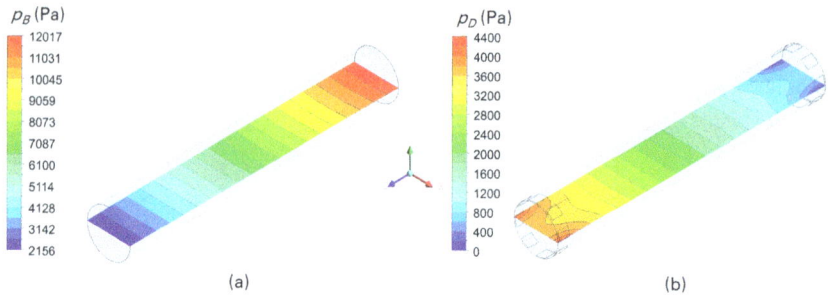

Figure 9.15: Color maps of pressure distribution in the *zx* mid-plane. (a) blood side; (b) dialysate side. Reproduced (adapted) from [105], with permission from Elsevier (2022).

9.5.6 Fluid flow and solute concentration distributions

The present section reports results obtained with the porous media model for a baseline scenario: blood and dialysate flow rates were set at 300 and 500 mL/min, respectively, with an ultrafiltration flow rate fixed at 10 mL/min. Membrane and fluids properties were as in Table 9.4 and Table 9.5, respectively. The oncotic pressure in the blood was set at 3,700 Pa (~28 mmHg as in typical human blood [110]). For the baseline scenario, the model predicts clearances of ~257 mL/min for urea and ~172 mL/min for B12 vitamin. Figure 9.15 illustrates the pressure distributions within both compartments of the module. Here, blood flows from right to left, while dialysate flows from left to right.

The pressure maps for both the blood and the dialysate sides display a linear gradient along most of the module length, consistent with observation by Osuga et al. [111]. The pressure drops between the inlets and outlets were ~9,860 Pa for blood and ~4,400 Pa for dialysate. This disparity arises from the differences in the fluid properties, blood being about 5 times more viscous than dialysate, and the variations in their respective axial Darcy permeabilities. The blood outlet pressure was set to 2,156 Pa to obtain an ultrafiltration flow rate of 10 mL/min.

Figure 9.16 reports the corresponding concentration distributions of urea and B12 vitamin. The maps show a mainly axial concentration stratification in both the blood and the dialysate, with a superimposed radial gradient. This gradient is most pronounced near the dialysate inlet and blood outlet regions, due to the peripheral locations of the dialysate inlet-outlet ports. These findings align qualitatively with the results reported by Ding et al. [104].

9.5.7 Parametric sensitivity assessment

A parametric analysis was performed to assess the sensitivity of the results to different parameters: the membrane's diffusive permeability, the oncotic pressure, the ultrafiltration and the dialysate flow rates.

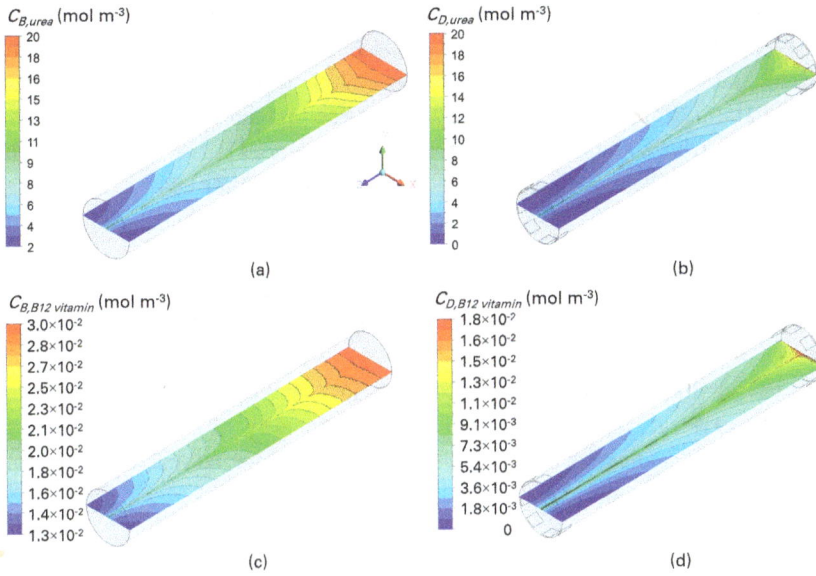

Figure 9.16: Color maps of solute concentration in the *zx* mid-plane. Left column: blood side; right column: dialysate side. Solute: (a, b) urea; (c, d) B12 vitamin. Reproduced (adapted) from [105], with permission from Elsevier (2022).

At first, a baseline scenario was simulated. Subsequently, the effect of varying each parameter individually, while keeping all other parameters constant, was assessed to determine its impact on the results.

The bar graphs in Figure 9.17 condense, in terms of solute clearance, the results of the parametrical study. For the two solutes, urea (a) and B12 vitamin (b), the baseline scenario result is represented by the white bar, while the other bars correspond to each variant analyzed.

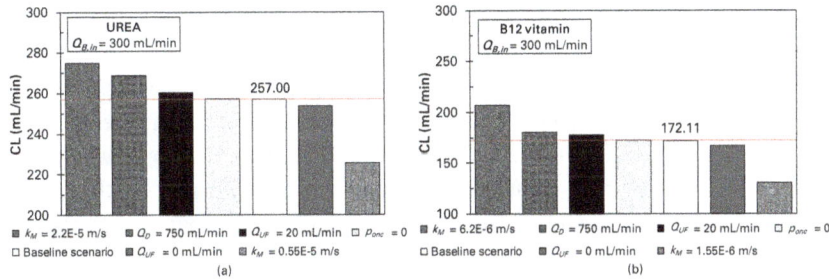

Figure 9.17: Values of the solute clearances obtained in the parametrical analysis. Solute: (a) urea; (b) B12 vitamin. Reproduced (adapted) from [105], with permission from Elsevier (2022).

The membrane's diffusive permeability, k_M, is the most effective parameter. Doubling k_M results in a clearance increase of ~7 % for urea and ~20 % for B12 vitamin. On the other hand, halving k_M leads to a reduction in solute clearances of ~12 % (urea) and ~24 % (B12 vitamin). The dialysate flow rate, Q_D, is the second most effective parameter. An increase in Q_D from 500 to 750 mL/min results in a roughly 4 % rise in clearance for both solutes. The ultrafiltration flow rate, Q_{UF}, has a relatively minor effect on clearance, even though it significantly affects hydrodynamics, particularly in term of backfiltration. A $\pm$ 10 mL/min change in Q_{UF} from the baseline value of 10 mL/min results in a clearance variation of ~ $\pm$ 1 % for urea and ~ $\pm$ 3 % for B12 vitamin. Including or excluding plasma proteins (oncotic pressure) in the blood had a negligible influence on solute clearance for both solutes.

Lastly, the possibility of enhancing a module performance by employing geometries alternative to the typical cylindrical one has been investigated by the present authors in a dedicated work [112] confirming the effectiveness of the commercial module design for the currently available membrane properties.

9.6 Conclusions and outlook

This chapter has provided an overview of the mathematical modelling approaches employed to study commercial haemodialyzers, which consist of cylindrical modules filled with hollow fiber.

A brief overview of healthy kidney function and its pathologies is provided to help the reader identify the essential functions that replacement treatment must replicate and the key reasons for its necessity. Subsequently, the chapter presents hollow fiber membrane processes for renal treatments of uremic patients, along with a classification of hemodialysis membranes based on the polymer material composition.

The discussion emphasized the importance of accurately representing fluid dynamics, solute transport and membrane characteristics to effectively predict haemodialyzer performance. Small-scale CFD models, which predict fluid flow and mass transfer in small domains, including either a single fiber (using a unit cell approach to simulate regular lattices of straight fibers) or a limited number of fibers, have been reported. These models represent the first level of a more complex multiscale modelling tool developed to understand fundamental fluid dynamics parameters and solute transport phenomena within a haemodialysis module. Additionally, simulations of small portions of the bundle can help investigate fluid flow and mass transfer in non-uniform fiber arrays. Simulations of random fiber arrangements are also briefly discussed, with evaluations of the relevant effects of randomness on hydrodynamics and mass transfer.

The porous media approach has been explored, highlighting its applications and current limitations. Sensitivity analysis demonstrates that parameters such as the membrane's diffusive permeability and the dialysate flow rate significantly influence solute clearance, whereas the impact of ultrafiltration flow rate and oncotic pressure is comparatively minor.

Current dialyzers are likely operating near their performance limits in terms of configurations and operating conditions, suggesting that optimizing these variables may be offer limited benefits. Future improvements in clearance performance will probably depend on the development of new membranes technologies with much higher diffusive permeability. The interpenetrating-fluid, porous-media model offers versatility and could be adapted for other processes involving heat or mass transfer between separated fluids.

Moving forward, future research could focus on refining model accuracy by incorporating more complex factors. The modelling tools presented in this chapter could serve as a foundation step for more advanced models. For example, developing flow conditions deserves more accurate investigations, and also simulations under the fully developed assumption are currently only partially complete, hindering a complete understanding. A thorough investigation of the effects of the bundle non-uniformity and a detailed parametric study of random fiber arrangements would be beneficial. Enhancing the porous media model with permeability and mass transfer correlations tailored for random distributions of hollow fibers could more accurately capture the complexities of real fiber bundles. Additionally, efforts are being made to account for the non-uniform porosity distribution in actual bundles, with a focus on radial variations. Simulating geometries with different local porosity values, directly derived from experimental cross-section images of real bundle, could better reproduce the behavior of actual bundles. This is increasingly feasible thanks to advancement in image acquisition techniques.

Another significant area of focus is the inclusion of fiber undulation effects, which impact hydraulic permeability and mass transfer coefficients, allowing for a more realistic simulation of the fluid dynamics within the dialysis module. Currently, many companies manufacturing haemodialysis modules are trending towards the use of self-structured (undulated) fiber bundles. These fiber bundles exhibit interesting behaviors, ensuring adequate clinical performance. An in–depth experimental investigation, beyond the current literature, is advisable to fully characterize modules using self-structured hollow fiber bundles. This exploration could provide valuable insights into their performance and help refine existing models for better predictive accuracy.

Therefore, through the synergistic integration of increasingly detailed modelling tools and advancements in membrane science technology, the objective of developing more accurate models could soon be realized.

Acknowledgments: The authors would like to thank the editors David Bogle and Tomasz Sosnowski for their guidance and review of this article before its publication.

References

1. Farquhar MG, Kanwar YS. Functional organization of the glomerulus: state of the science in 1979. In: Michael AF, Cummings N, editors. Immune mechanisms in renal disease. New York: Plenum Press; 1982:1–35 pp.

2. Huang W, Chen YY, He FF, Zhang C. Revolutionizing nephrology research: expanding horizons with kidney-on-a-chip and beyond. Front Bioeng Biotechnol 2024;12. https://doi.org/10.3389/fbioe.2024.1373386.
3. Navar LG, Bell PD, White RW, Watts, RL, Williams, RL. Evaluation of the single nephron glomerular filtration coefficient in the dog. Kidney Int 1977;12:137–49.
4. Van Damme M, Bergmann P, Lambert PP. A three layer model to estimate charge densities in the glomerular wall. In: Lambert PP, Bergmann P, Beauwens R, editors. The pathogenicity of cationic proteins. New York: Raven Press; 1983:223–36 pp.
5. Farquhar MG. The glomerulal basement membrane: a selective macromolecular filter. In: Hay ED, editor. Cell Biology of Extracellular Matrix. New York: Plenum Press; 1981:335–78 pp.
6. Farquhar MG, Courtoy PJ, Lemkin MC, Kanwar YS. Current knowledge of the functional architecture of the glomerular basement membrane. In: Kuhn K, Schone H, Timpl R, editors. New Trends in Basement Membrane Research. New York: Raven Press; 1982.
7. Caulfield JP, Farquhar MG. Distribution of anionic sites in the glomerular basement membranes. Their possible role in filtration and attachment. Proc Nat Acad Sci USA 1976;73:1646–50.
8. Kanwar YS, Farquhar MG. Anionic sites in the glomerular basement membrane. 'In vivo' and 'in vitro' localization to the laminae rarae by cationic probes. J Cell Biol 1979;81:137–53.
9. Venkatachalam MA, Rennke HG. Glomerular filtration of macromolecules: structural, molecular and functional determinants. In: Leaf A, Giebisch G, Bolis L, Cornini S, editors. Renal Pathophysiology. New York: Raven Press; 1980:43–56 pp.
10. Deen WM, Bridges CR, Brenner BM. Biophysical basis of glomerular permselectivity. J Memb Biol 1983;71: 1–10.
11. Bayliss LE, Tookey-Kerridge M, Russell DS. The excretion of protein by the mammalian kidney. J Physiol 1933;77:386–98.
12. Chang RLS, Ueki IF, Troy JL, Deen WM, Robertson CR, Brenner BM. Permselectivity of the glomerular capillary wall to macromolecules: II. Experimental observations in the rat. Biophys J 1975;15:887–906.
13. Rennke HG, Cotran RS, Venkatachalam MA. Role of molecular charge in glomerular permeability. Tracer studies with cationized ferritin. J Cell Biol 1975;67:638–46.
14. Rennke HG, Venkatachalam MA. Glomerular permeability: 'in vivo' tracer studies with polyanionic and polycationic ferritins. Kidney Int 1977;11:44–53.
15. Rennke HG, Venkatachalam MA. Glomerular filtration of proteins: clearance of anionic, neutral and cationic horseradish peroxidase in the rat. Kidney Int 1978;13:278–88.
16. Brenner BM, Lawrence WE. Modern concepts of glomerular permselectivity. In: Lambert PP, Bergmann P, Beauwens R, editors. The pathogenicity of cationic proteins. New York: Raven Press; 1983:183–205 pp.
17. Bohrer MP, Baylis C, Humes HD, Glassock RJ, Robertson CR, Brenner BM. Permselectivity of the glomerular capillary wall. Facilitated filtration of circulating polycations. J Clin Invest 1978;61:72–8.
18. Kanwar YS, Rosenzweig LJ. Altered glomerular permeability as a result of focal detachment of visceral epithelium. Kidney Int 1982;21:565–74.
19. Gregor HP, Gregor CD. Synthetic membrane technology. Sci Am 1978;239:112–28.
20. Jager KJ, Kovesdy C, Langham R, Rosenberg M, Jha V, Zoccali C. A single number for advocacy and communication-worldwide more than 850 million individuals have kidney diseases. Nephrol Dial Transplant 2019;34:1803–5.
21. United States Renal Data System. 2018 USRDS annual data report: epidemiology of kidney disease in the United States. Bethesda, MD: National Institutes of Health, National Institute of Diabetes and Digestive and Kidney Diseases; 2018.
22. Dialysis Market Size, Share & COVID-19 Impact Analysis, By type (products and services), by dialysis type (hemodialysis and peritoneal dialysis), by End user (dialysis centers & hospitals and home care), and regional forecast, 2020-2027, 2020.
23. Leaf A, Giebisch G, Bolis L, Gorini S, editors. Renal Pathophysiology. New York: Raven Press; 1980.

24. Arnaout MA, Rennke HG, Cotran RS. Membranous nephropathy. In: Stein JH, editor. Contemporary issues in nephrology. New York: Nephrotic Syndrome. Churchill Livingstone; 1982, vol 9:199–235 pp.
25. Olson JL, Rennke HG, Venkatachalam MA. Alterations in charge and size selectivity barrier of the glomerular filter in Aminonucleoside Nephrosis in rats. Lab Invest 1981;44:271–9.
26. Rennke HG. Charge and size selective properties of the glomerular capillary wall in normal rats and in experimentally induced Proteinuria. In: Lambert PP, Bergmann P, Beauwens R, editors. The Pathogenicity of Cationic Proteins. New York: Raven Press; 1983:272–80 pp.
27. Vernier RL, Papermaster BW, Good RA, Aminonucleoside Nephrosis I. Electron microscopic study of the renal lesions in rats. J Exp Med 1959;109:115–26.
28. Robson AM, Gianagiacomo J, Keinstra RA, Naqvi ST, Ingelfinger JR. Normal glomerular permeability and its modification by minimal change nephrotic syndrome. J Clin Invest 1974;54:1190–9.
29. Bohrer MP, Baylis C, Robertson CR, Brenner BM, Troy JL, Willis WT. Mechanism of puromycin–induced defects in the transglomerular passage of water and macromolecules. J Clin Invest 1977;60:152–61.
30. Weening JJ, Rennke HG. Glomerular permeability and polyanion in Adriamycin Nephrosis in the rat. Kidney Int 1983;24:152–9.
31. Barnes JL, Venkatachalam MA. Glomerular interactions of exogenous and endogenous polycations. In: Lambert PP, Bergmann P, Beauwens R, editors. The pathogenicity of cationic proteins. New York: Raven Press; 1983:281–93 pp.
32. Seiler MW, Rennke HG, Venkatachalam MA, Cotran RS. Pathogenesis of polycation-induced alterations ("Fusion") of glomerular eipithelium. Lab Invest 1977;36:48–61.
33. Chang RLS, Robertson CR, Deen WM, Brenner BM. Permselectivity of the glomerular capillary wall to macromolecules: I. Theoretical considerations. Biophys J 1975;15:861–86.
34. Eisenbach GM, vanLiew JB, Boylan JW, Manz N, Muir P. Effect of angiotensin on the filtration of protein in the rat kidney: a micropuncture study. Kidney Int 1975;8:80–7.
35. Baylis C, Deen WM, Myers BD, Brenner BM. Effects of some vasodilator drugs on transcapillary fluid exchange in renal cortex. Am J Phys 1976;230:1148–58.
36. Colton CK, Lysaght MJ. Membranes for hemodialysis. In: Replacement of renal function by dialysis. Dordrecht: Springer; 1996:103–13 pp.
37. Lysaght MJ. Hemodialysis membranes in transition. Contrib Nephrol 1988;61:1–17.
38. Lysaght MJ. Evolution of hemodialysis membranes. Contrib Nephrol 1995;113:1–10.
39. Clark WR, Hamburger RJ, Lysaght MJ. Effect of membrane composition and structure on solute removal and biocompatibility in hemodialysis. Kidney Int 1999;56:2005–15.
40. Klinkmann H, Vienken J. Membranes for dialysis. Nephrol Dial Transplant 1995;10:39–45.
41. Craddock PR, Fehr J, Dalmasso AP, Brigham KL, Jacob HS. Hemodialysis Leukopenia: pulmonary vascular leukostasis resulting from complement activation by dialyzer cellophane membranes. J Clin Invest 1977; 59:879–88.
42. Hakim RM, Fearon DT, Lazarus JM, Perzanowski CS. Biocompatibility of dialysis membranes: effects of chronic complement activation. Kidney Int Elsevier Masson SAS 1984;26:194–200.
43. Hakim RM. Clinical implications of hemodialysis membrane biocompatibility. Kidney Int 1993;44:484–94.
44. Ronco C, Clark WR. Haemodialysis membranes. Nat Rev Nephrol Spring US 2018;14:394–410.
45. Takeyama T, Sakai Y. Polymethylmethacrylate: one biomaterial for a series of membrane. Contrib Nephrol 1998;125:9–24.
46. Clark WR, Gao D, Ronco C. Membranes for dialysis: composition, structure and function. Contrib Nephrol 2002;137:70–7.
47. Cabasso I, Klein E, Smith JK. Polysulfone hollow fibers. I. Spinning and properties. J Appl Polym Sci 1976;20: 2377–94.
48. Xu ZL, Chung TS, Huang Y. Effect of polyvinylpyrrolidone molecular weights on morphology, oil/water separation, mechanical and thermal properties of polyetherimide/polyvinylpyrrolidone hollow fiber membranes. J Appl Polym Sci 1999;74:2220–33.

49. Ronco C, Neri M, Lorenzin A, Garzotto F, Clark WR. Multidimensional classification of dialysis membranes. Contrib Nephrol 2017;191:115–26.

50. Misra M. Basic mechanisms governing solute and fluid transport in hemodialysis. Hemodial Int 2008;12: 25–8.

51. Sam R. Hemodialysis: diffusion and ultrafiltration. Austin J Nephrol Hypertens 2014;1:1010.

52. Ronco C, Fabris A, Feriani M. Hemodialysis fluid composition. In: Jacobs C, Kjellstrand CM, Koch KM, editors. Replacement of renal function by dialysis. Dordrecht: Springer; 1996:256–76 pp.

53. Azar AT, Canaud B. Hemodialysis system. In: Azar AT, editor. Modeling and control of dialysis systems. Springer; 2013:144–7 pp.

54. Ronco C, Ghezzi PM, Brendolan A, Crepaldi C, La GG. The haemodialysis system: basic mechanisms of water and solute transport in extracorporeal renal replacement therapies. Nephrol Dial Transplant 1998; 13:3–9.

55. Kessler M, Canaud B, Pedrini LA. European best practice guidelines for haemodialysis (part 1): section II: haemodialysis adequacy. Nephrol Dial Transplant 2002;17:17–21.

56. Vanholder R, Smet RD, Argilés A, Baurmeister U, Brunet P. Review on uremic toxins: classification, concentration, and interindividual variability. Kidney Int 2003;63:1934–43. Glorieux G

57. Ofsthun NJ, Zydney AL. Importance of convection in artificial kidney treatment. Contrib Nephrol 1994;108: 53–70.

58. Lorenzin A, Neri M, Clark WR, Garzotto F, Brendolan A, Nalesso F, et al. Modeling of internal filtration in theranova hemodialyzers. Contrib Nephrol 2017;191:127–41.

59. Clark WR, Gao D, Neri M, Ronco C. Solute transport in hemodialysis: advances and limitations of current membrane technology. Contrib Nephrol 2017;191:84–99.

60. Ross SM, Uvelli DA, Babb AL. One-dimensional mathematical model of transmembrane diffusional and convective mass transfer in a hemodialyzer. Am Soc Mech Eng 1973:8. (73-WA/Bio-14).

61. Villarroel F, Klein E, Holland F. Solute flux in hemodialysis and hemofiltration membranes. Trans Am Soc Artif Intern Organs 1977;23:225–32.

62. Sargent JA, Gotch FA. Principles and biophysics of dialysis. In: Replacement of renal function by dialysis. Dordrecht: Springer; 1979:38–68 pp.

63. Jaffrin MY, Ding L, Laurent JM. Simultaneous convective and diffusive mass transfers in a hemodialyser. J Biomech Eng 1990;112:212–9.

64. Jaffrin MY. Convective mass transfer in hemodialysis. Artif Organs 1995;19:1162–71.

65. Waniewski J. Mathematical modeling of fluid and solute transport in hemodialysis and peritoneal dialysis. J Memb Sci 2006;274:24–37.

66. Ledebo I. Principles and practice of hemofiltration and hemodiafiltration. Artif Organs 1998;22:20–5.

67. Messer J, Mulcahy B, Fissell WH. Middle-molecule clearance in CRRT: in vitro convection, diffusion and dialyzer area. ASAIO J 2009;55:224–6.

68. Ronco C, Feriani M, Chiaramonte S, Brendolan A, Bragantini L, Conz P, et al. Backfiltration in clinical dialysis. Nature of the phenomenon and possible solutions. Contrib Nephrol 1990;77:96–105.

69. Rangel AV, Kim JC, Kaushik M, Garzotto F, Neri M, Cruz DN, et al. Backfiltration: past, present and future. Contrib Nephrol 2011;175:35–45.

70. Tamburini A, Renda M, Cipollina A, Micale G, Ciofalo M. Investigation of heat transfer in spacer-filled channels by experiments and direct numerical simulations. Int J Heat Mass Tran 2016;93:1190–205.

71. Miyagi T. Viscous flow at low Reynolds numbers past an infinite row of equal circular cylinders. J. Phys. Soc. Japan 1958;13:493–6.

72. Happel J. Viscous flow relative to arrays of cylinders. AIChE J 1959;5:174–7.

73. Sparrow EM, Loeffler AL. Longitudinal laminar flow between cylinders arranged in regular array. AIChE J 1959;5:325–30.

74. Ishimi K, Koroyasu S, Hikita H. Mass transfer in creeping flow past periodic arrays of cylinders. J Chem Eng Jpn 1987;20:492–8.

75. Cancilla N, Gurreri L, Marotta G, Ciofalo M, Cipollina A, Tamburini A, et al. CFD prediction of shell-side flow and mass transfer in regular fiber arrays. Int J Heat Mass Tran 2021;168. https://doi.org/10.1016/j.ijheatmasstransfer.2020.120855.

76. Magalhães HLF, Gomez RS, Leite BE, Nascimento JBS, Brito MKT, Araújo MV, et al. Investigating the dialysis treatment using hollow fiber membrane: a new approach by CFD. Membranes (Basel) 2022;12:710.

77. Yaqoob T, Ahsan M, Hussain A, Ahmad I. Computational fluid dynamics (CFD) modeling and simulation of flow regulatory mechanism in artificial kidney using finite element method. Membranes (Basel) 2020;10: 139.

78. Yaqoob T, Ahsan M, Farrukh S, Ahmad I. Design and development of a computational tool for a dialyzer by using computational fluid dynamic (CFD) model. Membranes (Basel) 2021;11:916.

79. Pozzobon V, Perré P. Mass transfer in hollow fiber membrane contactor: computational fluid dynamics determination of the shell side resistance. Sep Purif Technol 2020;241. https://doi.org/10.1016/j.seppur.2020.116674.

80. Skartsis L, Khomami B, Kardos JL. Resin flow through fiber beds during composite manufacturing processes. Part II: numerical and experimental studies of Newtonian flow through ideal and actual fiber beds. Polym Eng Sci 1992;32:231–9.

81. Larson RE, Higdon JJL. Microscopic flow near the surface of two-dimensional porous media. Part 1. Axial flow. J Fluid Mech 1986;166:449–72.

82. Winograd Y, Toren M, Solan A. Reverse osmosis in shell and tubes. Desalination 1974;14:173–87.

83. Ronco C, Scabardi M, Goldoni M, Brendolan A, Crepaldi C, La Greca G. Impact of spacing filaments external to hollow fibers on dialysate flow distribution and dialyzer performance. Int J Artif Organs 1997;20:261–6.

84. Li W, Liu J, He L, Liu J, Sun S, Huang Z, et al. Simulation and experimental study on the effect of channeling flows on the transport of toxins in hemodialyzers. J. Memb. Sci. 2016;501:123–33.

85. Bao L, Lipscomb GG. Mass transfer in axial flows through randomly packed fiber bundles with constant wall concentration. J. Memb. Sci. 2002;204:207–20.

86. Bao L, Lipscomb GG. Well-developed mass transfer in axial flows through randomly packed fiber bundles with constant wall flux. Chem Eng Sci 2002;57:125–32.

87. Sun L, Panagakos G, Lipscomb G. Effect of packing nonuniformity at the fiber bundle–case interface on performance of hollow fiber membrane gas separation modules. Membranes (Basel) 2022;12:1139.

88. Cancilla N, Gurreri L, Ciofalo M, Cipollina A, Tamburini A, Micale G. Hydrodynamics and mass transfer in straight fiber bundles with non-uniform porosity. Chem Eng Sci 2023;279. https://doi.org/10.1016/j.ces.2023.118935.

89. Cancilla N, Ciofalo M, Cipollina A, Tamburini A, Micale G. Straight fiber bundles with non-uniform porosity: shell-side hydrodynamics and mass transfer in cross flow. Chem Eng Sci 2024;291. https://doi.org/10.1016/j.ces.2024.119947.

90. Frank A, Lipscomb GG, Dennis M. Visualization of concentration fields in hemodialyzers by computed tomography. J. Memb. Sci. 2000;175:239–51.

91. Cancilla N, Ciofalo M, Cipollina A, Tamburini A, Micale G. Effects of shell-side non-ideal flow in hollow fibre membrane contactors operating in cross-flow. In: Proc 41st UIT Int. Heat Transfer Conf Naples, Italy; 2024: 19–21 pp.

92. Sangani AS, Mo G. Inclusion of lubrication forces in dynamic simulations. Phys Fluids 1994;6:1653–62.

93. Chen X, Papathanasiou TD. The transverse permeability of disordered fiber arrays: a statistical correlation in terms of the mean nearest interfiber spacing. Transp. Porous Med. 2008;71:233–51.

94. Matsumura Y, Jackson TL. Numerical simulation of fluid flow through random packs of cylinders using immersed boundary method. Phys Fluids 2014;26:043602.

95. Matsumura Y, Jackson TL. Numerical simulation of fluid flow through random packs of polydisperse cylinders. Phys Fluids 2014;26:123303.

96. Lemanski J, Lipscomb GG. Effect of shell-side flows on hollow-fiber membrane device performance. AIChE J 1995;41:2322–6.

97. Happel J, Brenner H. Low reynolds number hydrodynamics. Englewood Cliffs: Prentice-Hall; 1965.
98. Skartsis L, Kardos JL, Khomami B. Resin flow through fiber beds during composite manufacturing processes. Part I: review of Newtonian flow through fiber beds. Polym Eng Sci 1992;32:221–30.
99. Liao Z, Poh CK, Huang Z, Hardy PA, Clark WR, Gao D. A numerical and experimental study of mass transfer in the artificial kidney. J Biomech Eng 2003;125:472.
100. Eloot S, D'Asseler Y, De Bondt P, Verdonck P. Combining SPECT medical imaging and computational fluid dynamics for analyzing blood and dialysate flow in hemodialyzers. Int J Artif Organs 2005;28:739–49.
101. Łabęcki M, Piret JM, Bowen BD. Two-dimensional analysis of fluid flow in hollow-fibre modules. Chem Eng Sci 1995;50:3369–84.
102. Lemanski J, Lipscomb GG. Effect of shell-side flows on the performance of hollow-fiber gas separation modules. J. Memb. Sci. 2002;195:215–28.
103. Ding W, He L, Zhao G, Zhang H, Shu Z, Gao D. Double porous media model for mass transfer of hemodialyzers. Int J Heat Mass Tran 2004;47:4849–55.
104. Ding W, Li W, Sun S, Zhou X, Hardy PA, Ahmad S, et al. Three-dimensional simulation of mass transfer in artificial kidneys. Artif Organs 2015;39:E79–89.
105. Cancilla N, Gurreri L, Marotta G, Ciofalo M, Cipollina A, Tamburini A, et al. A porous media CFD model for the simulation of hemodialysis in hollow fiber membrane modules. J. Memb. Sci. 2022;646. https://doi.org/10.1016/j.memsci.2021.120219.
106. Cancilla N, Gurreri L, La Rosa M, Ciofalo M, Cipollina A, Tamburini A, et al. Influence of bundle porosity on shell-side hydrodynamics and mass transfer in regular fiber arrays: a computational study. Int J Heat Mass Tran 2023;203. https://doi.org/10.1016/j.ijheatmasstransfer.2022.123841.
107. Bergman T, Lavine A, Incropera F, Dewitt D. Fundamentals of heat and mass transfer, 7th ed. Hoboken, NJ: John Wiley & Sons; 2011.
108. Green DW, Perry RH. Perry's chemical engineers' handbook, 8th ed. New York: McGraw-Hill; 2008.
109. ANSYS CFX reference guide release 18.2. Canonsburg, PA, USA: ANSYS Inc., 2018.
110. Fournier RL. Basic transport phenomena in biomedical engineering, 4th ed. Boca Raton, FL: CRC Press, Taylor & Francis Group; 2017.
111. Osuga T, Obata T, Ikehira H, Tanada S, Sasaki Y, Naito H. Dialysate pressure isobars in a hollow-fiber dialyzer determined from magnetic resonance imaging and numerical simulation of dialysate flow. Artif Organs 1998;22:907–9.
112. Cancilla N, Gurreri L, Marotta G, Ciofalo M, Cipollina A, Tamburini A, et al. Performance comparison of alternative hollow-fiber modules for hemodialysis by means of a CFD-based model. Membranes (Basel) 2022;12:118.
113. Cancilla N, Nicolò G, Ciofalo M, Cipollina A, Tamburini A, Micale G. Cross flow hydrodynamics in regular and random fiber bundles in the Darcyan and non-Darcyan regimes. Chem Eng Sci 2025;301:120768.

Krystian Jędrzejczak, Arkadiusz Antonowicz, Krzysztof Wojtas,
Wojciech Orciuch, Malenka Bissell and Łukasz Makowski*

10 Chemical engineering methods in better understanding of blood hydrodynamics in atherosclerosis disease

Abstract: *Background/Objective*: Cardiovascular diseases are among the leading causes of death in the 21st-century society. One of the most common cardiovascular diseases is atherosclerosis, where the accumulation of plaque in blood vessels leads to blockages, increasing the risk of mechanical hemolysis or embolism. *Methods*: Recent advancements in clinical imaging technologies, including 4D MRI, allow for non-invasive assessments of both blood vessel conditions and blood flow hydrodynamics. Computational fluid dynamics (CFD) simulations of the cardiovascular system have also contributed to a deeper understanding of heart and blood vessel function. In addition to CFD simulations, 3D printing is increasingly used to create realistic models of the cardiovascular system based on medical imaging data, which can be used for further study and testing. *Results*: The integration of modern medical imaging techniques with CFD simulations offers new opportunities in diagnosing and planning treatment for cardiovascular diseases, including atherosclerosis. CFD simulations provide detailed insights into blood flow dynamics within arteries affected by plaque build-up, enabling a more precise understanding of disease progression. In this study, CFD results were validated against micro – particle image velocimetry (μPIV) measurements performed on 3D-printed models of the left coronary artery bifurcation. The comparison showed strong agreement between CFD simulations and PIV measurements, confirming the accuracy of CFD models in replicating real-world blood flow conditions. These results highlight the potential of combining 4D MRI, CFD simulations, and 3D printing for enhancing cardiovascular research and improving clinical outcomes. *Conclusion*: Modern imaging and CFD simulations offer effective non-invasive methods for diagnosing atherosclerosis-related complications, improving the accuracy of treatment planning.

Corresponding author: Łukasz Makowski, Faculty of Chemical and Process Engineering, Warsaw University of Technology, Waryńskiego 1, 00-645, Warsaw, Poland, E-mail: Lukasz.Makowski.ichip@pw.edu.pl
Krystian Jędrzejczak, Faculty of Chemical and Process Engineering, Warsaw University of Technology, Waryńskiego 1, 00-645, Warsaw, Poland; and Leeds Institute of Cardiovascular and Metabolic Medicine, University of Leeds, Leeds, UK
Arkadiusz Antonowicz, Faculty of Chemical and Process Engineering, Warsaw University of Technology, Waryńskiego 1, 00-645, Warsaw, Poland; and Eurotek International Sp.z o.o., Skrzetuskiego 6, 02-726, Warsaw, Poland
Krzysztof Wojtas and Wojciech Orciuch, Faculty of Chemical and Process Engineering, Warsaw University of Technology, Waryńskiego 1, 00-645, Warsaw, Poland
Malenka Bissell, Leeds Institute of Cardiovascular and Metabolic Medicine, University of Leeds, Leeds, UK

As per De Gruyter's policy this article has previously been published in the journal Physical Sciences Reviews. Please cite as: K. Jędrzejczak, A. Antonowicz, K. Wojtas, W. Orciuch, M. Bissell and Ł. Makowski "Chemical engineering methods in better understanding of blood hydrodynamics in atherosclerosis disease" *Physical Sciences Reviews* [Online] 2024. DOI: 10.1515/psr-2024-0061 | https://doi.org/10.1515/ 9783111394558-010

Keywords: atherosclerosis; hemodynamics; CFD; 4D MRI; µPIV

10.1 Introduction of physiology of the circulatory system

Despite ongoing advancements in medicine, cardiovascular diseases remain a significant challenge in modern society [1–3]. Today's lifestyle, characterized by insufficient physical activity and unhealthy dietary habits, frequently results in hypertension or atherosclerosis [4, 5]. Atherosclerosis is a key contributor to cardiovascular diseases, which can lead to stroke or heart attack. The accumulation of cholesterol deposits reduces the lumen of blood vessels, causing an increase in local shear stress. This elevated shear stress can damage erythrocytes [6–8].

As a result of local death of red blood cells due to hemolysis, endothelial and smooth muscle cells become impaired due to a decrease in NO and direct toxicity of hemoglobin and Fe^{2+} released from erythrocytes [9]. Damaged endothelium leads to exposure of the deeper layers of the artery wall, which are rich in collagen, affecting circulating platelets, which react with activation and clot formation. Hemolysis can occur in atherosclerosis at various stages, from very early stages to severe arterial stenosis [9]. The basis of treating atherosclerosis is to stop this pathological process as quickly as possible. Guidelines for endovascular interventions in cardiovascular disease mainly focus on the severity of arterial narrowing before angioplasty (i.e., internal carotid artery or coronary artery).

Currently, percutaneous endovascular intervention with balloon angioplasty followed by stent implantation is one of the most common methods of treating patients with advanced atherosclerosis of the carotid or coronary arteries. Research into the etiopathology of hemolysis in atherosclerosis may help develop new guidelines for interventions performed in the early stages of the disease. Due to the existing risk of complications, knowledge about the impact of stenosis on the hydrodynamics of blood flow in a given vessel is extremely valuable. Hence, there is an increased interest in non-invasive blood flow measurements combined with advanced clinical imaging such as 4D flow MRI [10–14] and computational fluid dynamics (CFD) for non-invasive diagnosis of atherosclerosis [10, 11].

4D flow MRI is a developing technique that allows the imaging of tissues and the determination of blood flow through a vessel over time. These studies can be conducted in both clinical and preclinical conditions, with the preclinical MRI scanners offering much larger electromagnetic fields up to 18 T [12]. The increase in the electromagnetic field translates into an increase in the signal-to-noise ratio, directly correlating with the imaging quality. In clinical comparison, the standard is magnetic resonance imaging with a field of 1.5 T or 3 T.

At the same time, the development of computer technology allowed for CFD analysis of complex geometries of the circulatory system [8, 10, 11, 13–33]. Over the years, new numerical methods and models of blood circulation have been developed [34]. On the other hand, even the best model without proper experimental verification raises doubts about whether it is correct. The problem of experimental verification is solved, among others, by combining the 4D flow MRI imaging method with CFD calculations [35], where the boundary conditions can be tailored to a given patient to analyze the flow and develop population-averaged models more precisely.

Moreover, due to the complex rheology of blood, it is important to consider non-Newtonian characteristics of blood. Many blood viscosity models consider the shear-thinning effect [36–42], but some models include thixotropic effects [8, 43–49]. Furthermore, selecting an appropriate flow turbulence model that applies to both laminar and transient flow observed in the zone after the stenosis is crucial. Besides the previously mentioned techniques, 3D printing can be used to create accurate cardiovascular phantoms that will be later used for experimental validation of CFD correctness. In previous articles, 3D-printed channel models and micro particle image velocimetry (μPIV) [10, 50] were used to validate the turbulence model used in the CFD simulations. μPIV techniques can be applied to various geometries as supplementary experiments to 4D flow MRI. μPIV can deliver significantly higher spatial and temporal resolution. Although it's difficult to obtain 3D information, it's still possible to use 3D PIV [51] or tomographic PIV [52].

Moreover, in the case of high shear stresses, it is also important to consider the hemolysis process in the calculations [6–8, 53–61]. There are many hemolysis models with varying degrees of accuracy and complexity, and it is important to strike a balance between increasing the model's prediction accuracy and increasing the required computing power.

10.2 Mathematical modeling

10.2.1 Mathematical flow formulation

The description of the hemodynamics of the circulatory system is complicated by the complex structure of blood vessels and the heart. Numerous branches of various dimensions and the pulsating work of the heart make a full description of the flow and pressure changes extremely complicated. In engineering applications, many models of the functioning of the circulatory system have been developed, both dimensionless models where analogies are used between electrical systems and the structure of the circulatory system [62], as well as one- [62] or two- [63] dimensional models where spatial dependencies are introduced for signals generated by individual components of the circulatory system [34]. In addition, 3D models are used where blood flow is analyzed locally. In the case of analyzing a section of the circulatory system, it is very important to select appropriate boundary conditions that can be personalized per patient and be average values for a representative patient. Boundary conditions can be given *a priori* or

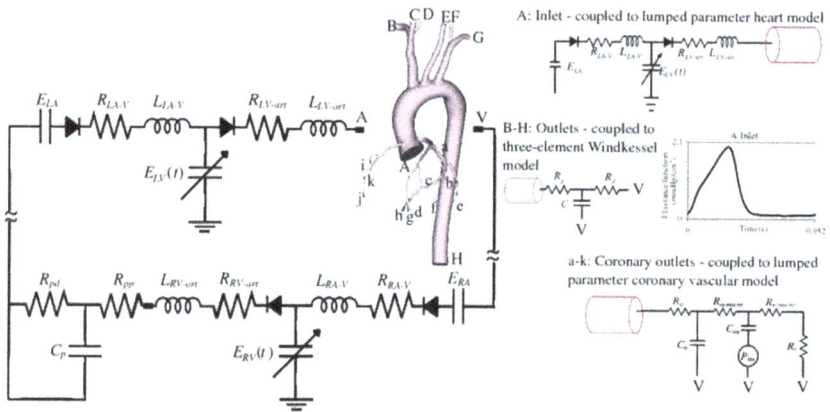

Figure 10.1: Problem specification of the inlet, upper branch vessels, the descending thoracic aorta, and coronary outlets for simulations of blood flow in a normal thoracic aorta model with coronary outlets [34]. Ann Biomed Eng, Patient-Specific Modeling of Blood Flow and Pressure in Human Coronary Arteries., 38, 2010, Kim, H.J.; Vignon-Clementel, I.E.; Coogan, J.S.; Figueroa, C.A.; Jansen, K.E.; Taylor, C.A. (0090-6964/10/ 1000-3195/0 © 2010 Biomedical Engineering Society) "With permission of Springer".

implemented as a hybrid model combining 3D modeling and reduced dimensionless models that reflect the operation of the remaining elements of the circulatory system [34] (Figure 10.1).

10.2.2 Rheology and hemolysis models

Blood is a mixture of plasma and cells suspended in it, as well as minerals and vitamins. When flowing through large vessels and the heart, the behavior of blood can be approximated using the Newtonian model. However, in the case of flow through smaller vessels, stenoses, or aneurysms, the assumption of constant blood viscosity is sometimes too simplistic. Over the years, many models have been developed to describe the relationship between blood viscosity and shear rate. Some of these models are based on previously known mathematical models, where constants in the equations were adjusted based on experimental data, such models as e.g. Cross, Casson, Carreau, Carreau–Yasuda, and Power-law [36–42]. In addition to simple mathematical models, more complex models were created that were additionally considered, such as blood hematocrit [64, 65]. Other approaches to the topic included taking into account the viscoelastic properties of blood [66] or trying to describe the behavior of blood from the microstructure perspective [8, 45]. The latter category is divided into two approaches: description from the point of view of a single blood cell or static description based on the balance of the red blood cell population.

It should also be borne in mind that red blood cells may undergo hemolysis under high shear stress. Over the years, many models have been developed to describe this phenomenon. There various models which have been developed so far such as Power-law equation model [6], Eulerian version of Power-law equation model [7, 67], empirical formulation for blood pumps [53], Lagrangian formulation of the Power-law [54], Lagrangian Power-law formulation for closed-loop circulations [55], viscoelastic Lagrangian model [56], strain-tensor-based Lagrangian models [57–59], strain-scalar-based Lagrangian model [60], Eulerian strain-tensor-based model [61], cell-resolved Lagrangian solver [68] and population balance based model [8].

10.2.3 Numerical schemes

Various numerical methods are used in *in silico* analysis; the most frequently used are the finite volume method and the finite element method. However, apart from it, there are others such as finite difference method, spectral methods [69], lattice Boltzmann method (LBM) [70, 71], arbitrary Lagrangian–Eulerian (ALE) methods [72], immerse boundary method (IBM) [73], particle methods [74] or hybrid models [75–77].

The finite volume method is based on mass, momentum, and energy balances in predefined control volumes. The values in the cell centers are calculated by iteration, and the values on the cell walls are interpolated using interpolation schemes of various orders, affecting the calculations' accuracy and stability. However, in the case of the finite element method, the values are calculated for the network nodes. The main advantage of the finite volume method is the fulfillment of the conservation equations of mass, momentum, and energy because convective flows compensate each other within the balance on the walls of the control volume. In contrast, in the case of the finite element method, additional stabilizing terms are necessary to ensure the preservation of these laws. On the other hand, the finite element method copes better with diffusive flows because it can accurately determine the gradients, which can sometimes be problematic in the case of the finite volume method. After all, the values on the walls are interpolated. Various software uses FVM, such as commercial ANSYS Fluent [8, 14, 15, 27] or open-source OpenFOAM [28], and for FEM, there are COMSOL Multiphysics [78] or Abaqus [79], both commercial.

In the case of other methods, there are, for example, spectral method based Nektar++ [69], LBM based Palabos [70, 71], ALE methods based LS-Dyna [72], IBM based IBAMR [73], Particle methods based DualSPHysics [74] or hybrid such as lifex-cfd [75], SimVascular [76] or ANSYS Fluent coupled with ANSYS Mechanical [77].

CFD simulations are one of the most frequently used tools in modeling the functioning of the circulatory system. There have been many works presenting the use of simulations in the circulatory system to model blood flow in vessels with stents, heart function, and other areas. One of the interesting applications of CFD in the circulatory system is the modeling of shear stresses on the wall. As part of one of the previous works, it was verified that the impact of the pulsating nature of the flow on the average stresses is relatively small, as can be seen in Figure 10.2, and it is possible to operate on a steady average flow with a good approximation [13].

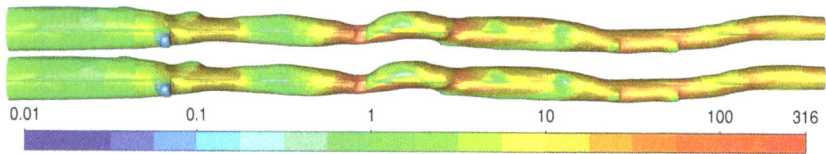

Figure 10.2: Comparison of the shear stresses (Pa) on the wall for the transient simulation (top) with the case for the mean velocity (bottom); (blood flows from left to right) [13].

Subsequent research examined, among other things, how the impact of exercise changes the hydrodynamics of flow in the carotid arteries, which directly affects the increase in shear stress and, consequently, a greater risk of hemolysis, which increases the risk of clot formation that can block further sections of the arteries. Figure 10.3 shows the influence of the increase in blood flow during exercise on the increase in the turbulent nature of the flow in the zone behind the stenosis [11]. This shows how important it is to take into account the change in the nature of flow from laminar to turbulent in arteries affected by atherosclerosis.

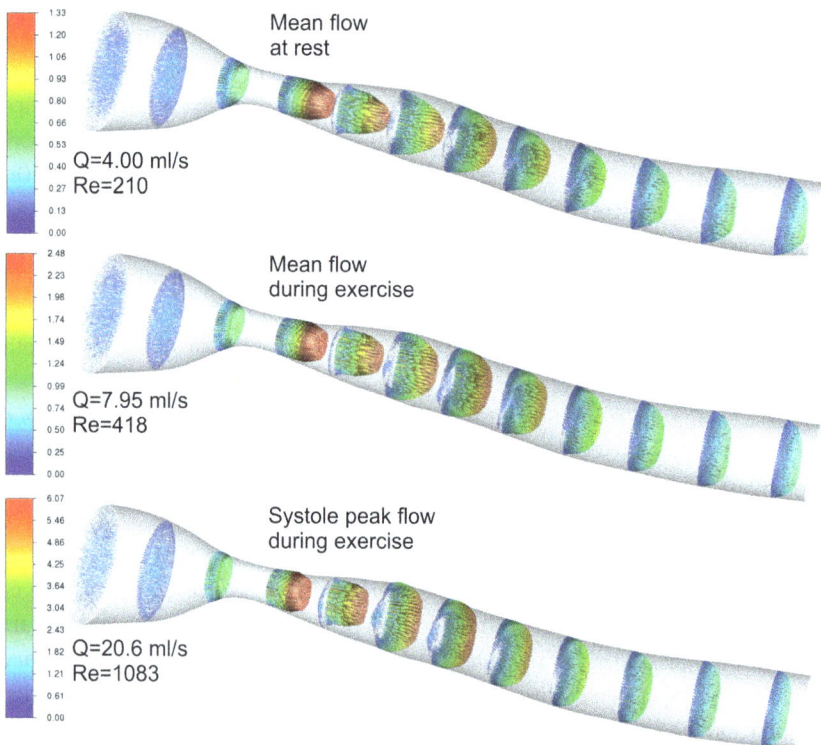

Figure 10.3: 3D velocity magnitude [m/s] profile results for carotid artery during rest and exercise [11].

10.3 Experimental techniques

10.3.1 Medical imaging

With the development of technology and medicine, many medical imaging methods have been created that allow obtaining high-resolution three-dimensional models. Well-known techniques commonly used in modeling the circulatory system are: optical coherence tomography [80–84], near-infrared spectroscopy [85], ultrasound imaging [86–89], computed tomography [90–96], and magnetic resonance imaging [96–102]. 4D flow MRI utilizes the same apparatus as classical MRI but can also reconstruct the velocity flow field using specialized commercial imaging software. It is also possible to analyze the 4D flow MRI data using an open-source Matlab toolbox developed by Prof. Sotelo et al. [103] 4D flow MRI can for example be very useful in analyzing complex blood flow profiles and quantifying the work of the heart; the results of 4D flow MRI are shown in Figures 10.4 and 10.5.

10.3.2 Experimental verification techniques

Experimental validation is crucial to ensure the correctness of CFD simulation. Particle image velocimetry is widely used to verify a fluid flow pattern. There are various different subtechniques such as 2D PIV [10, 50], Stereoscopic (2D3C) PIV [51], Tomographic PIV (3D3CPIV) [52], Echo PIV (EPIV) [105, 106], Smartphone-based PIV [107] or X-ray PIV [108]. 2D PIV uses one camera to measure 2 vector components of the local velocities in a plane perpendicular to the camera, illuminated by laser light, based on the displacement of particles between two consecutive frames. Smartphone-based PIV is similar but uses a smartphone instead of a typical camera. Stereoscopic PIV differs from 2D PIV because 2 cameras are required to correlate stereoscopic images to obtain 3rd component of velocity vectors instead of 2D velocity vectors in 2D PIV. It is worth mentioning that the calibration process for Stereoscopic PIV is more complex than for 2D PIV. Volumetric PIV is an extension of stereoscopic PIV because it measures the velocity field in volume instead of in-plane for previous techniques. Echo PIV differs from others because the echocardiography apparatus is used instead of a camera to create images. On the other hand, X-ray PIV, as the name says, uses X-ray images.

Previous studies compared CFD measurement results for coronary arteries with stenoses in both contour plots (Figure 10.6) and XY plots (Figure 10.7) [10]. It can be noted that the PIV and CFD results show very good agreement, which proves the correctness of the CFD simulation and that the quality of 3D printing allows for obtaining high-resolution phantoms of the circulatory system. The developed research methodology allows for the identification of dead zones and recirculation loops that increase the risk of blood clots.

During the latest research, a 2D µPIV was conducted. A µPIV system based on a New Wave Solo double-pulsed 532-nm laser with a <10-ns pulse duration and a Dantec

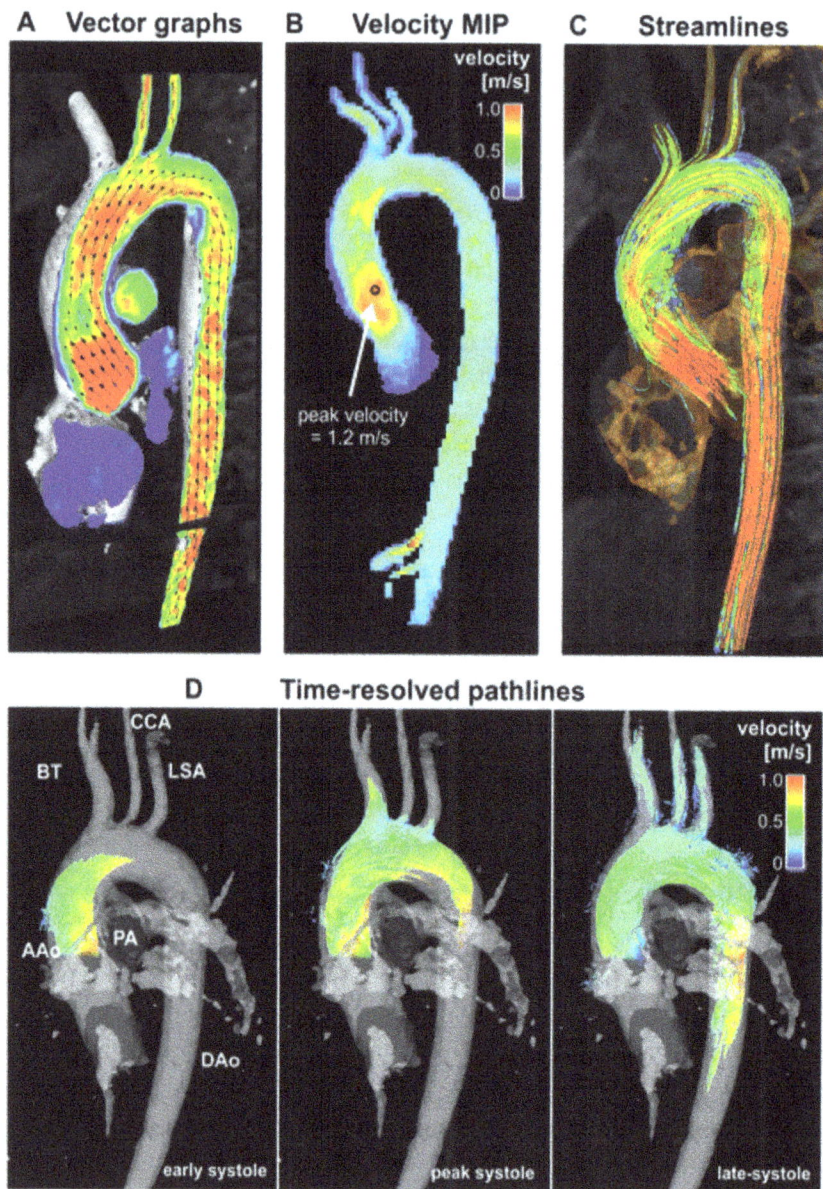

Figure 10.4: Examples of 4D Flow CMR visualization techniques. All examples are based on data acquired in the aorta of a healthy volunteer. In these examples, flow visualization is overlaid onto a segmentation of the aorta. (A) An oblique slice that transects the aorta has been color-coded by flow speed and combined with a graph of velocity vectors which here displays the speed and direction of blood velocity in black arrows at a coarser grid than the acquired voxels. This type of visualization provides a quick overview of velocity fields. (B) A maximum intensity projection (MIP) image of flow speed permits identification of areas of elevated velocity and the point of peak velocity while displaying the peak velocities of the whole volume projected onto this single slice image. (C) Streamlines are instantaneously tangent to the velocity vector field and are useful to visualize 3D velocity fields at discrete time points. Here, the peak systolic velocity field is shown. (D) Pathlines are the trajectories that massless fluid particles would follow through the dynamic velocity field. Pathlines are suitable for studies of the path of pulsatile blood flow

Dynamics FlowSense 4M MkII double-frame camera with a resolution of 2048 × 2048 pixels, 7.4 µm pixel size, and 12-bit pixel depth was used. For camera optics, a 60 mm macro lens with spacer rings were used to obtain the field-of-view below 10 × 10mm, and an Edmund Optics long-pass filter transmission of >90 % wavelength >538 nm (blocking laser light with optical density ≥6.0) was used. The system was managed using DynamicStudio v7.5 fluid measurement software and a Dantec Dynamics TimerBox TTL synchronization unit. Eurotek light sheet optics were used to generate a laser beam. The 3D-printed sample was placed on two Standa translation stages with a 150-mm travel range mounted perpendicularly and a micrometer screw for accurate positioning. Dantec Dynamics fluorescent polyamide particles with a 1–20 µm size distribution were added as seeding particles. A Legato 100 syringe pump forced a flow and was used in a closed loop. The flow rate was 2.31 mL/s, which was split into 2 canals, LAD and LCX, with a ratio near 1:1.1. Each measurement was started after the flow had stabilized. 280 images per sample position were acquired. Five fields-of-view were recorded to obtain the entire test geometry. Eurotek provided the calibration tool. The measurement system is schematically shown in Figure 10.8.

The average area represented by a single vector is around 145 × 145 µm. Temporal resolution was 7 Hz, but steady-state flow measurements were considered, so this had no impact on the results.

10.4 Results

CFD simulations were carried out using ANSYS Fluent 2023R2. For comparison with PIV measurements, the same dynamic viscosity and density as blood-like fluid was used to maintain the same kinematic viscosity as blood. Similarly to the previous simulation, the GEKO turbulence model with transitional flow options was adopted to be flexible between laminar and transitional flows [10, 11, 13]. Like PIV measurements, the blood flow on the inlet was set at 2.31 ml/s. The outflow condition was used for the outlets to maintain the 1:1.1 split ratio between the LAD and LCX arteries. The results of CFD simulation for 3 different geometries were presented in Figures 10.5–10.7. Each has a similar shape; the

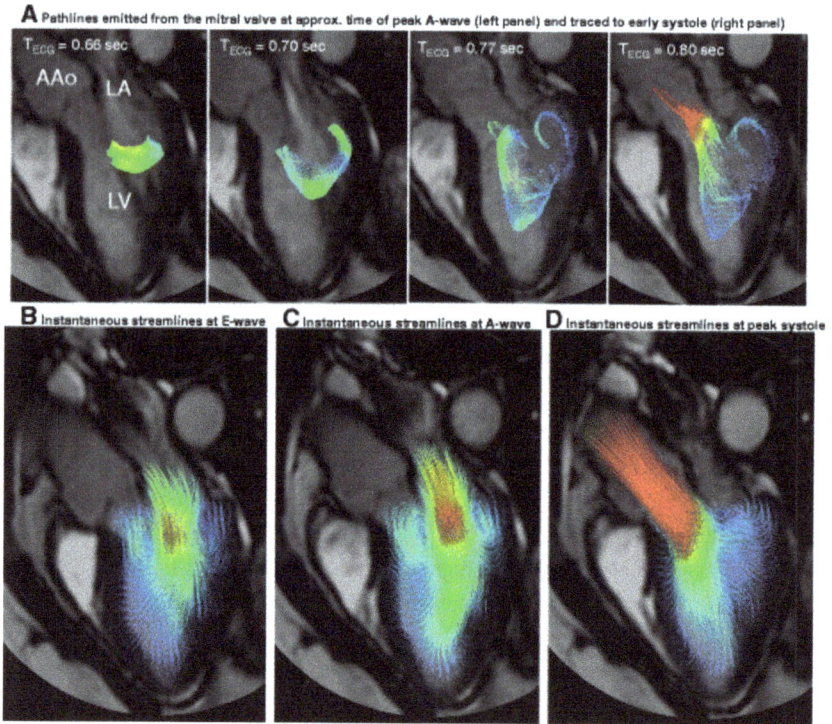

Figure 10.5: Examples of 4D flow CMR visualization techniques, demonstrated on intracardiac flow data acquired in a healthy volunteer. In these examples, flow visualization is overlaid onto a 2D bSSFP acquisition in a three-chamber view. (A) Pathlines are the trajectories that massless fluid particles would follow through the dynamic velocity field and are suitable for studies of the path of pulsatile blood flow over time. Here, the transit of blood through the left ventricle (LV) is shown by pathlines emitted from the mitral valve at the time point of peak A-wave and traced to the time point of early systole systole. The timing of the ECG (TECG) is included for reference. (B–D) Streamlines are instantaneously tangent to the velocity vector field and are useful to visualize 3D velocity fields at discrete time points. Here, streamlines generated in a long-axis plane show parts of the intracardiac velocity field at the time points of b peak early filling (E-wave), c peak late filling (A-wave), and d peak systole [104]. Journal of Cardiovascular Magnetic Resonance, 4D Flow Cardiovascular Magnetic Resonance Consensus Statement., 17, 72, 2015, Dyverfeldt, P.; Bissell, M.; Barker, A.J.; Bolger, A.F.; Carlhäll, C.J.; Ebbers, T.; Francios, C.J.; Frydrychowicz, A.; Geiger, J.; Giese, D.; et al. (© 2015 Dyverfeldt et al. This is an Open Access article distributed under the terms of the Creative Commons Attribution License (http://creativecommons.org/licenses/by/4.0), which permits unrestricted use, distribution, and reproduction in any medium, provided the original work is properly credited. The Creative Commons Public Domain Dedication waiver (http://creativecommons.org/publicdomain/zero/1.0/) applies to the data made available in this article, unless otherwise stated.) "With permission of Springer".

only difference is that atherosclerosis is asymmetrical and symmetrical and appears at the bifurcation area. Model A is free of diseases; model B has atherosclerosis on the LAD side of geometry, and model C has diseases on both the LAD and the LCX sides. All parameters measured together with PIV images are shown in Table 10.1.

a)

b)

| 0.00 | 0.04 | 0.08 | 0.12 | 0.16 | 0.20 | 0.24 | 0.28 | 0.32 | 0.36 | 0.40 |

c)

| 0.00 | 0.04 | 0.08 | 0.12 | 0.16 | 0.20 | 0.24 | 0.28 | 0.32 | 0.36 | 0.40 |

d)

| 0.00 | 0.30 | 0.60 | 0.90 | 1.20 | 1.50 | 1.80 | 2.10 | 2.40 | 2.70 | 3.00 |

e)

| 0.00 | 0.30 | 0.60 | 0.90 | 1.20 | 1.50 | 1.80 | 2.10 | 2.40 | 2.70 | 3.00 |

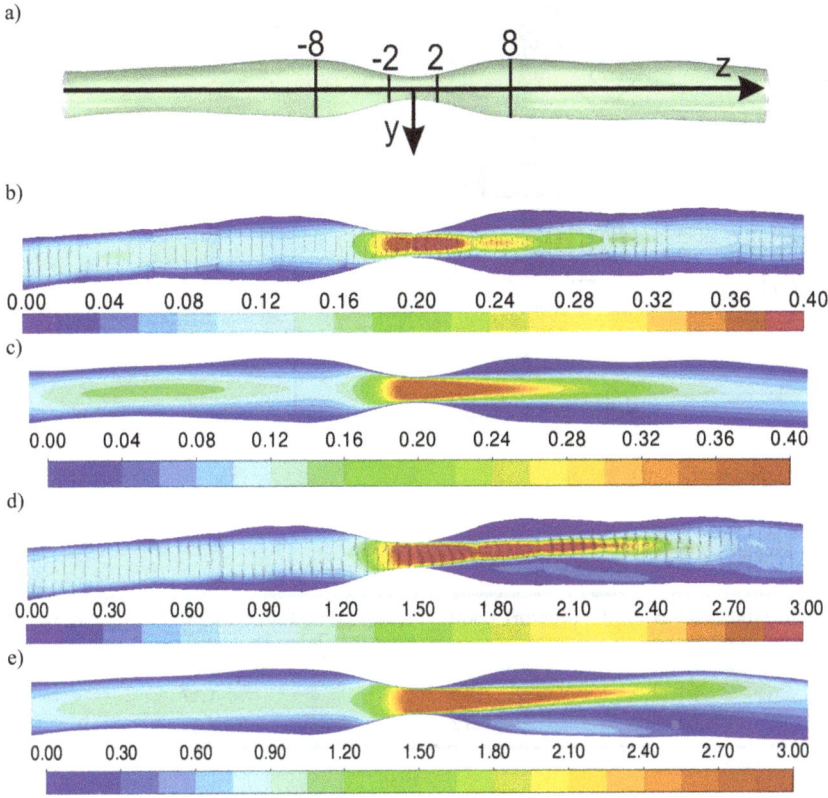

Figure 10.6: Analyzed geometry and comparison between CFD simulations and PIV experiments results. (a) 3D model with cross-sections for velocity profile comparison. The green cross-section is used for µPIV measurements and computational fluid dynamics comparison. (b) Contours of a velocity magnitude obtained from µPIV measurements for a flow rate of 0.625 mL/s. (c) Contours of a velocity magnitude obtained from computational fluid dynamics simulation for a flow rate of 0.625 mL/s. (d) Contours illustrating velocity magnitude obtained from µPIV measurements at a flow rate of 5 mL/s. (e) Contours illustrating velocity magnitude obtained from computational fluid dynamics simulation at a flow rate of 5 mL/s [10].

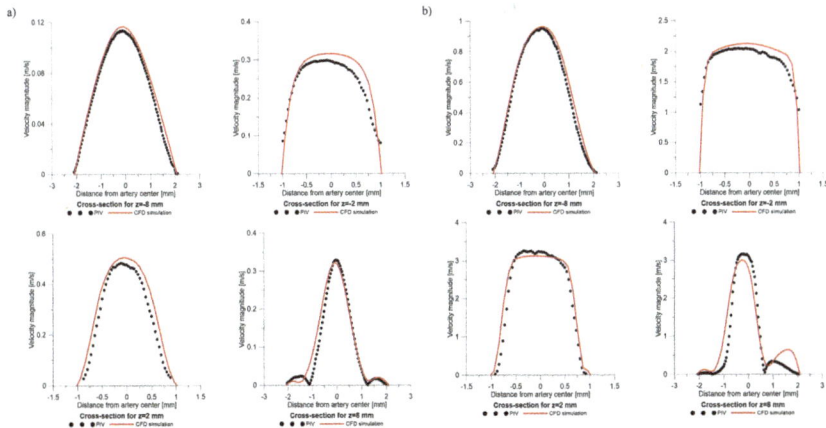

Figure 10.7: Comparison of µPIV measurements and CFD simulation at two different flow rates: (a) 0.625 mL/s (b) 5 mL/s [10].

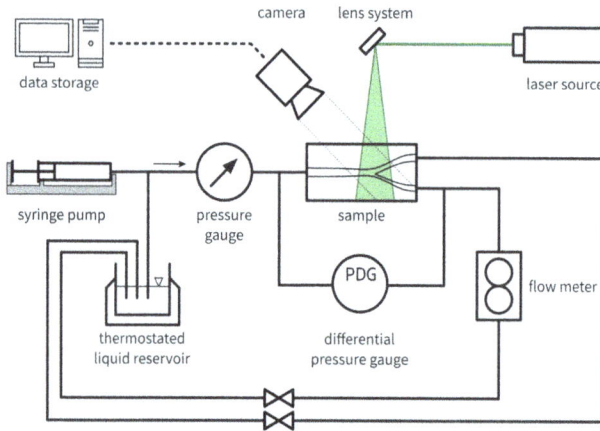

Figure 10.8: Experimental setup schematics.

Table 10.1: Experiment details.

Model	Split ratio LAD:LCX	Inlet pressure [kPa]	Pressure drop for LCX [kPa]	Temperature [°C]
A	1:1.15	35.6	1.03–1.04	24
B	1:1.12	34.9	1.16–1.17	24
C	1:1.08	36.3	2.09–2.10	24

Figure 10.9 presents the blood flow pattern for healthy bifurcation of the left coronary artery. It can be seen that there is a small stagnation zone after bifurcation in the proximal part of the LAD artery, which is visible for both the simulation and the PIV experiment. The values of velocity magnitude for both simulation and experiment are very similar.

Figure 10.10 shows the blood flow pattern for bifurcation of the left coronary artery with severe stenosis between the LAD and left main coronary arteries. There is a visible

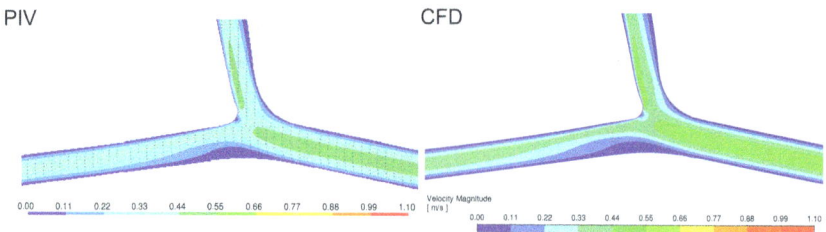

Figure 10.9: Comparison between PIV experiment and CFD simulation for the geometry of healthy coronary artery.

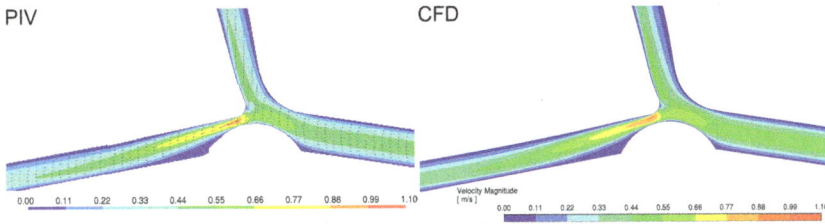

Figure 10.10: Comparison between the PIV experiment and CFD simulation for the geometry of coronary artery with stenosis on the LAD side of the bifurcation.

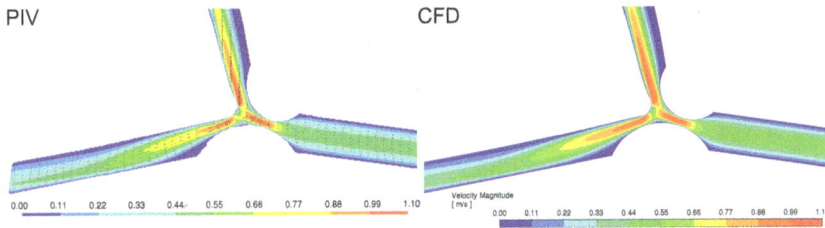

Figure 10.11: Comparison between the PIV experiment and CFD simulation for the geometry of coronary artery with stenoses on the LAD and LCX side of the bifurcation.

jet in the stenosis area and stagnation zone after stenosis on the opposite side of the artery wall. The results from both simulation and experiment are in excellent agreement.

Figure 10.11 depicts the blood flow pattern for bifurcation of the left coronary artery with severe stenosis between the LAD artery and the left main coronary artery and another between the LCX artery and the left main coronary artery. There are visible jets in the stenosis areas and stagnation zones after stenoses on the opposite side of the artery walls. The experiments and CFD simulation provide the same results, showing that PIV measurements can be applied to validated CFD simulations of cardiovascular flows.

10.5 Conclusions

Advances in 4D MRI and computational fluid dynamics (CFD) simulations have enabled non-invasive diagnostics for atherosclerosis, providing detailed insights into blood flow in plaque-affected arteries. These simulations can help clinicians assess wall shear stress and plan more precise treatments. The use of 3D-printed vascular models, combined with CFD and particle image velocimetry (PIV), allows for accurate validation of simulations, enabling realistic testing of patient-specific treatment strategies. Integrating modern imaging, CFD, and 3D printing offers a major step forward in diagnosing and treating cardiovascular diseases, improving both safety and effectiveness.

Acknowledgment: The authors would like to thank the editors David Bogle and Tomasz Sosnowski for their guidance and review of this article before its publication.

References

1. Alpert JS. A few unpleasant facts about atherosclerotic arterial disease in the United States and the world. Am J Med 2012;125:839–40.
2. Amini M, Zayeri F, Salehi M. Trend analysis of cardiovascular disease mortality, incidence, and mortality-to-incidence ratio: results from global burden of disease study 2017. BMC Publ Health 2021;21. https://doi.org/10.1186/s12889-021-10429-0.
3. Kim H, Kim S, Han S, Rane PP, Fox KM, Qian Y, et al. Prevalence and incidence of atherosclerotic cardiovascular disease and its risk factors in Korea: a nationwide population-based study. BMC Publ Health 2019;19. https://doi.org/10.1186/s12889-019-7439-0.
4. Spector R. New insight into the dietary cause of atherosclerosis: implications for pharmacology. J Pharmacol Exp Therapeut 2016;358:103–8.
5. Henning RJ. Obesity and obesity-induced inflammatory disease contribute to atherosclerosis: a review of the pathophysiology and treatment of obesity. Am J Cardiovasc Dis 2021;11.
6. Giersiepen M, Wurzinger LJ, Opitz R, Reul H. Estimation of shear stress-related blood damage in heart valve prostheses-in vitro comparison of 25 aortic valves. Int J Artif Organs 1990;13:300–6.
7. Lacasse D, Garon A, Pelletier D. Mechanical hemolysis in blood flow: user-independent predictions with the solution of a partial differential equation. Comput Methods Biomech Biomed Eng 2007;10:1–12.
8. Jędrzejczak K, Makowski Ł, Orciuch W. Model of blood rheology including hemolysis based on population balance. Commun Nonlinear Sci Numer Simul 2023;116:106802.
9. Michel JB, Martin-Ventura JL. Red blood cells and hemoglobin in human atherosclerosis and related arterial diseases. Int J Mol Sci 2020;21:1–20.
10. Jędrzejczak K, Antonowicz A, Makowski Ł, Orciuch W, Wojtas K, Kozłowski M. Computational fluid dynamics validated by micro particle image velocimetry to estimate the risk of hemolysis in arteries with atherosclerotic lesions. Chem Eng Res Des 2023;196:342–53.
11. Jędrzejczak K, Orciuch W, Wojtas K, Kozłowski M, Piasecki P, Narloch J, et al. Prediction of hemodynamic-related hemolysis in carotid stenosis and aiding in treatment planning and risk stratification using computational fluid dynamics. Biomedicines 2024;12. https://doi.org/10.3390/biomedicines12010037.
12. https://www.bruker.com/en/products-and-solutions/preclinical-imaging/mri/biospec/biospec-180-11.html [Accessed 24 Sep 2024].
13. Jędrzejczak K, Makowski Ł, Orciuch W, Wojtas K, Kozłowski M. Hemolysis of red blood cells in blood vessels modeled via computational fluid dynamics. Int J Numer Method Biomed Eng 2023;39. https://doi.org/10.1002/cnm.3699.
14. Wojtas K, Kozłowski M, Orciuch W, Makowski Ł. Computational fluid dynamics simulations of mitral paravalvular leaks in human heart. Materials 2021;14. https://doi.org/10.3390/ma14237354.
15. Kozłowski M, Wojtas K, Orciuch W, Smolka G, Wojakowski W, Makowski Ł. Parameters of flow through paravalvular leak channels from computational fluid dynamics simulations-data from real-life cases and comparison with a simplified model. J Clin Med 2022;11. https://doi.org/10.3390/jcm11185355.
16. Kozłowski M, Wojtas K, Orciuch W, Jędrzejek M, Smolka G, Wojakowski W, et al. Potential applications of computational fluid dynamics for predicting hemolysis in mitral paravalvular leaks. J Clin Med 2021;10. https://doi.org/10.3390/jcm10245752.
17. Gori F, Boghi A. Three-dimensional numerical simulation of blood flow in two coronary stents. Numeri Heat Transf A Appl 2011;59:231–46.

18. Albadawi M, Abuouf Y, Elsagheer S, Ookawara S, Ahmed M. Predicting the onset of consequent stenotic regions in carotid arteries using computational fluid dynamics. Phys Fluids 2021;33. https://doi.org/10.1063/5.0068998.

19. AL-Rawi M, AL-Jumaily AM, Belkacemi D. Non-invasive diagnostics of blockage growth in the descending aorta-computational approach. Med Biol Eng Comput 2022;60:3265–79.

20. Kopylova V, Boronovskiy S, Nartsissov Y. Approaches to vascular network, blood flow, and metabolite distribution modeling in brain tissue. Biophys Rev 2023;15:1335–50.

21. Viola F, Del Corso G, De Paulis R, Verzicco R. GPU accelerated digital twins of the human heart open new routes for cardiovascular research. Sci Rep 2023;13. https://doi.org/10.1038/s41598-023-34098-8.

22. Lodi Rizzini M, Candreva A, Mazzi V, Pagnoni M, Chiastra C, Aben JP, et al. Blood flow energy identifies coronary lesions culprit of future myocardial infarction. Ann Biomed Eng 2023;52:226–38.

23. Belkacemi D, Tahar Abbes M, Al-Rawi M, Al-Jumaily AM, Bachene S, Laribi B. Intraluminal thrombus characteristics in AAA patients: non-invasive diagnosis using CFD. Bioengineering 2023;10. https://doi.org/10.3390/bioengineering10050540.

24. Khan PM, Sharma SD, Chakraborty S, Roy S. Effect of heart rate on the hemodynamics in healthy and stenosed carotid arteries. Phys Fluids 2023;35. https://doi.org/10.1063/5.0153323.

25. Gils C, Hansen DL, Nybo M, Frederiksen H. Elevated hemolysis index is associated with higher risk of cardiovascular diseases. Clin Chem Lab Med 2023;61:1497–505.

26. Carbonaro D, Mezzadri F, Ferro N, De Nisco G, Audenino AL, Gallo D, et al. Design of innovative self-expandable femoral stents using inverse homogenization topology optimization. Comput Methods Appl Mech Eng 2023;416:116288.

27. Valentim MXG, Zinani FSF, da Fonseca CE, Wermuth DP. Systematic review on the application of computational fluid dynamics as a tool for the design of coronary artery stents. Beni Suef Univ J Basic Appl Sci 2023;12. https://doi.org/10.1186/s43088-023-00382-9.

28. Jayendiran R, Nour B, Ruimi A. Fluid-structure interaction (FSI) analysis of stent-graft for aortic endovascular aneurysm repair (EVAR): material and structural considerations. J Mech Behav Biomed Mater 2018;87:95–110.

29. Martin DM, Murphy EA, Boyle FJ. Computational fluid dynamics analysis of balloon-expandable coronary stents: influence of stent and vessel deformation. Med Eng Phys 2014;36:1047–56.

30. Rigatelli G, Zuin M, Dell'Avvocata F, Vassilev D, Daggubati R, Nguyen T, et al. Evaluation of coronary flow conditions in complex coronary artery bifurcations stenting using computational fluid dynamics: impact of final proximal optimization technique on different double-stent techniques. Cardiovasc Revascularization Med 2017;18:233–40.

31. Wüstenhagen C, Borowski F, Grabow N, Schmitz KP, Stiehm M. Comparison of stented bifurcation and straight vessel 3D-simulation with a prior simulated velocity profile inlet. Curr Directions Biomed Eng 2016;2:293–6.

32. Gundert TJ, Marsden AL, Yang W, LaDisa J, JF. Optimization of cardiovascular stent design using computational fluid dynamics. J Biomech Eng 2012;134. https://doi.org/10.1115/1.4005542.

33. Boite Y, Suaiden Klein T, de Andrade Medronho R, Wajnberg E. Numerical simulation of flow-diverting stent: comparison between branches in bifurcation brain aneurysm. Biomech Model Mechanobiol 2023;22:1801–14.

34. Kim HJ, Vignon-Clementel IE, Coogan JS, Figueroa CA, Jansen KE, Taylor CA. Patient-specific modeling of blood flow and pressure in human coronary arteries. Ann Biomed Eng 2010;38:3195–209.

35. Shahid L, Rice J, Berhane H, Rigsby C, Robinson J, Griffin L, et al. Enhanced 4D flow MRI-based CFD with adaptive mesh refinement for flow dynamics assessment in coarctation of the aorta. Ann Biomed Eng 2022;50:1001–16.

36. Razavi A, Shirani E, Sadeghi MR. Numerical simulation of blood pulsatile flow in a stenosed carotid artery using different rheological models. J Biomech 2011;44:2021–30.

37. Boyd J, Buick JM, Green S. Analysis of the Casson and Carreau-Yasuda non-Newtonian blood models in steady and oscillatory flows using the Lattice Boltzmann method. Phys Fluids 2007;19:93103.
38. Siauw WL, Ng EYK, Mazumdar J. Unsteady stenosis flow prediction: a comparative study of non-Newtonian models with operator splitting scheme. Med Eng Phys 2000;22:265–77.
39. Shibeshi SS, Collins WE. The rheology of blood flow in a branched arterial system. Appl Rheol 2005;15: 398–405.
40. Johnston BM, Johnston PR, Corney S, Kilpatrick D. Non-Newtonian blood flow in human right coronary arteries: transient simulations. J Biomech 2006;39:1116–28.
41. Doost SN, Zhong L, Su B, Morsi YS. The numerical analysis of non-Newtonian blood flow in human patient-specific left ventricle. Comput Methods Progr Biomed 2016;127:232–47.
42. Morbiducci U, Gallo D, Massai D, Ponzini R, Deriu MA, Antiga L, et al. On the importance of blood rheology for bulk flow in hemodynamic models of the carotid bifurcation. J Biomech 2011;44:2427–38.
43. Ionescu CM. A memory-based model for blood viscosity. Commun Nonlinear Sci Numer Simul 2017;45: 29–34.
44. Giannokostas K, Moschopoulos P, Varchanis S, Dimakopoulos Y, Tsamopoulos J. Advanced constitutive modeling of the thixotropic elasto-visco-plastic behavior of blood: description of the model and rheological predictions. Materials 2020;13:4184.
45. Jariwala S, Horner JS, Wagner NJ, Beris AN. Application of population balance-based thixotropic model to human blood. J Nonnewton Fluid Mech 2020;281:104294.
46. Owens RG. A new microstructure-based constitutive model for human blood. J Nonnewton Fluid Mech 2006;140:57–70.
47. Moyers-Gonzalez M, Owens RG, Fang J. A non-homogeneous constitutive model for human blood. Part 1. Model derivation and steady flow. J Fluid Mech 2008;617:327–54.
48. Moyers-Gonzalez MA, Owens RG. A non-homogeneous constitutive model for human blood: Part II. Asymptotic solution for large péclet numbers. J Nonnewton Fluid Mech 2008;155:146–60.
49. Moyers-Gonzalez MA, Owens RG, Fang J. A non-homogeneous constitutive model for human blood: Part III. Oscillatory flow. J Nonnewton Fluid Mech 2008;155:161–73.
50. Antonowicz A, Wojtas K, Makowski Ł, Orciuch W, Kozłowski M. Particle image velocimetry of 3D-printed anatomical blood vascular models affected by atherosclerosis. Materials 2023;16:1055.
51. Vergine F, Maddalena L. Stereoscopic particle image velocimetry measurements of supersonic, turbulent, and interacting streamwise vortices: challenges and application. Prog Aero Sci 2014;66:1–16.
52. Saaid H, Voorneveld J, Schinkel C, Westenberg J, Gijsen F, Segers P, et al. Tomographic PIV in a model of the left ventricle: 3D flow past biological and mechanical heart valves. J Biomech 2019;90:40–9.
53. Arvand A, Hormes M, Reul H. A validated computational fluid dynamics model to estimate hemolysis in a rotary blood pump. Artif Organs 2005;29:531–40.
54. Goubergrits L, Affeld K. Numerical estimation of blood damage in artificial organs. Artif Organs 2004;28: 499–507.
55. Gu L, Smith WA. Evaluation of computational models for hemolysis estimation. Am Soc Artif Intern Organs J 2005;51:202–7.
56. Arwatz G, Smits AJ. A viscoelastic model of shear-induced hemolysis in laminar flow. Biorheology 2013;50: 45–55.
57. Arora D. Computational hemodynamics: hemolysis and viscoelasticity. Houston, Texas, USA: Rice University; 2006.
58. Ezzeldin HM, de Tullio MD, Vanella M, Solares SD, Balaras E. A strain-based model for mechanical hemolysis based on a coarse-grained red blood cell model. Ann Biomed Eng 2015;43:1398–409.
59. Vitello DJ, Ripper RM, Fettiplace MR, Weinberg GL, Vitello JM. Blood density is nearly equal to water density: a validation study of the gravimetric method of measuring intraoperative blood loss. J Vet Med 2015;2015. https://doi.org/10.1155/2015/152730.

60. Chen Y, Sharp MK. A strain-based flow-induced hemolysis prediction model calibrated by in vitro erythrocyte deformation measurements. Artif Organs 2011;35:145–56.
61. Dirkes N, Key F, Behr M. Eulerian formulation of the tensor-based morphology equations for strain-based blood damage modeling. Comput Methods Appl Mech Eng 2024;426. https://doi.org/10.1016/j.cma.2024.116979.
62. Shi Y, Lawford P, Hose R. Review of zero-D and 1-D models of blood flow in the cardiovascular system. Biomed Eng Online 2011;10. https://doi.org/10.1186/1475-925x-10-33.
63. Boujena S, Kafi O, El Khatib N. A 2D mathematical model of blood flow and its interactions in an atherosclerotic artery. Math Model Nat Phenom 2014;9:46–68.
64. Trejo-Soto C, Hernández-Machado A. Normalization of blood viscosity according to the hematocrit and the shear rate. Micromachines 2022;13. https://doi.org/10.3390/mi13030357.
65. Ameenuddin M, Anand M, Massoudi M. Effects of shear-dependent viscosity and hematocrit on blood flow. Appl Math Comput 2019;356:299–311.
66. Pinto SIS, Romano E, António CC, Sousa LC, Castro CF. The impact of non-linear viscoelastic property of blood in right coronary arteries hemodynamics — a numerical implementation. Int J Non Lin Mech 2020; 123:103477.
67. Garon A, Farinas M-I. Fast three-dimensional numerical hemolysis approximation. Artif Organs 2004;28: 1016–25.
68. Rydquist G, Esmaily M. A cell-resolved, Lagrangian solver for modeling red blood cell dynamics in macroscale flows. J Comput Phys 2022;461:111204.
69. Cantwell CD, Moxey D, Comerford A, Bolis A, Rocco G, Mengaldo G, et al. Nektar++: an open-source spectral/hp element framework. Comput Phys Commun 2015;192:205–19.
70. Tan J, Sinno TR, Diamond SL. A parallel fluid–solid coupling model using LAMMPS and Palabos based on the immersed boundary method. J Comput Sci 2018;25:89–100.
71. Latt J, Malaspinas O, Kontaxakis D, Parmigiani A, Lagrava D, Brogi F, et al. Palabos: parallel Lattice Boltzmann solver. Comput Math Appl 2021;81:334–50.
72. Zhang Y, Adams J, Wang VY, Horwitz L, Tartibi M, Morgan AE, et al. A finite element model of the cardiac ventricles with coupled circulation: biventricular mesh generation with hexahedral elements, airbags and a functional mockup interface to the circulation. Comput Biol Med 2021;137:104840.
73. Griffith BE. Immersed boundary model of aortic heart valve dynamics with physiological driving and loading conditions. Int J Numer Method Biomed Eng 2012;28:317–45.
74. Crespo AJC, Domínguez JM, Rogers BD, Gómez-Gesteira M, Longshaw S, Canelas R, et al. DualSPHysics: open-source parallel CFD solver based on smoothed particle hydrodynamics (SPH). Comput Phys Commun 2015;187:204–16.
75. Africa PC, Fumagalli I, Bucelli M, Zingaro A, Fedele M, Dede' L, et al. Lifex-cfd: an open-source computational fluid dynamics solver for cardiovascular applications. Comput Phys Commun 2024;296: 109039.
76. Updegrove A, Wilson NM, Merkow J, Lan H, Marsden AL, Shadden SC. SimVascular: an open source pipeline for cardiovascular simulation. Ann Biomed Eng 2017;45:525–41.
77. Chimakurthi SK, Reuss S, Tooley M, Scampoli S. ANSYS workbench system coupling: a state-of-the-art computational framework for analyzing Multiphysics problems. Eng Comput 2018;34:385–411.
78. Sun L, Ding L, Li L, Yin N, Yang N, Zhang Y, et al. Hemodynamic characteristics of cardiovascular system in simulated zero and partial gravities based on CFD modeling and simulation. Life 2023;13. https://doi.org/10.3390/life13020407.
79. Zhao S, Wu W, Samant S, Khan B, Kassab GS, Watanabe Y, et al. Patient-specific computational simulation of coronary artery bifurcation stenting. Sci Rep 2021;11. https://doi.org/10.1038/s41598-021-95026-2.
80. Bouma BE, Tearney GJ, Yabushita H, Shishkov M, Kauffman CR, DeJoseph Gauthier D, et al. Evaluation of intracoronary stenting by intravascular optical coherence tomography. Heart 2003;89:317–20.

81. Jang I-K, Bouma BE, Kang D-H, Park S-J, Park S-W, Seung K-B, et al. Visualization of coronary atherosclerotic plaques in patients using optical coherence tomography: comparison with intravascular ultrasound. J Am Coll Cardiol 2002;39. https://doi.org/10.1016/s0735-1097(01)01799-5.

82. Dohad S, Zhu A, Krishnan S, Wang F, Wang S, Cox J, et al. Optical coherence tomography guided carotid artery stent procedure: technique and potential applications. Cathet Cardiovasc Interv 2018;91:521–30.

83. Schwindt AG, Bennett JG, Crowder WH, Dohad S, Janzer SF, George JC, et al. Lower extremity revascularization using optical coherence tomography-guided directional atherectomy: final results of the EValuation of the PantheriS optical COherence tomography ImagiNg atherectomy system for use in the peripheral vasculature (VISION) study. J Endovasc Ther 2017;24:355–66.

84. Araki M, Park SJ, Dauerman HL, Uemura S, Kim JS, Di Mario C, et al. Optical coherence tomography in coronary atherosclerosis assessment and intervention. Nat Rev Cardiol 2022;19:684–703.

85. Waxman S, Dixon SR, L'Allier P, Moses JW, Petersen JL, Cutlip D, et al. In vivo validation of a catheter-based near-infrared spectroscopy system for detection of lipid core coronary plaques. Initial results of the SPECTACL study. JACC Cardiovasc Imaging 2009;2:858–68.

86. Finn AV, Kolodgie FD, Virmani R. Correlation between carotid intimal/medial thickness and atherosclerosis: a point of view from pathology. Arterioscler Thromb Vasc Biol 2010;30:177–81.

87. Lal BK, Hobson RW, Pappas PJ, Kubicka R, Hameed M, Chakhtura EY, et al. Pixel distribution analysis of B-mode ultrasound scan images predicts histologic features of atherosclerotic carotid plaques. J Vasc Surg 2002;35:1210–17.

88. Noflatscher M, Hunjadi M, Schreinlechner M, Sommer P, Lener D, Theurl M, et al. Inverse correlation of cholesterol efflux capacity with peripheral plaque volume measured by 3D ultrasound. Biomedicines 2023;11:1918.

89. Hegner A, Wittek A, Derwich W, Huß A, Gámez AJ, Blase C. Using averaged models from 4D ultrasound strain imaging allows to significantly differentiate local wall strains in calcified regions of abdominal aortic aneurysms. Biomech Model Mechanobiol 2023;22:1709–27.

90. Moneta GL, Edwards JM, Chitwood RW, Taylor LM, Lee RW, Cummings CA, et al. Correlation of North American symptomatic carotid endarterectomy trial (NASCET) angiographic definition of 70% to 99% internal carotid artery stenosis with duplex scanning. J Vasc Surg 1993;17:152–9.

91. Josephson SA, Bryant SO, Mak HK, Johnston SC, Dillon WP, Smith WS. Evaluation of carotid stenosis using CT angiography in the initial evaluation of stroke and TIA. Neurology 2004;63:457.

92. Maurovich-Horvat P, Ferencik M, Voros S, Merkely B, Hoffmann U. Comprehensive plaque assessment by coronary CT angiography. Nat Rev Cardiol 2014;11:390–402.

93. Divakaran S, Cheezum MK, Hulten EA, Bittencourt MS, Silverman MG, Nasir K, et al. Use of cardiac CT and calcium scoring for detecting coronary plaque: implications on prognosis and patient management. Br J Radiol 2015;88. https://doi.org/10.1259/bjr.20140594.

94. Motoyama S, Ito H, Sarai M, Kondo T, Kawai H, Nagahara Y, et al. Plaque characterization by coronary computed tomography angiography and the likelihood of acute coronary events in mid-term follow-up. J Am Coll Cardiol 2015;66:337–46.

95. Maurovich-Horvat P, Hoffmann U, Vorpahl M, Nakano M, Virmani R, Alkadhi H. The napkin-ring sign: CT signature of high-risk coronary plaques? JACC Cardiovasc Imaging 2010;3:440–4.

96. Dweck MR, Williams MC, Moss AJ, Newby DE, Fayad ZA. Computed tomography and cardiac magnetic resonance in ischemic heart disease. J Am Coll Cardiol 2016;68:2201–16.

97. Akçakaya M, Basha TA, Chan RH, Manning WJ, Nezafat R. Accelerated isotropic sub-millimeter whole-heart coronary MRI: compressed sensing versus parallel imaging. Magn Reson Med 2014;71:815–22.

98. Ong WY, Im K, Anias EGD, Atthias M, Tuber S, Lamm CDF, et al. Coronary magnetic resonance angiography for the detection of coronary stenoses. N Engl J Med 2001;345.

99. Hatsukami TS, Ross R, Polissar NL, Yuan C. Visualization of fibrous cap thickness and rupture in human atherosclerotic carotid plaque in vivo with high-resolution magnetic resonance imaging. Circulation 2000;102:959–64.

100. Kerwin WS, Zhao X, Chun Y, Hatsukami TS, Maravilla KR, Underhill HR, et al. Contrast-enhanced MRI of carotid atherosclerosis: dependence on contrast agent. J Magn Reson Imag 2009;30:35–40.

101. Zhang J, Rothenberger SM, Brindise MC, Markl M, Rayz VL, Vlachos PP. Wall shear stress estimation for 4D flow MRI using Navier–Stokes equation correction. Ann Biomed Eng 2022;50:1810–25.

102. Nath R, Kazemi A, Callahan S, Stoddard MF, Amini AA. 4Dflow-VP-Net: a deep convolutional neural network for noninvasive estimation of relative pressures in stenotic flows from 4D flow MRI. Magn Reson Med 2023;90:2175–89.

103. Sotelo J, Mura J, Hurtado D, Uribe S. A novel MATLAB toolbox for processing 4D flow MRI data. USA: International Society of Magnetic Resonance in Medicine (ISMRM); 2019.

104. Dyverfeldt P, Bissell M, Barker AJ, Bolger AF, Carlhäll CJ, Ebbers T, et al. 4D flow cardiovascular magnetic resonance Consensus Statement. J Cardiovasc Magn Reson 2015;17:72.

105. DeMarchi N, White C. Echo particle image velocimetry. J Vis Exp 2012:4265. https://doi.org/10.3791/4265.

106. Voorneveld J, Saaid H, Schinkel C, Radeljic N, Lippe B, Gijsen FJH, et al. 4-D echo-particle image velocimetry in a left ventricular phantom. Ultrasound Med Biol 2020;46:805–17.

107. Caridi GCA, Torta E, Mazzi V, Chiastra C, Audenino AL, Morbiducci U, et al. Smartphone-based particle image velocimetry for cardiovascular flows applications: a focus on coronary arteries. Front Bioeng Biotechnol 2022;10. https://doi.org/10.3389/fbioe.2022.1011806.

108. Park H, Yeom E, Lee SJ. X-ray PIV measurement of blood flow in deep vessels of a rat: an in vivo feasibility study. Sci Rep 2016;6. https://doi.org/10.1038/srep19194.

Federico Galvanin*, Chun Fung Lee and Yuxuan Yang

11 On the development of pharmacokinetic models for the characterisation and diagnosis of von Willebrand disease

Abstract: Von Willebrand disease (VWD) is a metabolic disease characterised by a qualitative and/or quantitative deficiency of von Willebrand factor (VWF) a multimeric glycoprotein that mediates platelet adhesion in haemostatic processes. Pharmacokinetic (PK) models have been developed to characterise VWD metabolic pathways and to achieve a model-based diagnosis based on clinical data. However, current PK models cannot be calibrated from infusion tests data, and their calibration requires stressful 24-h long tests to be carried out on subjects to achieve a statistically satisfactory estimation of the individual haemostatic parameters. The objectives of this review chapter are the following: *i)* to provide a review on physiological modelling of VWD starting from the analysis of basic VWF mechanisms in the body; *ii)* to describe methods and modelling tools used to provide a model-based diagnosis of VWD and, consequently, a classification of complex VWD types; *iii)* to illustrate how model-based design of experiments (MBDoE) techniques can be applied to maximise the information that can be obtained from advanced clinical tests (DDAVP) but also from infusion tests used in VWD treatment where blood analogues are administered through single or multiple injections. Results show how PK models calibrated from clinical data can be used to estimate key haemostatic parameters in the diagnosis of the disease. Promising results on the application of MBDoE to design infusion tests show how the duration of clinical tests for the identification of key haemostatic parameters can significantly be reduced from 24 h to 2.5 h, with the potential to increase the acquired test information if multiple infusions can be managed.

Keywords: von Willebrand disease; pharmacokinetic models; model-based design of experiments

11.1 Introduction

Von Willebrand disease (VWD) is one of the most diffuse bleeding disorders in humans, caused by a modification of von Willebrand factor (VWF), a key multimeric glycoprotein present in the bloodstream and playing a crucial role in the haemostatic process [1]. VWF

*Corresponding author: Federico Galvanin, Department of Chemical Engineering, University College London, London, UK, E-mail: f.galvanin@ucl.ac.uk
Chun Fung Lee and Yuxuan Yang, Department of Chemical Engineering, University College London, London, UK

As per De Gruyter's policy this article has previously been published in the journal Physical Sciences Reviews. Please cite as: F. Galvanin, C. F. Lee and Y. Yang "On the development of pharmacokinetic models for the characterisation and diagnosis of von Willebrand disease" *Physical Sciences Reviews* [Online] 2024. DOI: 10.1515/psr-2024-0058 | https://doi.org/10.1515/9783111394558-011

mediates platelet aggregation and thrombus growth, and binds, transports and protects coagulation factor VIII. VWD-induced alteration of VWF in the bloodstream causes symptoms ranging from sporadic or prolonged bleeding episodes, nosebleeds, bleeding from small lesions in skin, mucosa or the gastrointestinal tract, menorrhagia and excessive bleeding after traumas, surgical interventions or childbirth [2, 3]. According to the 2019 survey from the World Federation of Hemophilia, there are approximately 80000 confirmed cases of VWD worldwide [4]. This value is far lower than the expectation of 1 % global prevalence, which historically leads to only 0.1 % of disease carriers being diagnosed [5]. The low diagnosis rate is generally attributed to the complexity of the standard diagnosis procedures. The diagnosis requires numerous laboratory tests requiring the clinician's interpretation [6]. Human error and bias could lead to mis-diagnoses with consequence that might be fatal, and this motivates the development of systematic approaches for VWD diagnosis. Diagnosis of VWD is a complex task due to the heterogeneous nature of the disorder, characterised by a number of VWD types and subtypes [7]. Subjects affected by VWD are usually classified into three VWD possible types on the basis of having a partial (type 1), total (type 3) quantitative defect or a qualitative deficiency in plasma VWF (type 2) [1]. Whilst VWD type 2 and type 3 are straightforward to diagnose, as they involve a variety of qualitative defects on VWF (VWD type 2) or the total absence of VWF (VWD type 3), the diagnosis of VWD type 1, which represents the most common VWD type (accounting for the 75 % of all cases), may become a long and very complicated task because of the elusive nature of the disease. Diagnosing type 1 VWD poses several challenges because of the strong heterogeneous nature of the disorder and the high intra-subject variability observed in the haemostatic laboratory findings. Recent studies involving 24 h 1-desamino-8-d-arginine vasopressin (DDAVP) tests carried out on a genetically categorised population of subjects underlined the importance of impaired VWF secretion and elimination from the body in modulating type 1 VWD and the key role of genetic mutations that are still not easily understood [8]. Type 2 VWD is characterised by different subtypes: 1) Type 2A, where the binding of VWF with platelets is reduced because of discriminatory deficiency of high molecular weight multimers, which has better ability in blood clotting, the potential cause being that specific mutations increase the susceptibility of large multimers to reduce to low mul-timers in plasma; 2) Type 2B, where VWF prematurely binds with the platelets, which enhance the removal of both platelet and VWF from plasma before reaching the wound; 3) Type 2M, where the binding between platelet and VWF is decreased, which reduces probability of platelets to clot in the injured site; 4) Type 2N, where as a result of a genetic mutation, the VWF binding with the protein Factor VIII is impaired, and this reduces the probability of blood clotting in the injured site.

Acquired von Willebrand syndrome (AVWS) is a rare heterogeneous bleeding dis-order [9] similar to inherited VWD that occurs in patients with no personal or family history of bleeding. AVWS is not a result of genetic defects but may be caused by un-derlying pathological conditions, including lympho- and myeloproliferative disorders, solid tumours, immune diseases, cardiovascular disorders, hypothyroidism, diabetes, and infectious diseases, or the side effects of drugs [10]. Subjects affected by AVWS present severe bleeding symptoms requiring urgent and often multiple treatment [9].

Pharmacokinetic (PK) models of different degree of complexity have been recently proposed for the characterisation of VWD, starting from algebraic models [11] to models described by differential and algebraic equations (DAEs) characterising the multimeric VWF patterns in VWD [12–15] and AVWS [10]. The calibration of these models is based on the estimation of subject-specific haemostatic parameters to elucidate the critical pathways involved in the disease characterisation and to assist model-based approaches to VWD diagnosis [13, 16]. However, the complexity of these models, defined by the number of state variables and subject-specific parameters, might require the execution of advanced, time-consuming (24 h long) and cumbersome non-routine tests like the DDAVP (desmopressin) response test to achieve a precise estimation of the individual haemostatic parameters. DDAVP test is a dynamic test where desmopressin is administered subcutaneously at a prescribed dose to patients (0.3–0.4 µg/kg body weight) [10, 17], and blood samples are collected at regular fixed times to characterise the subject's response. DDAVP is also used in the treatment of severe forms of VWD as desmopressin is capable of inducing a fast release of VWF stored in the Weibel Palade bodies of the endothelial cells. The time course of VWF antigen (VWF:Ag) and VWF collagen binding (VWF:CB) can be quantitatively analysed using dynamic kinetic models to characterise the time variation of VWF concentration in plasma [17]. VWF kinetics depend on three key factors: *i*) the amount of VWF released and the rate of release; *ii*) VWF proteolysis, i.e. the reduction of VWF multimeric chains into smaller multimeric forms as a result of the activity of a specific enzyme (ADAMTS-13); and *iii*) VWF elimination from the blood stream (clearance). As illustrated in Budde et al. [18], DDAVP administration is not suitable to treat all the types of VWD and is not recommended in patients with specific co-morbidities including atherosclerosis, heart failure or other conditions requiring diuretic treatment, as well as in very young children or in patients older than 65–70 years. For these reasons, plasma-derived VWF/FVIII analogues [19] are nowadays the current standard for controlling acute bleeding episodes or as prophylaxis for invasive or surgical procedures. Available VWF concentrates differ in their purification and pathogen removal as well as in VWF multimeric concentration and activity [20], all aspects which affect therapeutic safety and efficacy. So far there have been limited specific studies on models specifically developed to characterise the kinetics of exogenous VWF infusion of VWF concentrates [21] and to quantify the intrinsic information that can be obtained from infusion tests when different VWF concentrates are used. A key challenge in the identification of physiological models of VWD is the precise estimation of the set of subject-specific haemostatic parameters from potentially limited amount of data, and the evaluation of their 'estimability'. Estimability is strictly related to the level of information acquired from clinical tests and to the protocol used for dynamic model calibration [22].

This chapter is structured as follows: in Section 11.2, routine and advanced tests used in the clinical diagnosis of VWD are introduced; Section 11.3 presents the fundamental mechanisms involved in the disease characterisation; Section 11.4 provides an overview of procedures for model-based diagnosis, including PK model formulation (Section 11.4.1), the problem of estimating metabolic parameters from data (Section 11.4.2), and the development of new kinetic model including VWF exogenous infusion (Section 11.4.3). Section 11.5 illustrates results on the application of model-based diagnosis to subjects affected by VWD, while Section 11.6 illustrates fundamentals in the application of model-based design of experiments techniques (MBDoE) [23, 24] for the design of VWF infusion tests used in the treatment of VWD. Results reported in Section 11.7 on AVWS subjects show the potential of optimally designed infusion tests in drastically decreasing the time and effort required for a precise identification of the key set of haemostatic parameters. Section 11.8 draws some final conclusions on the research in the area and future challenges.

11.2 Clinical diagnosis of von Willebrand disease

A guidance publishes from the National Heart, Lung and Blood Institute [6] gives a standard procedure for diagnosing VWD. Since VWD is an inherited disease, the procedure begins with reviewing the medical history of the patient's family and relatives. Preliminary haemostasis tests are then carried out including platelet count, partial thromboplastin time and prothrombin time. If the haemostasis test result is negative, the patient should be referred to other specialists; otherwise, initial VWD assays will be performed to classify the type of VWD. VWD assays include four main items:

1. VWF antigen (VWF: Ag) assay: shows the total VWF concentration in plasma regardless of the multimer molecular weight.
2. VWF Ristocetin Cofactor Activity (VWF: RCo) assay: to measure the degree of platelet agglutination induced after the addition of ristocetin.
3. Factor VIII: a blood-clotting protein that is essential in the coagulation process.
4. VWF collagen-binding assay (VWF: CB): to measure the binding of VWF to type I and III collagens. High molecular weight multimers have a higher affinity to collagen, so VWF:CB represents a measure of the concentration of high molecular weight VWF multimers in plasma. All these tests are routine tests usually carried out at basal, stationary conditions. In diagnosing VWD, VWF: RCo assay can be partially replaced by the VWF: CB assay [25] because the VWF: RCo assay is time-consuming, and the result particularly difficult to reproduce [5]. Since the collagens favourably attaches to the larger multimer, the VWF: CB result is useful to discriminate the types of VWD that are insufficient in large multimers such as type 1, 2A and 2B. If all these tests failed to give a clear diagnosis, one or more *advanced laboratory tests* are required. These tests are very assorted, but there are some common options followed in the clinical practice [6]:

1. Measurement of multimer distribution patterns by gel electrophoresis;
2. The VWF Ristocetin Cofactor Activity (VWF: RCo);
3. The binding of factor VIII to VWF;
4. Desmopressin (DDVAP) test;
5. DNA sequencing.

The identification of the VWD type might become a long and cumbersome procedure, as it largely depends on the experience of the clinician and the subjective ability to systematically analyse the results from routine and advanced tests. When analysing the results, the clinician might potentially ask to repeat some of the tests if needed to then provide a clear identification of the disease through differential diagnosis.

11.3 From fundamental mechanisms to VWD modelling

Figure 11.1 describes the base mechanisms involved in the distribution of VWF in the bloodstream from the production to elimination [13]. After VWF is synthesised in the ethnophiles cell as ultra-large multimers, there are three basic mechanisms taking place:
1. VWF release: the ultra-large VWF multimers are released into the plasma.
2. VWF proteolysis: the enzyme ADAMTS13 splits the ultra-large multimers into shorter chains, which are the low molecular weight VWF multimers.
3. VWF elimination (even known as *VWF clearance*): all multimers are removed from plasma in the liver eventually with a mechanism that does not depend on multimer size.

Any irregularity in these steps can lead to low VWF levels or abnormal multimer distribution hence different types of VWD.

Figure 11.2a and 11.b shows an example of data collected from DDAVP clinical tests for O healthy subjects and a subject affected by AVWS in terms of VWF antigen (VWF:Ag) and VWF collagen binding (VWF:CB). Clinical data have from DDAVP been supplied by the Hospital of Padua. DDAVP (1-desamino-8-ᴅ-argine vasopressin; Emosint, Sclavo, Italy) was

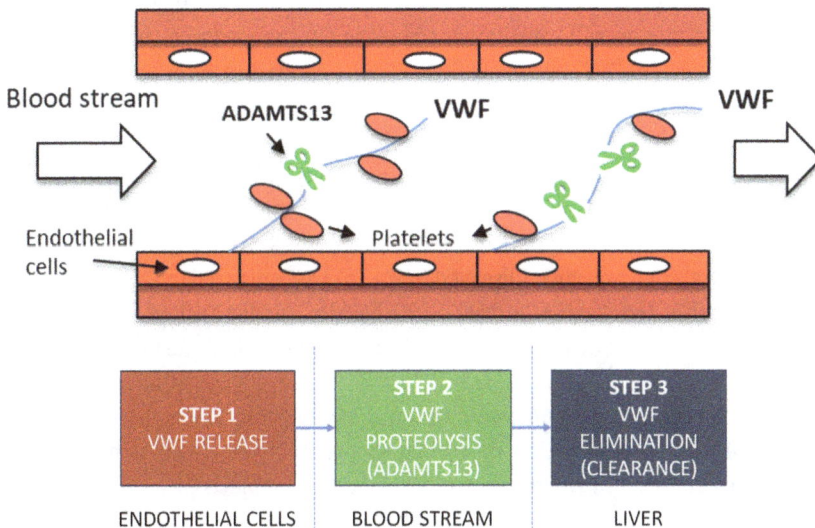

Figure 11.1: Base mechanisms involved in the distribution of VWF in the bloodstream.

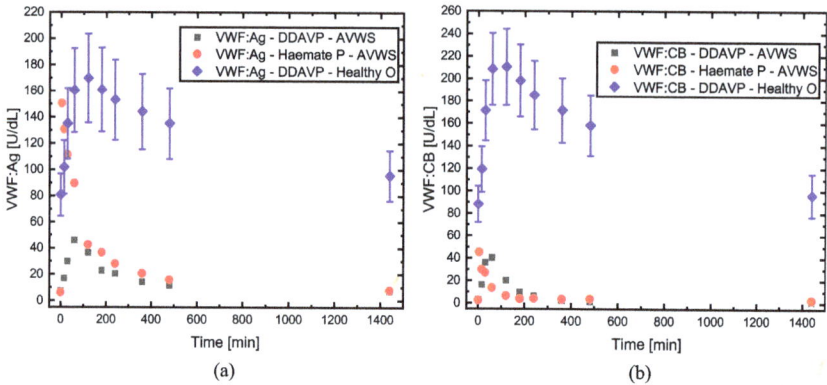

Figure 11.2: Examples of (a) VWF:Ag and (b) VWF:CB measurements after DDAVP administration to healthy O (blue diamonds), AVWS subject (black squares) and after VWF analogue (Haemate P) administration for a subject affected by AVWS (red circles) [21].

administered subcutaneously at a dose of 0.3 µg kg^{-1}. Blood samples were collected before and 15, 30, 60, 120, 180, 240, 480 min and 24 h after administering DDAVP for a pool of health subjects (O/non-O blood group) and for a subject affected by AVWS. AVWS patient and normal subjects were studied in accordance with the Helsinki Declaration, after obtaining their written informed consent, and our ethical board's approval of the study. The same subject was also treated with exogenous intravenous administration of Haemate P, a VWF concentrate commonly used in the treatment of VWD. After administering 2,000 U of Haemate P (a VWF analogue) (Behring GMBH, Hattersheim am Main, Germany), blood samples were collected at 4, 15, 30, 60, 120, 180, 240, 360, 480 min and at 24 h. In clinical practice, sampling points are concentrated at the beginning of the test, as intravenous administration produces faster dynamics in VWF as compared to subcutaneous DDAVP administration. As VWF exists across a multimeric range, VWF:Ag represents a measure of the overall VWF amount in plasma for the subjects, including high and low molecular weight VWF species, while VWF:CB is a measure of the amount of high molecular weight species only.

There are several important aspects to observe from Figure 11.2:

– All curves show a peak that corresponds to the maximum in VWF release in overall terms (VWF:Ag, Figure 11.2a) and in terms of high molecular weight multimers (VWF:CB, Figure 11.2b)

– After the peak, a slower decay is observed in VWF:Ag as compared to VWF:CB caused by the proteolytic activity (i.e. a fraction of high molecular weight multimers is reduced to multimers with shorter chains). This is valid for both healthy O subjects and subjects affected by AVWS.

– AVWS is characterised by significantly reduced VWF:Ag and VWF:CB levels before and after DDAVP administration (levels are considerably low also at basal state, i.e. see values at $t = 0$ min when compared to healthy O subjects);

- The infusion of Haemate P in the AVWS patient prompted a sudden increase in low molecular weight species (see VWF:ag peak in the first observation after 4 min) but produced a limited release of high multimeric species (relatively low VWF:CB levels) during the test;
- For the AVWS patient, very low VWF:CB levels are observed both after DDAVP and after Haemate P infusion;
- The infusion of Haemate P forces a very fast dynamic VWF response, i.e. by 240 min after the administration most of the VWF:CB was no longer detectable.

Since high molecular weight multimers are more active in the coagulation process, and their deficiency leads to prolonged bleeding in subjects even after small lesions or scars. It is of primary importance to understand: *i)* if and how infusion tests can be used for the identification of subject-specific metabolic parameters; *ii)* if infusion tests can be more or less informative than a standard DDAVP test, i.e. if this test can provide a more precise and accurate estimation of haemostatic parameters; *iii)* if the infusion protocol can be personalised and optimally designed; *iv)* given that a conventional DDAVP requires 24 h to be execute, if the overall test duration can be shortened by adopting infusion tests, preserving at the same time the required level of information.

11.4 Model-based diagnosis of VWD

A model-based procedure for VWD diagnosis based on the quantitative characterisation of the metabolic pathways involved in post-DDAVP and VWF infusion studies is illustrated in Figure 11.3. Given the availability of historical data for each subject class, the variance of the population can be characterised by estimating the parameters of a

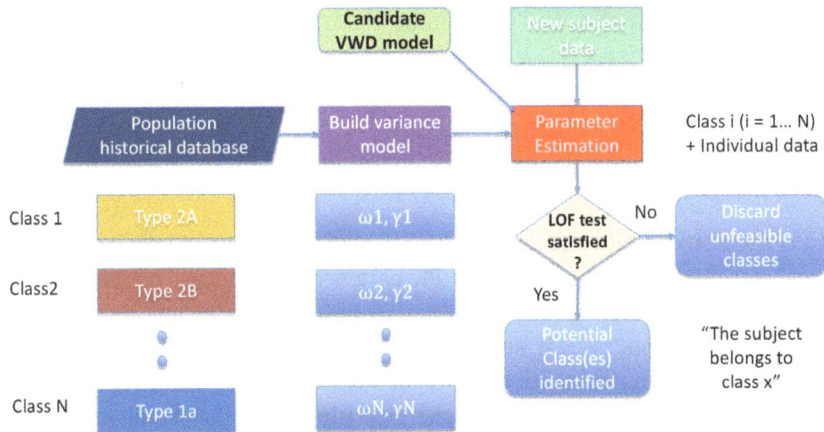

Figure 11.3: Procedure used for model-based diagnosis.

heteroscedastic model (see Section 11.4.2, equation (11.15)). When test data are available for the unknown subject, a parameter estimation is carried out to estimate the set of kinetic parameters of a candidate model, based on both historical data from each subject's class and individual data [13]. The class providing the lowest lack-of-fit (LOF) statistics represents the class of belonging, as it evaluates both the deviation between model predictions and individual test data (residuals, see Section 11.4.2, equation (11.15)) and the distance from the population data.

The following sections contain a description of the pharmacokinetic models used for model-based diagnosis (Section 11.3.1) and the identification of metabolic parameters from DDAVP data (Section 11.3.2) and exogenous infusion data (Section 11.3.3).

11.4.1 Pharmacokinetic models of VWD

One-compartmental models with first order input and output kinetics are used to investigate the time course of VWF:Ag (or VWF:CB) concentration after DDAVP administration [26]. These models take the algebraic form

$$y^{AG} = A\left(e^{-k_e(t-\tau)} - e^{-k_0(t-\tau)}\right) + B \tag{11.1}$$

where y^{AG} is the VWF:Ag concentration ([U/dL]), A represents the intercept ([U/dL]) and B ([U/dL]) the VWF baseline calculation, while k_0 and k_e are the release and elimination parameters, respectively. A lag time phase in both release and elimination does exist and is represented by the constant τ. The relevant pharmacokinetic (PK) parameters that can be obtained from (1) are the amount of VWF:Ag released after DDAVP administration (Q), the elimination half-life ($T_{1/2}$, [h]), plasma clearance (CL, [mL/kg/h]) and velocity of release (V_{re} [U/kg/h]). Their expressions are

$$Q = AV_d\frac{(k_0 - k_e)}{k_0} \tag{11.2}$$

$$T_{1/2} = \ln 2/k_e \tag{11.3}$$

$$CL = k_eV_d \tag{11.4}$$

$$V_{re} = Bk_eV_d \tag{11.5}$$

where V_d is the distribution volume evaluated following Menache and coworkers [27] (V_d = 40 mL/kg). Average values for (2–5) PK parameters are usually expressed as means ± standard error of the mean. The model has been applied in clinical practice to quantitatively analyse both VWF:Ag and VWF:CB data from clinical trials and provided useful insights on pharmacokinetics of different VWD types [26]. However, a strong limitation of the model (1) is that it aims at characterising either the overall amount of VWF (defined by VWF:Ag) or the amount of high molecular weight multimers (VWF:CB) by simply modelling the balance between the release of VWF from endothelial cells and its removal from the blood circulation. The model does not provide any information about the relative abundancy of high or low molecular weight multimers in the blood stream defining the multimeric distribution of VWF in plasma and conditioning the haemostatic activity of the subject affected by the disease. The extent of modification of VWF multimer distribution reflects the competition between clearance and proteolysis by means of ADAMTS13.

A mechanistic PK model for the description of VWD was first proposed by Galvanin et al. [13] to describe the proteolysis mechanism and to quantify the distribution and relative concentration of different multimeric species in subjects affected by VWD. A model scheme is reported in Figure 11.4a. After DDAVP administration, a three-step mechanism is known to occur [27]:

1. Release of super ultra large multimers (SUL); the release rate and amount are subject-dependent;
2. Proteolysis of SUL to smaller species by means of ADAMTS13: SUL multimers can be cleaved to high (HMW), ultra-large (UL) or low (LMW) molecular weight multimers;
3. Clearance (i.e. multimer elimination from plasma), taking place at the liver level and independent of the multimer size.

For each subject, the release rate is determined by the value of k_0 [min^{-1}]; the rate of proteolysis of SUL, UL and HMW to lower molecular weight species is described by parameters k_i, while the elimination rate for both UL, HMW and LMW is defined by k_e [min^{-1}].

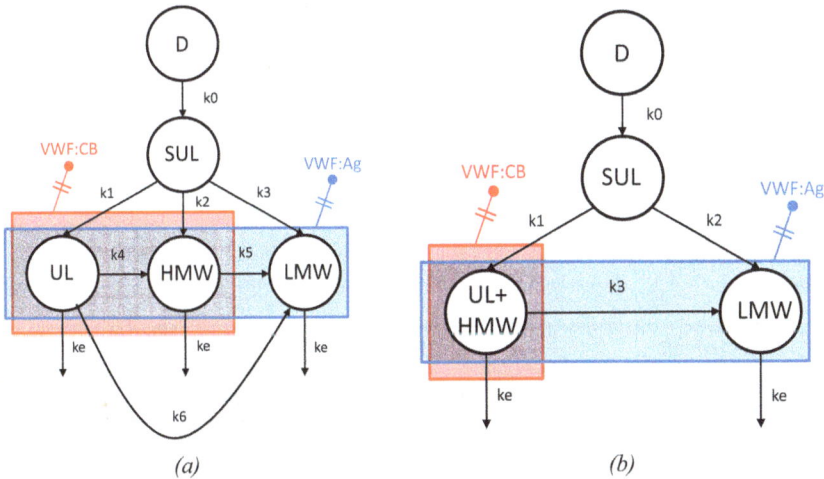

Figure 11.4: Structure of the mechanistic models used for model-based VWD diagnosis: a) original model by Galvanin et al. [13]; b) simplified model. VWF:Ag and VWF:CB measurements are indicated by the blue and red box, respectively.

The model was remarkably efficient to represent the variability observed in healthy subjects, 2A, 2B and Vicenza subjects and allowed to perform a model-based diagnosis based on estimated model parameters [13]. However, it required multimeric assays using gel electrophoresis to quantify the amount of UL in plasma after DDAVP. This measurement is essential for a precise estimation of the proteolytic parameters for a single subject, as parameters k_1 and k_4 are not identifiable from VWF:Ag and VWF:CB data only. Data from multimeric analysis are usually difficult and expensive to obtain, as they require a specific knowledge on the electrophoresis techniques and a significant effort in terms of analytical resources. For this reason, the model complexity was reduced to develop the model represented in Figure 11.4b. The simplified model was developed under the following physiological assumptions:

a) At the basal state, both HMW and LMW multimers are present, but SUL concentration is zero;

b) SUL multimers cannot be measured directly from VWF measurements, and their release is only a consequence of DDAVP administration;

c) Only a compartment quantifying the sum of UL and HMW can be fully characterised, and these multimers can be cleaved to LMW multimers.

It is assumed that only the sum of HMW and LMW multimers can be evaluated from VWF:Ag measurements, while VWF:CB measurements are exclusively imputed to the (UL + HMW) amount. The proposed mechanistic model allows for the evaluation of standard pharmacokinetic parameters including Q, $T_{1/2}$, CL, V_{re} and the evaluation of the velocity of VWF removal V_{el} [U/kg/h] as in equations (11.1)–(11.5). More importantly, it allows the quantitative evaluation of VWF levels involved in the proteolytic channels thanks to the estimation of k_1, k_2 and k_3 parameters. The model was extremely efficient on identifying subjects affected by VWD for well-characterised subjects (see Table 11.1) aligning with the results from differential diagnosis, but failed to clearly distinguish between borderline healthy cases (see shaded area in the table), particularly when parameters k_1 and k_2 were estimated with large uncertainty.

Table 11.1: Example of model-based diagnosis results using the simplified model reported in Galvanin et al. [13]. Columns represent the values of chi-square obtained from the LOF related to each class. Minimum chi-square value for each identified class is indicated in bold. Shaded cells indicate uncertainty in classification.

Test subject	Differential diagnosis	LOF test (χ^2 test)				Model-based diagnosis
		0	Non-O	2B	Vicenza	
C	Vicenza	107	102	133	**35**	Vicenza
D	Non-O	1236	**1229**	1958	5083	Non-O
E	Non-O	5350	**3409**	7268	9148	Non-O
F	2B	92	87	**20**	177	2B

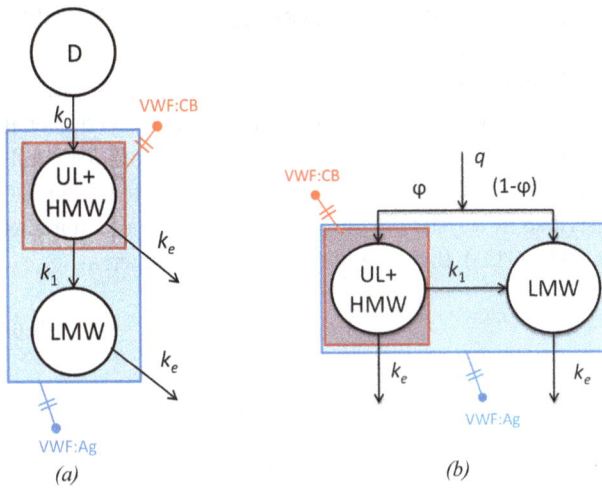

Figure 11.5: Simplified compartmental models of VWD. (a) Structure of the post-DDAVP model of VWD proposed by Ferrari et al. [14] representing the distribution of ultralarge + high (UL + HMW) and low molecular weight (LMW) multimers in the blood; (b) structure of the model proposed by Galvanin et al. [21] including exogenous VWF infusion, where q is the infusion rate [U/min] and φ is an effective partition constant defining the split between (UL + HMW) and LMW. Accessible compartments through VWF:Ag and VWF:CB measurements are indicated by the blue and red box, respectively.

The Ferrari and coworkers [14] dynamic model represents a further simplification of the original model and has been developed to represent the evolution in time of different multimeric species after DDAVP administration from VWF:Ag and VWF:CB data. The model assumes that i) the proteolysis of SUL is extremely fast, so that the SUL compartment can be neglected; ii) SUL can only decompose to (UL + HMW). The model is a simplification of the model by Galvanin et al. [13] but, unlike the original model, is structurally identifiable from VWF:Ag and VWF:CB data, i.e. model parameters can always be precisely estimated from DDAVP clinical data. This makes the model more suitable to investigate heterogeneous VWD forms, such as type 1 VWD, where the probability of incurring into false negatives during a differential diagnosis is higher. This model structure is illustrated in Figure 11.5a and the mathematical details are reported in Section 11.4.2.

The model of Ferrari and coworkers [14] can only represent release after subcutaneous DDAVP administration, and assumes that all the VWF is released from endothelial cells after a standard DDAVP dose is administered. To overcome this limitation, a new pharmacokinetic model has been proposed by Galvanin et al. [21] to explicitly include exogenous VWF administration as reported in Figure 11.5b. In this model, the partition constant φ is introduced to consider the possibility to administer different VWF analogues, characterised by a different relative concentration of (UL + HMW) and LMW multimers. This model is detailed in Section 11.4.3.

11.4.2 Identification of haemostatic parameters from DDAVP tests

The model assumes that after DDAVP administration, both high molecular weight (HMW) and ultralarge molecular weight (UL) VWF multimers are released from the endothelial cells. Then, HMW and UL multimers are cleaved to low molecular weight (LMW) multimers by the metalloprotease ADAMTS-13 before being finally eliminated from the bloodstream. This model is described by a system of differential and algebraic equations (DAEs)described by equations (11.6)–(11.11). Differential equations are written as

$$\frac{dx^{\text{UL+HMW}}}{dt} = k_0 D e^{-k_0(t-t_{\max})} - k_1\left(x^{\text{UL+HMW}} - x_b^{\text{UL+HMW}}\right) - k_e\left(x^{\text{UL+HMW}} - x_b^{\text{UL+HMW}}\right) \tag{11.6}$$

$$\frac{dx^{\text{LMW}}}{dt} = k_1\left(x^{\text{UL+HMW}} - x_b^{\text{UL+HMW}}\right) - k_e\left(x^{\text{LMW}} - x_b^{\text{LMW}}\right) \tag{11.7}$$

where $x^{\text{UL+HMW}}$ and x^{LMW} are the amount of UL + HMW and LMW multimer units [U] contained in the plasma; the subscript b refers to the basal state (i.e. the state of the subject before the DDAVP test starts); t is the test execution time and $t_{\max}$ is the time at which the release profile peaks. In the kinetic model, k_0 [min^{-1}] represents the kinetics of VWF release from endothelial cells; k_1 [min^{-1}] the proteolytic conversion of large and ultra-large VWF multimers into LMW multimers and k_e [min^{-1}] represents the clearance of VWF from the circulation, which is assumed to be the same for both the UL + HMW multimers and the LMW multimers [28]. The amount of VWF released, Q^{DDAVP} [U], can be calculated from

$$Q^{\text{DDAVP}} = \int_0^\tau k_0 D e^{-k_0(t-t_{\max})} dt \tag{11.8}$$

where D [U/dL] is a release parameter and τ is the overall test duration [min]. It is important to notice that, for a given subject, parameter k_0 quantifies the rate of release, while D is related to the amount of VWF released from the endothelial cells after a standardised DDAVP dose of 0.3 µg/kg body weight. A limitation of this model is that it does not include the amount of DDAVP administered to the subject as explicit variable. The measured responses are the antigen concentration y^{AG} [U/dL] and collagen binding concentration y^{CB} [U/dL], which are defined, respectively, by the following algebraic equations:

$$y^{AG} = \frac{x^{\text{UL+HMW}} + x^{\text{LMW}}}{V_d} \tag{11.9}$$

$$y^{CB} = \frac{x^{\text{UL+HMW}}}{V_d} \tag{11.10}$$

It is assumed that VWF:CB measurements can quantify the amount of UL and HMW multimers in plasma, while VWF:Ag measurements quantify the overall amount of VWF multimers (i.e. UL + HMW + LMW). A correction was introduced in the definition of the collagen binding measurements in order to account for the different affinity of multimers to collagen observed in clinical tests using the following algebraic equation:

$$y^{CB'} = ky^{CB}\frac{y_b^{AG}}{y_b^{CB}} \tag{11.11}$$

where k is a correction factor to be estimated from data, and y_b^{AG} and y_b^{CB} are antigen and collagen binding concentration measurements [U/dL] determined at basal state. In (11.9) and (11.10), $V_d = 40$ mL/kg$_{bw}$ is the approximate distribution volume again evaluated according to Menache et al. [27]. Initial conditions for differential state variables (i.e. at $t = 0$) can be calculated from basal antigen and collagen binding concentrations:

$$x(0) = \left[x_b^{UL+HMW} x_b^{LMW} \right] = \left[y_b^{CB} V_d y_b^{AG} V_d - y_b^{CB} V_d \right] \tag{11.12}$$

The full set of model parameters to be estimated from available post-DDAVP VWF:Ag and VWF:CB measurements is $\theta^{DDAVP} = [k_0 \quad k_1 \quad k_e \quad D \quad k \quad y_b^{CB} \quad t_{max}]$. The DDAVP test needs to be carried out on each single subject [14] to achieve a statistically precise estimation of the individual kinetic parameters to accurately quantify the rate of VWF release, proteolysis and elimination from plasma. Nonlinear parameter estimation results are assessed in terms of estimated values and a-posteriori statistics including t-values and confidence intervals. For a statistically precise estimation, the t-value for each model parameter is calculated from

$$t_i = \frac{\widehat{\theta}_i}{\sigma_{\theta_i}} i = 1 \dots N_\theta \tag{11.13}$$

where $\widehat{\theta}_i$ represents the estimated value from maximum likelihood parameter estimation and σ_{θ_i} the corresponding standard deviation. Each t-value calculated from (11.13) is compared against a tabulated reference t-value related to $(N - N_\theta)$ degrees of freedom and 95 % confidence level, where N is the total number of test samples and N_θ the total number of model parameters. A t-value higher than the reference t-value indicates a precise parameter estimation. Model adequacy is evaluated using a lack-of-fit (LOF) χ^2 test, by comparing the calculated chi-square

$$\chi^2 = \sum_{i=1}^{N} \frac{r_i^2}{\sigma_i^2} \tag{11.14}$$

with a tabulated reference chi-square at a 95 % confidence level for $(N - N_\theta)$ degrees of freedom (χ_{ref}^2) [29]. In (11.14), r_i and σ_i^2 are, respectively, the residual (difference between measured value and model prediction) for the i-th observation and the corresponding variance of measurement error. If $\chi^2 < \chi_{ref}^2$, the model is adequate to represent the test data. The heteroscedastic relative variance model equation

$$\sigma^2 = \omega^2 (y^2)^\gamma \tag{11.15}$$

is used to estimate the variability in the test response y (VWF:Ag or VWF:CB) at each time point. The variance is quantified at the level of the single individual and of the population of subjects (for the population y represents the average response for each class of subjects), by estimating parameters ω and y directly from data.

11.4.3 Models including exogenous infusion of VWF concentrates

In the infusion models, VWF is distributed among the (UL + HMW) and LMW compartments, and the release from endothelial cell is assumed to be negligible, as illustrated in Figure 11.5b. The model is represented by the following differential equations

$$\frac{dx^{UL+HMW}}{dt} = \varphi q - k_1 \left(x^{UL+HMW} - x_b^{UL+HMW} \right) - k_e \left(x^{UL+HMW} - x_b^{UL+HMW} \right) \tag{11.16}$$

$$\frac{dx^{LMW}}{dt} = (1 - \varphi)q + k_1 \left(x^{UL+HMW} - x_b^{UL+HMW} \right) - k_e \left(x^{LMW} - x_b^{LMW} \right) \tag{11.17}$$

where φ is the effective partition constant, representing the relative amount of high and low molecular weight multimers that are present in the injected dose, which is specific for each VWF concentrate and can be calculated from the specific collagen binding capacity

$$\varphi = \frac{VWF:CB^{IV}}{VWF:Ag^{IV}} \tag{11.18}$$

where $VWF:CB^{IV}$ and $VWF:Ag^{IV}$ are collagen binding and antigen VWF measurements carried out on the infused VWF concentrate. Intravenous administration is modelled through the infusion rate q [U/min]:

$$q = \begin{cases} D^{IV} & t \leq t_{inj} \\ 0 & t_{inj} < t \leq \tau \end{cases} \tag{11.19}$$

In (11.19), D^{IV} is the discrete injection rate [U/min] and t_{inj} is the injection time [min]. The model is subject to the following additional constraint on infusion dose:

$$Q^{IV} = \int_0^\tau q \, dt \tag{11.20}$$

where Q^{IV} is the actual injected dose of VWF concentrate [U]. The full model is constituted by the system of differential and algebraic equations (11.16)–(11.20) including (9-10) and (11) to be solved with the initial conditions provided by (11.12). For this model, the full set of model parameters to be estimated from VWF:CB and VWF:Ag data is

$$\theta^{IV} = \left[k_1 k_e D^{IV} k y_b^{CB} t_{inj} \right] \tag{11.21}$$

The parameter sets in both models (i.e. θ^{DDAVP} and θ^{IV}) are determined for each subject by iteratively solving a nonlinear optimisation problem based on maximum likelihood parameter estimation [30] following the procedure described in Taverna et al. [15] and carried out using the commercial software gPROMS® ModelBuilder [31]. VWF:Ag and VWF:CB measurements are assumed to be normally distributed with a standard deviation of 2 U/dL as evaluated from repeated measurements on the AVWS subject, as reported in Galletta et al. [10].

11.5 Model-based diagnosis of VWD subjects

Given the availability of VWD:Ag and VWF:CB historical data, it is possible to characterise the variability in the population by estimating the parameters of the heteroscedastic variance model (15) as reported in Table 11.2. Results show a significantly higher variability in healthy subjects characterised by O blood group, as indicated by the higher value of ω. Results reported in Table 11.3 show the estimated values of PK parameters using the Ferrari et al. [14] model for healthy subjects with O and non-O blood group, 2A,

Table 11.2: Estimated parameter values of the heteroscedastic variance model used to describe the population of subjects as in equation (11.15).

Response	Parameter	Healthy O	Healthy non-O	Vicenza	2B
VWF: Ag	ω	0.63	5.51	0.59	0.48
	γ	0.5	0.18	0.66	0.67
VWF: CB	ω	0.28	2.55	0.24	0.2
	γ	0.69	0.34	0.89	1.08

Table 11.3: Estimation of PK parameters for the Ferrari et al. [14] model from population data obtained for healthy subjects (O, non-O), 2A, 2B and Vicenza subjects. Values in bold indicate critical values for selected VWD types.

Model parameter	Subject's class				
	Healthy O	Healthy non-O	2B	Vicenza	2A
D	17.586	117.912	716.066	682.427	821.996
k	1.0382	0.9317	0.2399	0.6453	0.2451
k_0	0.0233	0.0260	0.0045	0.0093	0.0023
k_1	0.0003	0.0001	**0.0077**	**0.0121**	**0.0061**
k_e	0.0016	0.0007	0.0094	**0.0335**	0.0115
t_{max}	124.244	47.837	77.990	57.818	264.468
y_b^{CB}	57.5759	85.1613	25.8928	4.7951	21.9648
$\chi2\ (\chi_{ref}^2)$	13.2603	3.6782	6.5063	2.51614	0.610841
	(24.9958)	(24.9958)	(24.9958)	(24.9958)	(24.9958)

2B and Vicenza subjects. Results reflect the physiological profile of the different VWD types: i) Vicenza subjects (a specific type 1 form) show highly increased elimination and proteolytic activity (k_e and k_1 parameters, respectively), as well as reduced release (low k_0 value) compared to healthy subjects; ii) 2A and 2B subjects show increased proteolysis, with subjects 2A being characterised by an extremely low release rate (low k_0) and high elimination (high k_e). This underlines the severity of 2A forms, as the subjects are characterised by very low VWF levels in the blood stream

As illustrated in Figure 11.6a, the quantification of key haemostatic parameters CL (clearance, equation (11.4)) and Q (amount of VWF released, equation (11.8)) shows a clear distinction between healthy subjects and 2A, 2B and Vicenza subjects, while for type 1 VWD subjects, classification results show a more fragmented behaviour. It is also important to observe the proximity of some type 1 subjects to healthy subjects, which makes the classification particularly challenging. The analysis can be extended by including genetic information on specific mutations of VWF genes characterising each subject (Figure 11.6b), which allows to identify mutations (C1130, 1534–3) that are responsible of increased elimination from the blood stream (high clearance).

The availability of a subject-specific calibrated model allows for the quantification of the amount of (UL + HMW) and LMW released after a DDAVP test. This can be quantified by the area under the x^L and $x^{UL + H}$ curves. Interestingly, this analysis underlines the existence of clear data clusters, as reported in Figure 11.7, in the definition of type 1 VWD subtypes. Three specific clusters could be identified:

1. Type 1A (purple balls): characterised by low levels of VWF released and low concentrations of both HMW and LMW multimers in plasma, higher than normal VWF clearance (associated with mutations R1205H, C1130G/F/R, W1144G);

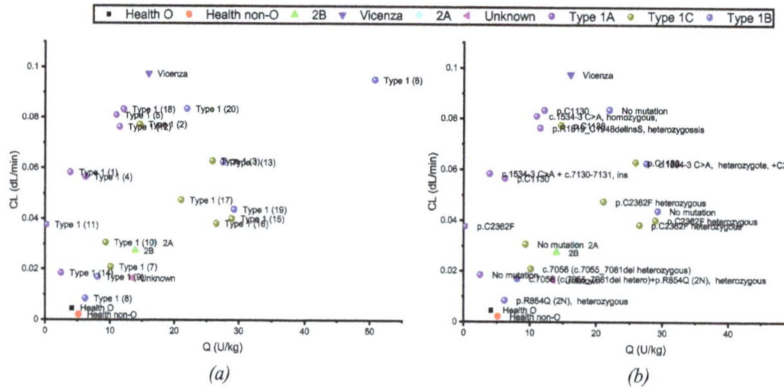

Figure 11.6: Clearance (CL) Vs amount of VWF released (Q) for (a) healthy subjects, 2A, 2B, Vicenza and selected type 1 individual subjects and (b) graphs including specific subjects mutations. Type 1 subjects are labelled in three distinct subtypes: type 1A, 1B and 1C.

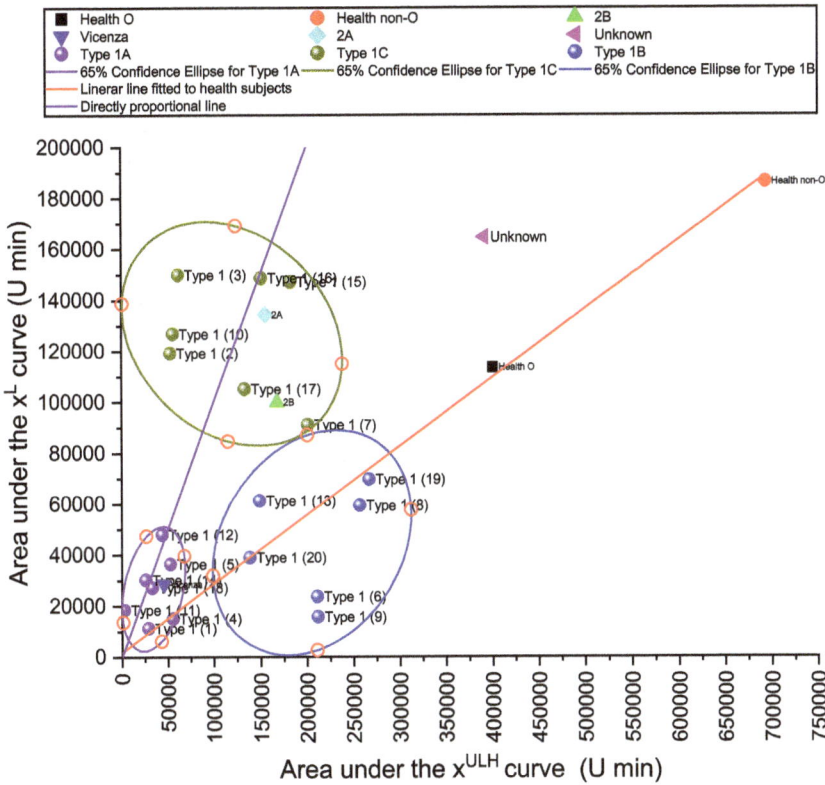

Figure 11.7: Analysis of the area under the curve (AUC) for LMW and (UL + HMW) multimers as computed by the Ferrari et al. [14] model. Lines show proportionality relationships between AUCs in selected classes.

2. Type 1B (blue balls): characterised by higher VWF levels and quasi-normal multimeric distribution, normal proteolytic activity but high clearance (associated with mutations R1205H, C1130G/F/R, W1144G);

3. Type 1C (green balls): characterised by high VWF levels but limited amount of HMW multimers, increased release (mutations G160W, N166I, L2207P), increased clearance (mutations R1205H, C1130G/F/R, W1144G) and accelerated proteolysis (mutation C1584).

The understanding of the relationship between PK parameters and mutations in type 1 VWD [32, 33] represents an open area of research, because mechanistic models have the potential to clarify and quantify the prevalent metabolic pathways involved in each type 1 subtype.

11.6 Model-based design of clinical tests

Information content analysis can be executed on both the post-DDAVP models of VWD (see Section 11.4.2) and on PK models of VWD including exogenous infusion (Section 11.4.3) with the following goals: *i*) study the distribution of information during clinical tests and evaluate the impact of information distribution on the overall test duration required to precisely estimate the set of PK parameters; *ii*) suggest the optimal infusion policy and/or allocation of sampling times for VWF:Ag and VWF:CB measurements; *iii*) quantify and rank the relative information that can be obtained using different VWF concentrates. The metric that is used to evaluate the overall information content of a clinical test is the trace of dynamic Fisher Information Matrix (FIM), which is defined by

$$I_d\left(\hat{\boldsymbol{\theta}}, t\right) = tr\left[\mathbf{H}_\theta\left(\hat{\boldsymbol{\theta}}, t\right)\right] \tag{11.22}$$

In Equation (11.22), $\mathbf{H}_\theta$ is the dynamic FIM calculated at the estimated value of model parameters, which are calculated from

$$\mathbf{H}_\theta\left(\hat{\boldsymbol{\theta}}, t\right) = \left[\mathbf{V}_\theta\left(\hat{\boldsymbol{\theta}}, t\right)\right]^{-1} \cong \sum_{j=1}^{N_m}\left[\frac{1}{\sigma_j^2}\left(\frac{\partial \hat{y}_j\left(\hat{\boldsymbol{\theta}}, t\right)}{\partial \theta_k} \frac{\partial \hat{y}_j\left(\hat{\boldsymbol{\theta}}, t\right)}{\partial \theta_l}\right)\right]_{k,l=1...N_\theta} \tag{11.23}$$

In Equation (11.23), the FIM, which is the inverse of the variance-covariance matrix of model parameters $\mathbf{V}_\theta$, is expressed as the product of the sensitivity of the *j*-th output variable with respect to each of the N_θ parameter in the conditions investigated in the *i*-th test, divided by the corresponding variance of measurement error (σ_j^2) for the *j*-th measured response (VWF:Ag or VWF:CB). Sensitivity coefficients appearing in (11.23) are calculated by integrating the sensitivity equations alongside the model equations as described in Bard [30]. Information from (11.23) can be decomposed to analyse the contribution to the information related to the estimation of the *i*-th model parameter (h_{ii}):

$$I_d\left(\hat{\boldsymbol{\theta}}, t\right) = tr\left[\mathbf{H}_\theta\left(\hat{\boldsymbol{\theta}}, t\right)\right] = \sum_{i=1}^{N_\theta} h_{ii}\left(\hat{\boldsymbol{\theta}}, t\right) \tag{11.24}$$

A maximum in I_d defines the most informative time points to take samples during the clinical test. When this maximum is located at the end of the test, information acquisition is favoured by long test durations. If an information peak is located at the very beginning of the test, samples can be concentrated in the first few hours of test execution and the test duration can significantly be reduced. Optimal sampling allocation can be obtained by solving the following optimal model-based design of experiments (MBDoE) problem [34]:

$$\mathbf{t}^{sp} = \mathrm{argmin}\psi\,[\mathbf{V}_\theta] = \mathrm{argmin}\psi\left[\left(\sum_{i=1}^{N_{sp}}\mathbf{H}_\theta\,(\theta,t_i)\right)^{-1}\right] \tag{11.25}$$

where $\mathbf{t}^{sp} = \begin{bmatrix} t_1 & t_2 & \dots & t_{N_{sp}} \end{bmatrix}$ is the optimal vector of sampling times and ψ [.] is a metric function of the variance-covariance matrix of model parameters, identifying the chosen experimental design criterion. Popular choices for ψ are the determinant (D-optimality), the trace (A-optimality), the largest eigenvalue (E-optimality) of $\mathbf{V}_\theta$ [35]. The optimisation in (11.25) is carried out considering practical constraints on sampling points allocation in time, including, for fixed number of samples N_{sp}: i) minimum time between consecutive measurements; ii) test duration. This set of constraints $\mathbf{C} = [C_{1i}\ C_2]$ are formulated as

$$C_{1i} = \Delta t_i = t_i - t_{i-1} \geq MTBM\ i = 1\dots N_{sp} \tag{11.26}$$

$$C_2 = \sum_{i=1}^{N_{sp}} \Delta t_i \leq \tau^{MAX} \tag{11.27}$$

where MTBM is the minimum time between consecutive measurements (here set to 15 min to propose a practical, clinically feasible test) and τ^{MAX} is the maximum allowed duration for the test (here fixed to 24 h, which is the maximum duration of a standard DDAVP test). If multiple infusion is considered, the optimal experimental design problem can be written as

$$\{\mathbf{t}^{sp}, \mathbf{D}^{IV}, \mathbf{t}_{inj}\} = \mathrm{argmin}\psi\,[\mathbf{V}_\theta] = \mathrm{argmin}\psi\left[\left(\sum_{i=1}^{N_{sp}}\mathbf{H}_\theta\,(\theta,t_i)\right)^{-1}\right] \tag{11.28}$$

and the objective is to determine the optimal experimental decision variables (elements of the experimental design vector) including optimal sampling times ($\mathbf{t}^{sp}$), injection times ($\mathbf{t}_{inj}$) and infusion rates ($\mathbf{D}^{IV}$). The optimisation (25) or (28) subject to (20) and (21) and the model equations (11.8)–(11.10) including (4–6) and (11) is carried out using the gPROMS ModelBuilder software [31] using a sequential quadratic programming (SQP) optimisation solver with multiple shooting to solve the resulting NLP problem.

11.7 Design of single and multiple infusion tests for the treatment of AVWS

11.7.1 Preliminary parameter estimation from DDAVP and VWF infusion tests data

Data available for a subject affected by AVWS have been used to calibrate the DDAVP model by Ferrari and coworkers [14] and the Galvanin et al. [21] models including VWF

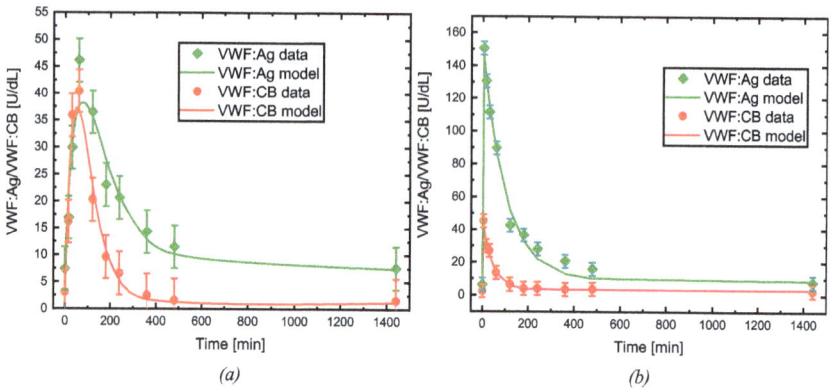

Figure 11.8: Model identification results from AVWS data using (a) the post-DDAVP model proposed by Ferrari et al. [14] and (b) the model proposed by Galvanin et al. [21] including exogenous VWF infusion. VWF:Ag and VWF:CB measurements are indicated, respectively, by green diamonds and red circles; error bars indicate the standard deviation in the data.

infusion. Results after model identification are illustrated in Figure 11.8a (post-DDAVP test) and Figure 11.8b (Haemate P administration test).

Parameter estimation results are reported in Table 11.4. Results show that both models are adequately fitting the available clinical data, providing very limited deviations from the measured VWF:Ag and VWF:CB concentrations, as underlined by the corresponding low χ^2 values reported in Table 11.4. A more detailed analysis of residuals reveal that the post-DDAVP model has some minor limitations on representing the initial VWF:Ag peak observed in the clinical test, while the infusion model tends to underestimate the observed VWF:Ag decay realised after 5–8 h from VWF infusion. Results from

Table 11.4: Estimated values of model parameters and a-posteriori statistics, including 95 % confidence intervals, t-test and χ^2 lack of fit test results for the post-DDAVP model and Haemate P infusion model. Asterisk* and bold values indicate parameters failing the t-test [21].

	Post-DDAVP model			Haemate P infusion model			
Model parameters	Estimated value	Confidence interval	t-value (Ref: 1.75)	Model parameters	Estimated value	95 % Confidence interval	t-value (Ref: 1.73)
k_1	0.01092	0.0044	2.13	k_1	0.01248	0.0049	2.53
k_e	0.00845	0.0042	2.49	k_e	0.00990	0.0005	18.60
k_0	0.02051	0.0095	1.98	D_{IV}	1658.254	8913.9784	**0.186***
D	1304.1110	762.5731	**1.71***	t_{inj}	2.7228	14.4830	**0.188***
t_{max}	219.6	10980.0105	**0.02***	–	–	–	–
χ^2	23.3	χ^2_{ref}	26.3	χ^2	25.5	χ^2_{ref}	28.9

parameter estimation (Table 11.4) show that the available clinical data allow a precise estimation of the key haemostatic parameters for the description of proteolysis (parameter k_1) and elimination (parameter k_e) pathways, as confirmed by the low 95 % confidence intervals. However, the description of release parameters D and t_{max} (post-DDAVP model) and infusion parameters D_{IV} and t_{inj} (Haemate P infusion model) is more difficult, due to the strong correlation and the limited amount of data points available to capture the initial transient behaviour observed after drug administration. Interestingly, the Haemate P infusion test allows for a more precise estimation of the elimination parameter k_e compared to a standard DDAVP test, while there are no significant differences when comparing the precision in the estimate for proteolytic parameter k_1.

By analysing the estimates for key parameters k_1 and k_e (Figure 11.9), it is apparent that the estimated parameter values obtained from the two different tests (DDAVP and Haemate P infusion) are very similar, and undistinguishable considering the uncertainty in parameter estimates. As illustrated in the figure, the AVWS subject shows accelerated proteolysis and elimination pathways compared to healthy control subjects, resulting in a lack of high molecular weight species in the blood stream and, consequently, a reduced haemostatic activity. A precise estimation of k_e and k_1 (minimum variance in the estimation of these parameters) is crucial for the model-based diagnosis of the subject and to achieve a clear distinction between AVWS subjects and subjects affected by other types of VWD.

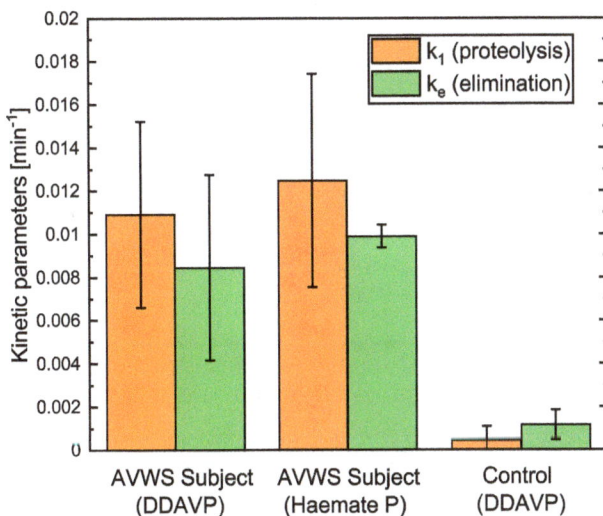

Figure 11.9: Parameter estimation results for key haemostatic parameters related to proteolysis (k1) and elimination (k_e) of VWF from plasma for the AVWS subject after DDAVP and Haemate P infusion, and comparison with healthy (O + non-O) control subjects. Bars on columns indicate 95 % confidence intervals [21].

11.7.2 Optimal design of Haemate P administration tests including single and multiple infusion

Results from parameter estimation illustrated in Section 11.7.1 showed a limitation of current infusion protocols to estimate the full set of model parameters (k_e, k_1 and D_{IV}) precisely. To overcome this limitation, a D-optimal MBDoE has been carried out to design alternative infusion protocols:

- **Protocol 1**: design of single infusion test where the objective is to optimise the allocation of sampling points, while the infusion rate is estimated to deliver a dose of q = 4500 U;
- **Protocol 2**: design of a multiple infusion test where the objective is to determine the optimal allocation of sampling points (t^{sp}) in time, time for three injections (t_{inj}) and corresponding infusion rates for the injections ($\mathbf{D}^{IV}$).

For Protocol 1 and Protocol 2, the corresponding optimal experimental design optimisation problems are defined by equations (11.25) and (11.28), respectively, subject to (20) and (21) and the model equations (11.8)–(11.10) including (11.4–11.6) and (11.11). In the everyday clinical procedures, there is a non-negligible uncertainty in the definition of each sample measurement, as it is impractical to sample with a resolution in time lower than 10 min. Therefore, a conservative constraint on the minimum time between measurements of 15 min has been assumed in the MBDoE optimisation. Optimal experimental design results are illustrated in Table 11.5 in terms of experimental design variables and test duration. Figure 11.10 shows the simulated VWF:Ag and VWF:CB profiles and the optimal allocation of samples determined by MBDoE for Protocol 1. As expected, given the faster information dynamics realised in infusion experiments, the sampling points are

Table 11.5: Allocation of sampling points in time and duration for DDAVP, Haemate P infusion and D-optimal designed Haemate P infusion tests.

Test protocol	Administration	Experimental design variables	Test duration [h]
DDAVP	**Standard dose DDAVP**	t^{sp} = [0 15 30 60 120 180 240 360 480 1440] [min]	24
Haemate P infusion	**Standard Haemate P dose single infusion**	t^{sp} = [0 4 15 30 60 120 180 240 360 480 1440] [min]	24
D-optimal MBDoE Haemate P infusion	**Optimised Haemate P dose single infusion**	t^{sp} = [0 15 30 45 60 75 90 105 120 135 150] [min]	2.50
D-optimal MBDoE Haemate P infusion	**Optimised Haemate P doses multiple infusion**	t^{sp} = [0 17 33 48 63 78 93 108 123 138 153] [min] t_{inj} = [0 42 83] [min] $\mathbf{D}^{IV}$ = [1407 1418 1416] [U/min]	2.54

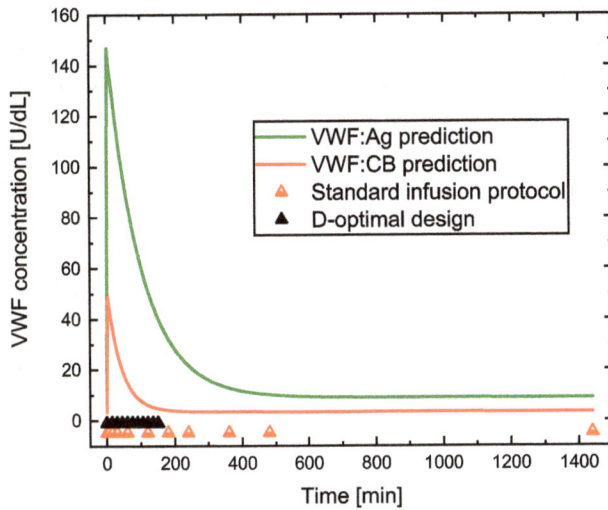

Figure 11.10: Protocol 1: predicted profiles of VWF:Ag and VWF:CB and allocation of sampling points as obtained from the D-optimal designed test (black triangles) as compared to the original allocation of sampling points in standard Haemate P infusion tests (red circles) [21].

concentrated at the very beginning of the test. Albeit not shown for the sake of conciseness, this result does not change significantly if different experimental design criteria are used (i.e. A- or E-optimal).

Results in terms of parameter estimation for Protocol 1 are reported in Table 11.6. It is interesting to verify that, if we assume that a precise injection time can be guaranteed during the infusion, i.e. by fixing the infusion time at $t_{inj} = 3$ min, a precise estimation of all key parameters k_1, k_e and D_{IV} can be achieved. Results show that Protocol 1 is more efficient to precisely estimate the kinetic parameters k_1 and k_e when compared to the original sampling used in Haemate P infusion tests (see Table 11.4), as demonstrated by the reduced confidence intervals in D_{IV}, while preserving a similar value in the other estimated parameters. Most importantly, note that this optimal sampling schedule (as the

Table 11.6: Protocol 1: estimated values of model parameters and a-posteriori statistics, including 95 % confidence intervals, t-test and χ^2 lack of fit test results obtained from the D-optimally designed Haemate P infusion test assuming a fixed injection time (t_{inj} = 3 min) [21].

Haemate P infusion model after MBDoE (Protocol 1)			
Model Parameters	**Estimated value**	**95 % Confidence Interval**	**t-value (Ref: 1.73)**
k_1	0.0140	0.0078	1.80
k_e	0.0099	0.0020	4.99
D_{IV}	1658.2500	159.9083	10.37
χ^2	23.7	χ^2_{ref}	28.9

286 —— 11 Development of PK models for VWD characterisation and diagnosis

one realised in Protocol 2) would require a considerably shorter test than the currently adopted infusion protocol (150 min–2.5 h against 24 h of the currently proposed infusion test), maintaining the same level of information for the determination of key PK parameters. Results show that a small variation in the injection time from 2.7 s (as reported in Table 11.4) to 3 s does not affect the estimated values of model parameters, but it slightly affects the precision of the estimates for parameters k_1 and k_e while the LOF test is passed and does not change significantly if t_{inj} is affected by uncertainty, as the test kinetics are very fast during the intravenous drug administration of Haemate P.

Results for Protocol 2 are reported in terms of infusion rate (Figure 11.11a) and VWF concentration profiles (Figure 11.11b). If a multiple administration of Haemate P is optimally designed using MBDoE, the injection times are concentrated in the first 1.2 h of the test and the design suggests a similar infusion rate for the three Haemate P injections.

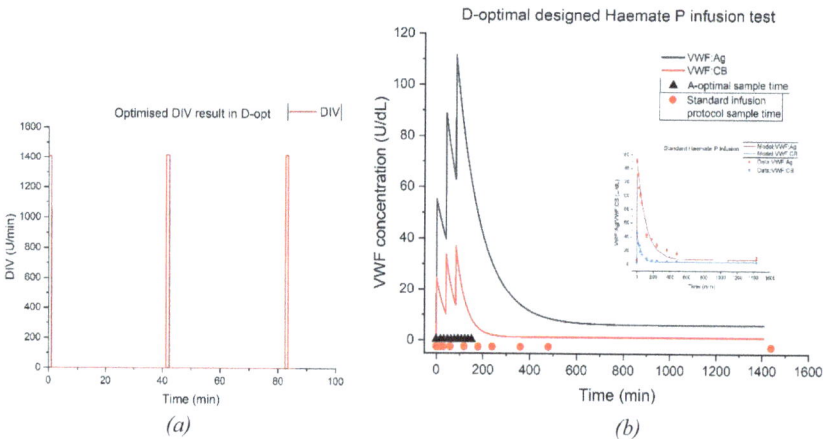

Figure 11.11: Protocol 2: (a) profile of Haemate P infusion rate as obtained from a D-optimal MBDoE optimisation; (b) predicted profiles of VWF:Ag and VWF:CB and allocation of sampling points as obtained from the D-optimal designed test (black triangles) as compared to the original allocation of sampling points in standard Haemate P infusion tests (red circles and inset figure).

Table 11.7: Protocol 2: estimated values of model parameters and a-posteriori statistics, including 95 % confidence intervals, t-test and χ^2 lack of fit test results obtained from the D-optimally designed Haemate P infusion test including multiple infusion assuming a fixed injection time (t_{inj} = 3 min).

Haemate P infusion model after MBDoE (Protocol 2)			
Model parameters	Estimated value	95 % Confidence interval	t-value (Ref: 1.73)
k_1	0.0145	0.0022	6.38
k_e	0.0094	0.0003	36.3
χ^2	21.7	χ^2_{ref}	28.9

Results from parameter estimation (Table 11.7) show a significant improvement in terms of precision of the estimates (compare Table 11.7 with Table 11.6) in the identification of k_1 and k_e parameters. However, this protocol requires an accurate administration of the VWF analogue and represents a more invasive procedure for the subject. These factors should be taken into account when implementing this optimally designed test in clinical facilities.

11.8 Conclusions

VWD is a very heterogeneous disease whose diagnosis requires a significant number of tests and experience, particularly when subjects are affected by specific VWD forms. The availability of PK models that can be tailored to the specificity of the single subject affected by VWD represents a key opportunity to achieve a quantitative description of the VWF multimer distribution for a faster and more effective diagnosis from clinical data. Model-based diagnosis has shown very promising results on identifying subjects affected by main VWD types, with type 1 VWD still offering a major challenge in the classification of VWD subtypes, given the strong heterogeneity of this specific VWD type. However, kinetic models can be affected by several limitations: i) often their calibration requires a 24 h-long tests (DDAVP test for example) to achieve a statistically satisfactory estimation of the PK metabolic parameters for each subject; ii) so far most of the PK models have been developed based on a fixed drug administration dose, while models including exogenous infusion of VWF concentrates, which represent the main form of treatment for severe forms of VWD, have found (so far) limited clinical application. New VWD models including exogenous VWF infusion have been recently proposed to bridge this research gap [21] and to provide a precise identification of haemostatic parameters from treatment tests. It has been shown that MBDoE techniques can be used to redesign currently adopted Haemate P infusion tests by optimally allocating the sampling points to maximise the information acquired during an infusion test. Results show that using MBDoE new clinically feasible sampling protocols can be designed where the test duration can successfully be reduced from 24 h to 2.5 h and where the injection time can be controlled to precisely estimate the full set of individual PK parameters. The possibility to reduce test duration associated to a conventional infusion test is a remarkable achievement. It allows patients to undergo a less stressful clinical procedure and facilitates clinical management in terms of both economical and organisational aspects. The precise estimation of individual haemostatic parameters allows to obtain a subject-specific calibrated model that can be used for personalised disease monitoring to improve the dosage of VWF concentrates, a key aspect to address when treating severe forms of VWD. Future work will aim to i) extend the applicability of the infusion models to other VWD types by implementing new MBDoE-optimised protocols in clinical facilities and estimating key PK parameters for new subjects affected by VWD; ii) design clinical tests that are more flexible and less stressful for the subjects; iii) consider the effect of model mismatch in the optimal experimental design formulation [36] so that the feasibility of the MBDoE-designed test [37] can be guaranteed even in scenarios of clinical uncertainty.

Acknowledgements: The authors would like to thank the editors David Bogle and Tomasz Sosnowski for their guidance and review of this article before its publication.

References

1. Lillicrap D, Budde U, Jessat U, Zimmerman R, Simon M, Kätzel R, et al. Von Willebrand disease-phenotype versus genotype: deficiency versus disease. Thromb Res 2007;87:57–64.
2. Sadler JE. Von Willebrand disease type 1: a diagnosis in search of a disease. Blood 2003;101:2089–93.
3. Sadler JE, Mannucci PM, Berntorp E, Bochkov N, Boulyjenkov V, Ginsburg D, et al. Impact, diagnosis and treatment of von Willebrand disease (2000). Thromb Haemost;84:160–74. https://doi.org/10.1055/s-0037-1613992.
4. World Federation of Haemophilia (WFH). Report on the annual global survey. WFH Reports 2020.
5. Rodeghiero F, Castaman G, Dini E. Epidemiological investigation of the prevalence of von Willebrand's disease. Blood 1987;69:454–9.
6. National Institute of Health. The Diagnosis, Evaluation and Management of von Willebrand Disease. National Institute of Health Reports 2008.
7. Groot E, Fijnheer R, Sebastian S, De Groot P, Lenting P. The active conformation of von Willebrand factor in patients with thrombotic thrombocytopenic purpura in remission. J Thromb Haemostasis 2009;7:962–9.
8. Atiq F, Heijdra J, Snijders F, Boender J, Kempers E, van Heerde WL, et al. Desmopressin response depends on the presence and type of genetic variants in patients with type 1 and type 2 von Willebrand disease. Blood Adv 2022;6:5317–26.
9. Tiede A, Rand JH, Budde U, Ganser A, Federici AB. How I treat the acquired von Willebrand syndrome. Blood 2011;117:6777–85.
10. Galletta E, Galvanin F, Bertomoro A, Daidone V, Casonato A. Acquired von Willebrand syndrome in patients with monoclonal gammopathy of undetermined significance investigated using a mechanistic approach. Blood Transfus 2021. https://doi.org/10.2450/2021.0121-21.
11. Casonato A, Daidone V, Padrini R. Assessment of von Willebrand factor propeptide improves the diagnosis of von Willebrand disease. Semin Thromb Hemost 2011;37:456–63.
12. Gezsi A, Budde U, Deak I, Nagy E, Mohl A, Schlammadinger A, et al. Accelerated clearance alone explains ultra-large multimers on von Willebrand disease Vicenza. J Thromb Haemostasis 2010;8:1273–80.
13. Galvanin F, Barolo M, Padrini R, Casonato A, Bezzo F. A model-based approach to the automatic diagnosis of von Willebrand disease. AIChE J 2014;60:1718–27.
14. Ferrari M, Galvanin F, Barolo M, Daidone V, Padrini R, Bezzo F, et al. A Mechanistic Model to Quantify von Willebrand Factor Release, Survival and Proteolysis in Patients with von Willebrand Disease. Thromb Haemost 2018;118:309–19.
15. Taverna B, Casonato A, Bezzo F, Galvanin F. A framework for the optimal design of a minimum set of clinical trials to characterize von Willebrand disease. Comput Methods Progr Biomed 2019;179:104989.
16. Castaldello C, Galvanin F, Casonato A, Padrini R, Barolo M, Bezzo F. A model-based protocol for the diagnosis of von Willebrand disease. Can J Chem Eng 2018;96:628–38.
17. Casonato A, Pontara E, Sartorello F, Cattini MG, Gallinaro L, Bertomoro A, et al. Identifying type Vicenza von Willebrand disease. J Lab Clin Med 2006;147:96–102.

18. Budde U, Metzner HJ, Muller HG. Comparative analysis and classification of von Willebrand factor/factor VIII concentrates: impact on treatment of patients with von Willebrand disease. Semin Thromb Hemost 2006;32:626–35.
19. Berntorp E. Haemate P/Humate-P: a systematic review. Thromb Res 2009;124:S11–4.
20. Auerswald G, Kreuz W. Haemate P/Humate-P for the treatment of von Willebrand disease: considerations for use and clinical experience. Haemophilia 2008;14:39–46.
21. Galvanin F, Galletta E, Bertomoro A, Daidone V, Casonato A. Optimal design of infusion tests for the identification of physiological models of acquired von Willebrand syndrome. Chem Eng Sci 2024:119660. https://doi.org/10.1016/j.ces.2023.119660.
22. Villaverde AJ, Pathirana D, Fröhlich F, Hasenauer J, Banga JR. A protocol for dynamic model calibration. Briefings Bioinf 2022;23:1–19.
23. Franceschini G, Macchietto S. Novel anticorrelation criteria for model-based experiment design: theory and formulations. AIChE J 2008;54:1009–24.
24. Chakrabarty A, Buzzard GT, Rundell AE. Model-based design of experiments for cellular processes. Syst Biol Med 2013;5:181–203.
25. Favaloro EJ, Thom J, Patterson D, Just S, Dixon T, Koutts J, et al. Desmopressin therapy to assist the functional identification and characterisation of von Willebrand disease: differential utility from combining two (VWF: CB and VWF:RCo) von Willebrand factor activity assays? Thromb Res 2009;123:862–8.
26. Casonato A, Gallinaro L, Cattini MG, Sartorello F, Pontara E, Padrini R, et al. Type von Willebrand disease due to reduced von Willebrand factor synthesis and/or survival: observations from a case study. Transl Res 2010;155:200–8.
27. Menache D, Aronson DL, Darr F, Montgomery RR, Gill JC, Kessler CM, et al. Pharmacokinetics of von Willebrand factor and factor VIIIC in patients with severe von Willebrand disease (type 3 VWD): estimation of the rate of factor VIIIC synthesis. Br J Haematol 1996;94:740–5.
28. Casonato A, Pontara E, Sartorello F, Cattini MG, Sartori MT, Padrini R, et al. Reduced von Willebrand factor survival in type Vicenza von Willebrand disease. Blood 2002;99:180–4.
29. Snedecor GW, Cochran WG. Statistical methods, 8th ed. Ames: Iowa State University Press; 1989.
30. Bard Y. Nonlinear parameter estimation. Cambridge, USA: Academic Press; 1974.
31. Siemens Process Systems Enterprise. gPROMS 2023. https://www.siemens.com/global/en/products/automation/industry-software/gproms-digital-process-design-and-operations.html.
32. Goodeve AC. The genetic basis of von Willebrand disease. Blood Rev 2010;24:123–34.
33. Goodeve A. Genetics of type 1 von Willebrand disease. Curr Opin Hematol 2007;14:444–9.
34. Fedorov V, Leonov S. Optimal design for nonlinear response models. Boca Raton: Taylor & Francis Group; 2014.
35. Pukelsheim F. Optimal design of experiments. Boca Raton, USA: Chapman & Hall; 1995.
36. Galvanin F, Barolo M, Macchietto S, Bezzo F. Optimal design of clinical tests for the identification of physiological models of type 1 diabetes in the presence of model mismatch. Med Biol Eng Comput 2011;49: 263–77.
37. Galvanin F, Bezzo F. Advanced techniques for the optimal design of experiments in pharmacokinetics. Comput Aided Chem Eng 2018;42:65–83.

Part IV: **Pharmacokinetics and drug delivery**

Roberto A. Abbiati* and Cesar Pichardo

12 An introduction to quantitative systems pharmacology for chemical engineers

Abstract: Quantitative systems pharmacology (QSP) is a discipline that integrates experimental and mathematical modelling practice to perform a variety of analysis in the pharmaceutical research and development space. As the pharma industry strives for leaner product development, reduction of time and costs, and the implementation of the personalized medicine ambition, modeling and simulation approaches are recognized as pivotal components to achieve these goals. Since there are notable similarities between chemical engineering modelling approaches and those of QSP, our aspiration for this chapter is setting the stage for further contribution by engineers in this space. To this end, we provide a concise overview of the various modelling applications currently employed across the pharmaceutical research and development value chain. We then focus on QSP, detailing specific research areas that benefit from its use, the relevant mathematical modelling techniques, and emphasizing its parallels with chemical engineering modelling. Finally, we illustrate two concrete examples of QSP applications in oncological drug development.

Keywords: quantitative systems pharmacology; QSP; chemical engineering; modelling and simulation; drug development; pharma

12.1 Introduction to pharma R&D

Pharmaceutical research and development (R&D) is one of the most challenging technical-scientific endeavors an organization can face in the modern days. It requires cutting edge scientific expertise, modern infrastructures and facilities, billions of dollars of investments, thousands of contributors working across the most diverse disciplines and decades of work.

In this book chapter we substantiate these daring statements elucidating the main activities of pharmaceutical R&D, with specific focus on those challenges that are being addressed with mathematical modeling-based approaches. Recent years have seen increasing focus on data analytics and modelling in an attempt to modernize the drug

*Corresponding author: Roberto A. Abbiati, Roche Pharma Research and Early Development, Predictive Modeling and Data Analytics, F. Hoffmann-La Roche Ltd, Grenzacherstrasse 124, 4070 Basel, Switzerland, E-mail: roberto.abbiati@roche.com. https://orcid.org/0000-0002-6052-5736
Cesar Pichardo, AstraZeneca R&D, Systems Medicine, Clinical Pharmacology & Quantitative Pharmacology, The Discovery Centre, 1 Francis Crick Avenue, Cambridge, CB2 0AA, UK

As per De Gruyter's policy this article has previously been published in the journal Physical Sciences Reviews. Please cite as: R. A. Abbiati and C. Pichardo "An introduction to quantitative systems pharmacology for chemical engineers" *Physical Sciences Reviews* [Online] 2024. DOI: 10.1515/psr-2024-0066 | https://doi.org/10.1515/9783111394558-012

development paradigm and reduce attrition [1] as pharmaceutical products grow more sophisticated and complex to develop.

Traditionally, drug development activities begin with the identification of a lead molecule, which showed some effect in the modulation of disease relevant biological mechanisms in *in vitro* experiments. Lead identification activities involve primarily chemistry techniques and high-throughput screenings, while computational techniques are increasingly applied for molecular-structure based design of lead compounds. Next, a lead compound is optimized in order to maximize either its potential to interact and modulate its biological target or its expected overall properties in an *in vivo* scenario (e.g., solubility, elimination half-life, immunogenicity). This implies modifying the chemical structure of the molecules to enhance potency, selectivity, and safety profiles. Here mathematical modelling can be applied to project the expected *in vivo* effect of molecular characteristics thereby informing decisions making on which changes to pursue [2–4].

The following early development phase consists of non-clinical toxicology studies conducted to assess *in vivo* safety, potential side effects and explore efficacy in preparation for clinical experimentation [5]. Here, mathematical models are used to estimate what could be a safe initial dose for entry in human based on animal data. The focus is both on safety and on the assessment of probability of successful clinical development. In fact the following human studies are extremely complex, long and costly so it is crucial to carefully assess the chances of success and take informed decisions about any further development.

At this stage is conducted a major model based activity, consisting in the characterization of how drugs are absorbed, distributed, metabolized, and eliminated in the body (i.e. pharmacokinetics or PK), as well as how they produce an effect on the modulation of a disease condition (i.e., pharmacodynamics or PD). The related computational models enable researchers to study dosing and project efficacy in humans. One of the key uses of preclinical PK/PD modelling is estimating the first in human (FIH) dose for a Phase I clinical study [6]. These activities require the modelling of animal PK and some extrapolation to humans (e.g., via allometric scaling) by taking into account factors such as body weight, drug metabolism, and safety margins.

As a drug candidate moves into clinical trials, mathematical modelling continues to play a vital role. In Phase I trials, which involve a small number of healthy volunteers, models are used to analyze the pharmacokinetic data and refine dosing regimens. In Phase II trials, conducted in patients, modelling is applied to assess the drug efficacy and to optimize the dose. In Phase III trials, large-scale studies are conducted to confirm the drug safety and efficacy, and modelling can help interpret the complex data generated.

It is in the translation from preclinical to clinical and primarily along with clinical Phases I and II that mathematical modelling has demonstrated its major impact. It provides quantitative evidence to support analysis on dose selection, efficacy criteria, and safety margins, thereby facilitating internal decision making as well as the interactions with regulatory agencies [7–9].

12.2 Quantitative systems pharmacology

From this extremely succinct summary of pharmaceutical R&D, it should be apparent that *in silico* modelling and experimental activities are tightly connected and in this very aspect lies the foundation of a modelling discipline called quantitative systems pharmacology (QSP). This is a recently established field of pharmaceutical sciences defined as a mechanism-based approach to translational medicine integrating experimental and computational methods to elucidate pharmacological concepts [10, 11]. QSP was defined after years of different groups applying mathematical modelling and systems pharmacology in the context of quantitative pharmacology [12] and currently deeply rooted in the longer standing discipline of pharmacometrics but still being applied in early stages of drug development [13, 14]. Chemical engineers have begun to be involved in QSP, as shown by Manca's 2018 book [15] and the examples in the core reaction engineering textbook by Fogler [16].

Elaborating more on QSP, its application space can be quite broad, for example it can be applied for the mathematical representation of the biological mechanism and physiological processes that concur in the disease phenotype, for the analysis of intracellular trafficking of drug molecules, or even to capture the activity of cell therapies like CAR-T cells (chimeric antigen receptor T-cells) at a tumor site. The variety of the opportunities for QSP application and the complexity of its implementation have made it challenging to really provide a unified definition and this has also proved a hurdle for communication with stakeholders involved in the drug development process. In this chapter, rather than focusing on each and every possible QSP application, we will aim at understanding what type of analysis can benefit from this methodology and what are the implementation requirements. The panorama of QSP application opportunities will be a natural consequence of this understanding.

QSP models are typically multi-scale, coherently with the fact that disease mechanisms are initiated at the molecular level but are eventually observed clinically as an organ or tissue dysfunction. Similarly when disease models are integrated with drug PK/PD, the processes of interest occur at different scale-levels. For example, post administration of a drug dose, disposition is described initially at the whole body level, but eventually is important to capture the drug concentration at the target site and the molecular process of target engagement. For these reasons QSP models are most commonly defined as bottom-up, meaning that they start by examining the individual components of a system and then integrate them to recreate a holistic representation. Interestingly, these model are not just multi-scale from a spatial point of view, but also with respect to the time scale, in fact while drug molecular activity with the target is in the fraction of a second, drug disposition in the body can take hours or days, whereas changes in disease progression is typically observed in months or years.

One prominent benefit of QSP is the possibility to integrate knowledge, thereby enabling extrapolation of model-based analysis results. Typically, these models allow us to combine a wide range of data from *in vitro* or animal experiments to make projections for humans. Further, we utilize clinical data to refine the model and possibly characterize the variability observed across the patient population. This possibility to combine knowledge generated by different research groups, across diverse experiments conducted over multiple years, makes QSP invaluable for clinical decision-making and sets it apart from other modelling applications.

12.3 QSP application space

We now discuss some concrete pharmaceutical R&D scenarios in which QSP can be adopted, next we detail how these models look from a technical perspective.

12.3.1 Disease progression

QSP can be applied to rationalize mechanistic understanding of disease genesis and progression [17, 18]. For example, multifaceted conditions like chronic kidney disease (CKD) or metabolic disfunction-associated steatotic liver disease (MASLD) are initiated by a multiplicity of concurring factors whose effect over time can lead to disease onset and progression to a variety of phenotypes. For a rational drug development initiative is crucial to understand the underlying disease dynamics, possibly considering diverse scenarios. Investigators may want to study the factors driving a slow versus fast disease progression, or what are the different treatments needed for a condition tackled in an early onset phase rather than in an advanced stage. Here modelling offers the opportunity to formalize our understanding of the disease progression dynamic in a unified and quantitative representation, that we can utilize to explore hypotheses and project the effect of hypothetical treatments, in collaboration with clinical expert opinion leaders.

In line with the previous example, one may ask the question of which of multiple potential targets is holding the highest disease modulation potential. For example, thinking at the above mentioned CKD or MASLD conditions, the therapeutic focus could be on preventing disease onset, or on downstaging of the early inflammatory process, or on slowing down fibrotic dynamics in advanced disease. Selecting the right target is crucial, both for a successful drug development but also for asset differentiation, in a market where ideally different classes of drugs will be available to the doctors and to the patients to optimally treat the need of each idiosyncratic condition. For example, given a QSP model, we can apply sensitivity analysis to identify the disease progression mechanism to which the outcome of interest is most sensitive to, thereby advising our development colleagues on which therapeutic option carries the highest success potential.

Beyond the sole focus on disease models, it eventually becomes crucial to combine drug specific properties. This is typically achieved by integrating PK and PD models with the disease model. Here we can ask questions like, what is the most suitable dosing schedule, what drug transport processes control drug disposition or what covariates should be taken into account.

12.3.2 Biomarkers

Another important application of QSP modelling is the study of biomarkers and their link to clinical endpoints. We define biomarkers as measurable indicators of biological state or condition [19]. For example, biomarkers could be protein levels, cell counts, physiological parameters, diagnostic images or gene expression measurements. Biomarkers are valuable when we can relate them to clinical status or events [20, 21].

The choice of the right biomarker to be monitored and the understanding of its role in a disease condition is of capital importance for the success of the clinical drug development activity. Since the relationship between a biomarker and an endpoint of interest is generally non-linear and variable across patients and disease stages, it is advisable to adopt QSP to describe the main processes that regulate biomarker level and how they are linked to the clinical endpoints [21, 22]. These models can predict the time course of the biomarker level as a disease progresses and as it is treated. They can also define a functional relationship between biomarkers and endpoints.

12.3.3 Patient variability and virtual populations

Variability is another important aspect in biology. All patients included in a study, despite having a common condition, are diverse in terms of their physiological status and their biological traits. In most cases we can expect the same disease to progress differently across the patient population and, similarly, we observe different efficacy levels of the medications.

It is very important to understand which are the main drivers of the observed variability and there is a multiplicity of methods that are applied to this end. Even here, QSP modelling has a role. We can adapt the parameterization of our models to cover a range of baseline conditions or the differences in progression dynamics [23–25]. In this case we create so-called virtual patients (VPs), which ultimately are specific parameterizations of a QSP model.

The parameter value distribution functions used to characterize the VPs can be directly based on measured biomarkers or can be based on regression via model fit. VPs analysis could focus on the general patient population and the overall observed variability, or could focus on an individual patient for which we may need to conduct a series of *in silico* analysis, in this case the model-version of an individual is called digital-twin.

Virtual populations are increasingly used in QSP since there is growing appetite for personalized medicine and optimized treatment, rather than the more obsolete approach of one-medication equal for everyone.

12.4 Mathematical characteristics of QSP models

QSP models are generally based on differential equations, most typically ordinary differential equations (ODE) generated from mass balances applied to the system of interest, where the only independent variable is time [26]. Here the integrated variables can be either biomarkers (thereby creating a direct model-based representation of measurable biological entities, e.g., a protein concentration in plasma), non-measurable entities (for example in case it is not practically possible to sample a biomarker *in vivo*, e.g., the density of a membrane receptor in a tumor mass), or even purely mathematical definitions without a real counterpart (in this case the variable is typically accessory to an abstraction or a simplification applied to the model in absence of sufficient knowledge or data).

In case, besides time dependency, we wish to describe spatial dependency, QSP models can also be based on partial differential equations (PDE), or can be Agent-Based models. These applications are less common due to the increased technical complexity and the data requirements [27, 28].

Focusing on ODE models, these are usually based on a compartmental approach. In such an approach, the system of interest is simplified and represented as a set of interacting variables. Each variable corresponds to a compartment and the relationship among them is based on some kind of functional form, often based on standard formulations of zero, first, or second order. For example, the transport of a species between compartments or simple chemical reactions are based on the law of mass action, whereas the kinetics of saturable processes are often based on Michaelis-Menten [29] or Hill [30] equations.

The model parameterization is ideally based on direct measurements (from dedicated *in vitro*/*in vivo* experiments or from scientific literature), or alternatively parameter values are estimated via regression and model fitting.

When QSP models describe very large systems, for example a disease condition with a multiplicity of biological processes, we call them platform-models. These models are valuable because they capture the complexity of the disease biology and allow for a wide-spectrum of analysis, however these are usually difficult to develop and require substantial time and resources.

When a model is more focused at answering a single, specific question minimizing the need for assumption or speculation, we call them fit-for-purpose models. These models are often preferred to maximize short-term value of model simulation and to minimize the risk of extrapolation inaccuracies.

12.5 Chemical engineering modelling theory affinities to QSP

Most ODE-based QSP models incorporate idealized chemical-reactor concepts such as the continuous stirred-tank reactors (CSTR) to capture the kinetics of drug disposition and chemical reactions. For example, the CSTR concept is suitable to model any drug metabolism site (e.g., liver, the main body site where molecules are metabolized) or the transport process of drug molecules across body regions, as long as tissue heterogeneity can be neglected for a given application.

Mass transport phenomena, including diffusion, convection, and active transport, are ubiquitous in human biology and the underlying mathematical theory is applied to depict the movement of drugs across cellular membranes and within different body tissues. Small molecules can generally diffuse across cell membranes driven by a concentration gradient, whereas active transport mechanisms are found for large molecules or hydrophilic molecules that require energy-dependent transporters. For example, active transport is found in the intestine (SGLT1), in the kidneys (Na^+/K^+-ATPase), in the liver (OATPs), in the brain (P-gp), just to cite a few.

Further, theories for receptor binding, competitive binding, saturation, and adsorption are crucial to represent a variety of ligand-receptor interactions and constitute the foundation of biochemical signal transduction. These are essential for understanding drug efficacy and toxicity. In most cases, PD models can assume proportionality between drug-receptor complex formation and effects, however this relationship is generally nonlinear, for example in case of competitive binding or receptor-saturation. Chemical engineers can recognize extensive similarities to the theories for chemical reaction kinetics in presence of solid catalysts.

Even if less frequently applied and not always explicitly defined as QSP models, fluid dynamics play an important role for applications in the medical space. For example, complex flow patterns have been modeled for the cardiovascular systems, the respiratory system, the urinary tract, the peritoneal cavity or for interstitial fluid pressure in solid tumors [31–36]. This offers plenty of opportunities for engineers to apply fluid dynamic theories and finite element analysis.

Finally, it is worth mentioning that numerical methods play a crucial role in QSP. Differential equation models can grow quite large and exhibit stiff behavior, therefore numerical integration techniques are essential for accurately solving these complex systems. Model optimization and parameter regression techniques are widely employed due to the difficulties in model parameterization due to inherent system uncertainties, as well as the technical and ethical challenges of experimentally conducting measurements *in vivo*. Model identifiability and sensitivity analysis are frequently utilized to characterize the structure of the models and to study their behavior under various conditions. Identifiability analysis helps in determining which parameters can be uniquely estimated from the available data, while sensitivity analysis assesses how changes in model parameters affect the model output. These techniques are invaluable for understanding the robustness and reliability of the models.

12.6 Examples of the application of QSP modelling in drug development

12.6.1 Development of bispecifics antibodies

Mechanistic modelling (e.g. QSP) has been used successfully to describe and understand the pharmacokinetics and pharmacodynamics of monoclonal antibodies (mAbs) [37, 38]. A natural extension of the approach has been applied to more complex molecules, designed to recognize two targets, commonly called bispecific antibodies (bsAbs) (see Figure 12.1).

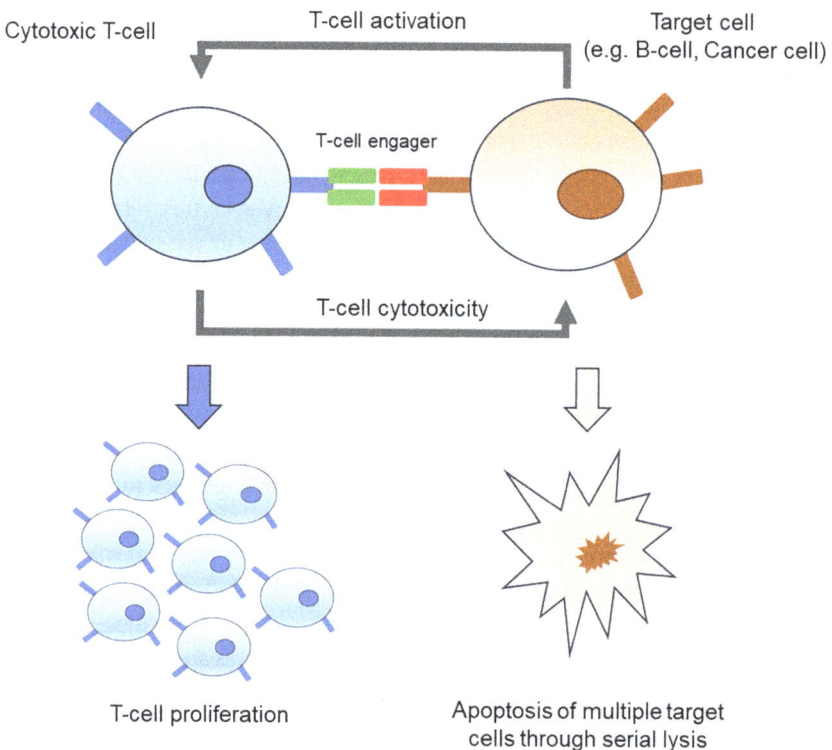

Figure 12.1: Bispecific T-cell engager antibody attaches to T cells (top left) and target cells (top right), enabling T cells to find and destroy cancer cells (bottom right). During this process, T cells are activated, creating more killer T cells (bottom left) [39, 40].

In a similar way to mAbs, a useful modelling approach for bsAbs can be based in a mass balance in physiological compartments (e.g. blood, lymph nodes, tumour, etc.) which should include the kinetics related to the formation of different complexes, i.e. complexes formed when the bsAbs binds to one or two targets, often called dimers and trimers respectively. Similarly to other modalities, QSP models of bsAbs can include different levels of complexity based on the biology and chemistry of the molecule, however, increasing the granularity in the modelling also requires a larger number of model parameters, which values might not be possible to get from experimental or clinical data.

Recent QSP work has shown the utility of the physiological (or mass balance) approach for bsAbs [41–44] and how this has been helpful to understand the mode of action of the molecule in terms of efficacy, in particular affecting tumor growth, and safety.

12.6.2 QSP modelling of T-cell engagers

The example shown here is based on a generic bispecific T-cell engager targeting two proteins: CD3 and C19, commonly expressed on the surface of T-cells and B-cells respectively, a good example of this type of compound is Blinatumomab (commercially known as Blincyto®) which was the first bsAbs approved by the American Food and Drug Administration (FDA) on 2014 to effectively treat hematological malignancies [45].

After several years of research and given its success as a first in class bsAbs to treat cancer, there have been various QSP modelling efforts used to describe the PK and PD of blinatumomab [46–49].

As an illustrative example of how a QSP model can be developed to explore the efficacy of a bsAbs we shown here the development of a model for CD3/CD19 bsAbs assuming is used to treat patients with diffuse large B cell lymphoma (DLBLC), a type of non-Hodgkin lymphoma (NHL).

12.6.2.1 Model assumptions

The following assumptions are made for model development as an illustrative example here:

- The bsAbs model will be based on a mass balance in two different physiological compartments: central (representing plasma and well perfused tissues) and the lymph system, also called tumor considering this is the compartment where malignant B-cells are expanding due to DLBCL.
- Each compartment is assumed to have constant volume and be well stirred.
- Changes in the tumor volume are negligible for the timescales considered in the simulations meaning the number of T- and B-cells is also constant, also assuming that each cell expressed the same number of receptors (CD3 and CD19) on their surface.

- All chemical reactions (e.g. for complex formation and dissociation) follow a mass-action law.
- Trimeric complex concentration is considered to be the main driver of efficacy and safety (model presented here was developed to explore the dynamics of complex formation after drug administration).
- IV infusion of bsAbs is assumed to be a zero order process (i.e. constant infusion rate during the time of infusion).

12.6.2.2 Model formulation

The model describes the changes in concentration of antibody and the two targets in all compartments as described in the diagram shown in Figure 12.2. The model equations are based on a mass balance in each compartment:

$$\text{Accumulation} = \text{Input} - \text{Output} - \text{Reaction}_{\text{Complex formation}} + \text{Reaction}_{\text{Dissociation}} \quad (12.1)$$

As mentioned previously, the kinetics related to the chemical reactions is assumed to follow the mass action law, with k_{on} and k_{off} the kinetic rate constants for complex formation and dissociation, respectively. Under these assumptions the following system of differential equations can be generated:

Central blood compartment:

$$\frac{dm_{\text{bsAbs}}^{\text{Blood}}}{dt} = \text{Infusion rate of bsAbs} + \text{mass flow}_{\text{bsAbs}}^{\text{Tumor to central}} - \text{mass flow}_{\text{bsAbs}}^{\text{Central to tumor}}$$

$$- \text{Reaction}_{\text{Complex formation}} + \text{Reaction}_{\text{Dissociation}} \quad (12.2)$$

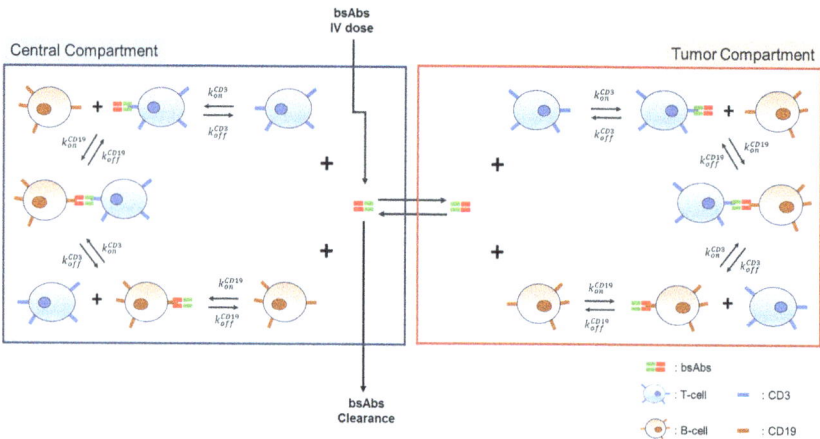

Figure 12.2: Model diagram for the mechanistic model of bsAbs. Model formulation assumed that the bsAbs will interact with T- and B-cells in circulation (central compartment) and in the lymph system (tumor compartment). Model equations are based on the mass accumulation of bsAbs and the two targets, CD3 and CD19.

$$V_{\text{Central}} \frac{d\,[\text{bsAbs}]^{\text{Blood}}}{dt} = R_{\text{infusion}} + \text{mass flow}_{\text{bsAbs}}^{\text{Tumor to central}} - \text{mass flow}_{\text{bsAbs}}^{\text{Central to tumor}}$$
$$- V_{\text{Central}} \left(k_{\text{on}}^{\text{CD3}}\, [\text{bsAbs}]^{\text{Blood}}\, [\text{CD3}]^{\text{Blood}} \right)$$
$$- V_{\text{Central}} \left(k_{\text{on}}^{\text{CD19}}\, [\text{bsAbs}]^{\text{Blood}}\, [\text{CD19}]^{\text{Blood}} \right) \qquad (12.3)$$
$$+ V_{\text{Central}} \left(k_{\text{off}}^{\text{CD3}}\, [\text{bsAbs.CD3}]^{\text{Blood}} \right)$$
$$+ V_{\text{Central}} \left(k_{\text{off}}^{\text{CD19}}\, [\text{bsAbs.CD19}]^{\text{Blood}} \right) - V_{\text{Central}}\, \text{kel}\, [\text{bsAbs}]^{\text{Blood}}$$

$$V_{\text{Central}} \frac{d\,[\text{CD3}]^{\text{Blood}}}{dt} = -V_{\text{Central}} \left(k_{\text{on}}^{\text{CD3}}\, [\text{bsAbs}]^{\text{Blood}}\, [\text{CD3}]^{\text{Blood}} \right)$$
$$- V_{\text{Central}} \left(k_{\text{on}}^{\text{CD3}}\, [\text{bsAbs.CD19}]^{\text{Blood}}\, [\text{CD3}]^{\text{Blood}} \right)$$
$$+ V_{\text{Central}} \left(k_{\text{off}}^{\text{CD3}}\, [\text{bsAbs.CD3}]^{\text{Blood}} \right) \qquad (12.4)$$
$$+ V_{\text{Central}} \left(k_{\text{off}}^{\text{CD3}}\, [\text{bsAbs.CD3.CD19}]^{\text{Blood}} \right)$$

$$V_{\text{Central}} \frac{d\,[\text{CD19}]^{\text{Blood}}}{dt} = -V_{\text{Central}} \left(k_{\text{on}}^{\text{CD19}}\, [\text{bsAbs}]^{\text{Blood}}\, [\text{CD19}]^{\text{Blood}} \right)$$
$$- V_{\text{Central}} \left(k_{\text{on}}^{\text{CD19}}\, [\text{bsAbs.CD3}]^{\text{Blood}}\, [\text{CD19}]^{\text{Blood}} \right)$$
$$+ V_{\text{Central}} \left(k_{\text{off}}^{\text{CD19}}\, [\text{bsAbs.CD19}]^{\text{Blood}} \right) \qquad (12.5)$$
$$+ V_{\text{Central}} \left(k_{\text{off}}^{\text{CD19}}\, [\text{bsAbs.CD3.CD19}]^{\text{Blood}} \right)$$

$$V_{\text{Central}} \frac{d\,[\text{bsAbs.CD3}]^{\text{Blood}}}{dt} = V_{\text{Central}} \left(k_{\text{on}}^{\text{CD3}}\, [\text{bsAbs}]^{\text{Blood}}\, [\text{CD3}]^{\text{Blood}} \right)$$
$$- V_{\text{Central}} \left(k_{\text{off}}^{\text{CD3}}\, [\text{bsAbs.CD3}]^{\text{Blood}} \right) \qquad (12.6)$$
$$+ V_{\text{Central}} \left(k_{\text{off}}^{\text{CD19}}\, [\text{bsAbs.CD3.CD19}]^{\text{Blood}} \right)$$

$$V_{\text{Central}} \frac{d\,[\text{bsAbs.CD19}]^{\text{Blood}}}{dt} = V_{\text{Central}} \left(k_{\text{on}}^{\text{CD19}}\, [\text{bsAbs}]^{\text{Blood}}\, [\text{CD19}]^{\text{Blood}} \right)$$
$$- V_{\text{Central}} \left(k_{\text{off}}^{\text{CD19}}\, [\text{bsAbs.CD19}]^{\text{Blood}} \right) \qquad (12.7)$$
$$+ V_{\text{Central}} \left(k_{\text{off}}^{\text{CD3}}\, [\text{bsAbs.CD3.CD19}]^{\text{Blood}} \right)$$

$$V_{\text{Central}} \frac{d\,[\text{bsAbs.CD3.CD19}]^{\text{Blood}}}{dt} = V_{\text{Central}} \left(k_{\text{on}}^{\text{CD19}}\, [\text{bsAbs.CD3}]^{\text{Blood}}\, [\text{CD19}]^{\text{Blood}} \right)$$
$$+ V_{\text{Central}} \left(k_{\text{on}}^{\text{CD3}}\, [\text{bsAbs.CD19}]^{\text{Blood}}\, [\text{CD3}]^{\text{Blood}} \right) \qquad (12.8)$$
$$- V_{\text{Central}} \left(k_{\text{off}}^{\text{CD10}}\, [\text{bsAbs.CD3.CD19}]^{\text{Blood}} \right)$$
$$- V_{\text{Central}} \left(k_{\text{off}}^{\text{CD3}}\, [\text{bsAbs.CD3.CD19}]^{\text{Blood}} \right)$$

Tumor compartment:

$$\frac{dm_{\text{bsAbs}}^{\text{Tumor}}}{dt} = -\text{mass flow}_{\text{bsAbs}}^{\text{Tumor to central}} + \text{mass flow}_{\text{bsAbs}}^{\text{Central to tumor}}$$
$$- \text{Reaction}_{\text{Complex formation}} + \text{Reaction}_{\text{Dissociation}} \tag{12.9}$$

$$V_{\text{Tumor}}\frac{d[\text{bsAbs}]^{\text{Tumor}}}{dt} = -\text{mass flow}_{\text{bsAbs}}^{\text{Tumor to central}} + \text{mass flow}_{\text{bsAbs}}^{\text{Tumor to peripheral}}$$
$$- V_{\text{Tumor}}\left(k_{\text{on}}^{\text{CD3}}[\text{bsAbs}]^{\text{Tumor}}[\text{CD3}]^{\text{Tumor}}\right)$$
$$- V_{\text{Tumor}}\left(k_{\text{on}}^{\text{CD19}}[\text{bsAbs}]^{\text{Tumor}}[\text{CD19}]^{\text{Tumor}}\right)$$
$$+ V_{\text{Tumor}}\left(k_{\text{off}}^{\text{CD3}}[\text{bsAbs.CD3}]^{\text{Tumor}}\right) \tag{12.10}$$
$$+ V_{\text{Tumor}}\left(k_{\text{off}}^{\text{CD19}}[\text{bsAbs.CD19}]^{\text{Tumor}}\right)$$

$$V_{\text{Tumor}}\frac{d[\text{CD3}]^{\text{Tumor}}}{dt} = -V_{\text{Tumor}}\left(k_{\text{on}}^{\text{CD3}}[\text{bsAbs}]^{\text{Tumor}}[\text{CD3}]^{\text{Tumor}}\right)$$
$$- V_{\text{Tumor}}\left(k_{\text{on}}^{\text{CD3}}[\text{bsAbs.CD19}]^{\text{Tumor}}[\text{CD3}]^{\text{Tumor}}\right)$$
$$+ V_{\text{Tumor}}\left(k_{\text{off}}^{\text{CD3}}[\text{bsAbs.CD3}]^{\text{Tumor}}\right) \tag{12.11}$$
$$+ V_{\text{Tumor}}\left(k_{\text{off}}^{\text{CD3}}[\text{bsAbs.CD3.CD19}]^{\text{Tumor}}\right)$$

$$V_{\text{Tumor}}\frac{d[\text{CD19}]^{\text{Tumor}}}{dt} = -V_{\text{Central}}\left(k_{\text{on}}^{\text{CD19}}[\text{bsAbs}]^{\text{Tumor}}[\text{CD19}]^{\text{Tumor}}\right)$$
$$- V_{\text{Tumor}}\left(k_{\text{on}}^{\text{CD19}}[\text{bsAbs.CD3}]^{\text{Tumor}}[\text{CD19}]^{\text{Tumor}}\right)$$
$$+ V_{\text{Tumor}}\left(k_{\text{off}}^{\text{CD19}}[\text{bsAbs.CD19}]^{\text{Tumor}}\right) \tag{12.12}$$
$$+ V_{\text{Tumor}}\left(k_{\text{off}}^{\text{CD19}}[\text{bsAbs.CD3.CD19}]^{\text{Tumor}}\right)$$

$$V_{\text{Tumor}}\frac{d[\text{bsAbs.CD3}]^{\text{Tumor}}}{dt} = V_{\text{Tumor}}\left(k_{\text{on}}^{\text{CD3}}[\text{bsAbs}]^{\text{Tumor}}[\text{CD3}]^{\text{Tumor}}\right)$$
$$- V_{\text{Tumor}}\left(k_{\text{off}}^{\text{CD3}}[\text{bsAbs.CD3}]^{\text{Tumor}}\right) \tag{12.13}$$
$$+ V_{\text{Tumor}}\left(k_{\text{off}}^{\text{CD19}}[\text{bsAbs.CD3.CD19}]^{\text{Tumor}}\right)$$

$$V_{\text{Tumor}}\frac{d[\text{bsAbs.CD19}]^{\text{Tumor}}}{dt} = V_{\text{Tumor}}\left(k_{\text{on}}^{\text{CD19}}[\text{bsAbs}]^{\text{Tumor}}[\text{CD19}]^{\text{Tumor}}\right)$$
$$- V_{\text{Tumor}}\left(k_{\text{off}}^{\text{CD19}}[\text{bsAbs.CD19}]^{\text{Tumor}}\right) \tag{12.14}$$
$$+ V_{\text{Tumor}}\left(k_{\text{off}}^{\text{CD3}}[\text{bsAbs.CD3.CD19}]^{\text{Tumor}}\right)$$

$$V_{\text{Tumor}}\frac{d[\text{bsAbs.CD3.CD19}]^{\text{Tumor}}}{dt} = V_{\text{Tumor}}\left(k_{\text{on}}^{\text{CD19}}[\text{bsAbs.CD3}]^{\text{Tumor}}[\text{CD19}]^{\text{Tumor}}\right)$$
$$+ V_{\text{Tumor}}\left(k_{\text{on}}^{\text{CD3}}[\text{bsAbs.CD19}]^{\text{Tumor}}[\text{CD3}]^{\text{Tumor}}\right)$$
$$- V_{\text{Tumor}}\left(k_{\text{off}}^{\text{CD19}}[\text{bsAbs.CD3.CD19}]^{\text{Tumor}}\right) \tag{12.15}$$
$$- V_{\text{Tumor}}\left(k_{\text{off}}^{\text{CD3}}[\text{bsAbs.CD3.CD19}]^{\text{Tumor}}\right)$$

with: $R_{Central}$ = IV infusion rate of bsAbs [nanomole/day]; $V_{Central}$ = volume of central compartment [l]; V_{Tumor} = volume of tumor compartment [l]; $[bsAbs]^{Blood}$ = concentration of bsAbs in blood [nanomolarity]; $[bsAbs]^{Blood}$ = concentration of bsAbs in tumor [nanomolarity]; $[CD3]^{Blood}$ = concentration of CD3 in blood [nanomolarity]; $[CD3]^{Tumor}$ = concentration of CD3 in tumor; $[CD19]^{Blood}$ = concentration of CD19 in blood [nanomolarity]; $[CD19]^{Tumor}$ = concentration of CD19 in tumor [nanomolarity]; $[bsAbs.CD3]^{Blood}$ = concentration of the dimer formed between bsAbs and CD3 in blood [nanomolarity]; $[bsAbs.CD3]^{Tumor}$ = concentration of the dimer formed between bsAbs and CD3 in tumor [nanomolarity]; $[bsAbs.CD19]^{Blood}$ = concentration of the dimer formed between bsAbs and CD19 in blood [nanomolarity]; $[bsAbs.CD19]^{Tumor}$ = concentration of the dimer formed between bsAbs and CD19 in tumor [nanomolarity]; $[bsAbs.CD3.CD19]^{Blood}$ = concentration of trimer complex in blood [nanomolarity]; $[bsAbs.CD3.CD19]^{Tumor}$ = concentration of trimer complex in tumor [nanomolarity];

12.6.2.3 Simulations and results

The ODE model was implemented in the Simbiology Toolbox of Matlab (http://www.mathworks.com) using the parameter values shown in Table 12.1.

Table 12.1: QSP model parameters for a CD3/CD19 T-cell engager.

Parameter	Value	Units	Description	Source
$V_{Central}$	4.52	l	Volume of the central compartment	[50]
CL	2.71	l/h	bsAbs clearance	[50]
kel	0.6	1/h	bsAbs elimination rate	Calculated as: kel = CL/$V_{Central}$
R_{Tumor}	1	cm	Tumor volume	Assumed, as in [51]
CD3	1e+5	Receptors/cells	Initial concentration of CD3 in blood	[52, 53]
CD19	2e+4	Receptors/cells	Initial concentration of CD19 in blood	[54]
k_{on}^{CD3}	3.85e−6	1/(nM * s)	Kinetic rate constant for CD3 complex formation	Calculated as: $k_{on}^{CD3} = k_{off}^{CD3}/K_D^{CD3}$
K_D^{CD3}	260	nM	CD3 binding affinity	[55]
k_{off}^{CD3}	1e−3	1/s	Kinetic rate constant for CD3 dissociation	Assumed, as in [56]
k_{on}^{CD19}	6.71e−4	1/(nM * second)	Kinetic rate constant for CD19 complex formation	Calculated as: $k_{on}^{CD19} = k_{off}^{CD19}/K_D^{CD19}$
K_D^{CD19}	1.49	nM	CD19 binding affinity	[55]
k_{off}^{CD19}	1e−3	1/s	Kinetic rate constant for CD19 dissociation	Assumed, as in [56]

As seen in Figures 12.3 and 12.4, model simulations can help to explore different dosing in terms of the pharmacokinetics and the formation of different complexes.

A very important outcome when using mechanistic models for bsAbs is that through simulation we can obtain a bell-shaped curve when plotting the concentration of trimers for different doses. This kind of plot is particularly useful to find optimal doses

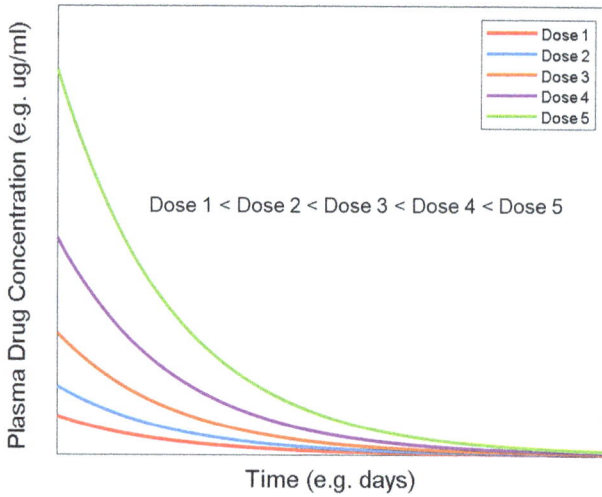

Figure 12.3: QSP model simulations: pharmacokinetics of a generic bsAbs. Initial drug concentration and exposure increase with higher doses.

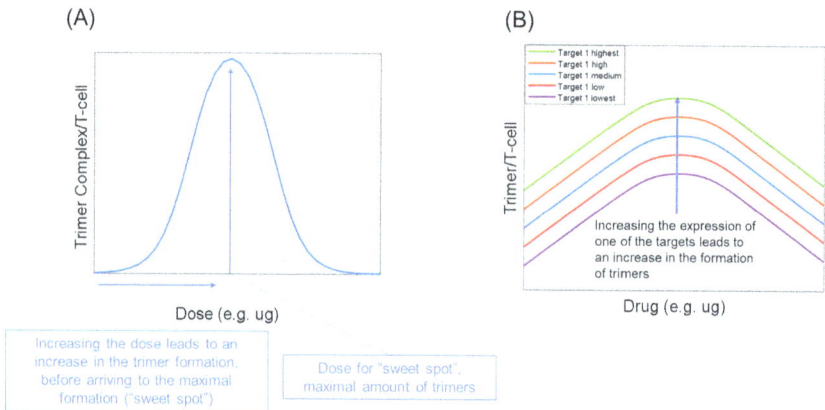

Figure 12.4: QSP model simulations: formation of trimeric complex. (A) A "bell-shaped" curve is obtained when plotting the trimer levels for different doses. There is a dose where the trimer formation is maximal ("sweet spot"); (B) QSP model can be used to explore the sensitivity of the trimer formation to variation in specific parameter values, here it is shown (in log-scale) how the trimer formation increases when the expression levels of one of the targets ("target 1") is increased.

maximising the trimer formation ("sweet spot"), increasing the dose beyond this point will saturate the targets forming mainly dimers and leaving less space to create trimers when the concentration of bsAbs is high. This result is very important for bsAbs and other modalities with molecules forming trimeric complexes, e.g. proteolysis targeting chimera (PROTAC), showing the utility of QSP modelling for dose optimisation.

12.6.3 Model-based analysis of neutropenia to explore clinical dosing schedule options

Neutropenia is a state of low blood neutrophil count and it is a toxic side-effect of some cancer medications. During clinical development of avadomide, an immunomodulatory drug developed for lymphoma, neutropenia severity was found to be a dose-limiting toxicity, which posed challenges in optimizing dosing regimens for patients [57].

A model-based strategy was designed to link clinical neutrophil dynamics to avadomide PK and PD, in order to characterize the pattern of neutropenia, and investigate dose levels and schedules which could minimize the occurrence of severe neutropenia while allowing for sufficient drug exposure [58].

The full model includes several components (Figure 12.5), the core element is the model for neutrophil life-cycle, which consists of sequential compartments representing the formation of the neutrophil cell line in the human bone marrow. Progenitor cells which are committed to this hematopoietic lineage undergo sequentially to proliferation, progressive maturation, storage within the bone marrow and eventually release to blood

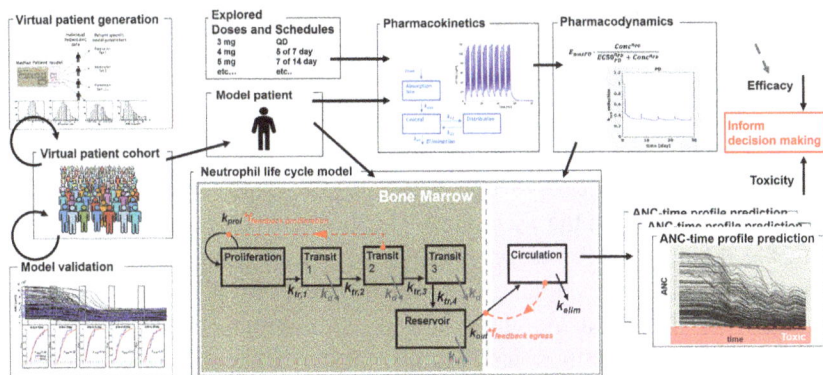

Figure 12.5: Overview of the QSP model workflow. The full model consists of a combination of three components: (i) neutrophil life-cycle, (ii) avadomide pharmacokinetics, (iii) avadomide pharmacodynamics. Their integrated simulation computes the neutrophil count in blood given various avadomide administrations. To qualify the model for its context of use, the simulation outputs were compared to relevant clinical data to demonstrate consistency. The model was applied to explore the neutrophil count dynamics for virtual cohorts of patients with different characteristics receiving various avadomide dosing schedules [58].

circulation. Mathematically, this is implemented as a sequence of compartments (which are equivalent to the CSTR idealization in chemical engineering) where immature cells from upstream compartments are converted to the following maturation step. In addition, to mimic important control mechanisms that regulate the cell maturation process in the human bone marrow, dedicated functions are introduced to modulate the proliferation of progenitor cells and the egress from the reservoir pool into peripheral circulation. These functions are needed to maintain a physiological behavior, but due to the complexity of the underlying biological regulatory loops, their mathematical formulation is semi-empiric. This approach is sometimes adopted in QSP, when we seek for a balance between the complexity of the system and the focus on the objective of the analysis. As introduced previously, such models are defined fit-for-purpose [59], meaning that they should be appropriate and adequate for their intended use, rather than being overly complex.

Along with the neutrophils life-cycle model, two more elements are included to integrate the effect of the drug. The PD model establishes the functional relationship between drug concentration in plasma and the perturbation induced to the system, which for avadomide consists in the induction of a block along the neutrophil maturation sequence [57, 60].

While PD models can take various forms [61], one common choice is the Hill function, which utilizes three parameters to modulate the shape of a sigmoidal curve [62]. In this case, the Hill function is used to reduce the transfer rate between the neutrophil transit compartments in an avadomide concentration-dependent manner.

The PK model describes the concentration-time profile of avadomide in plasma, which is the input to the PD model. In this case a simple two-compartment model was adopted, however PK models exist in various forms and complexities [63–65]. For avadomide, the PK model accounts for the processes of drug absorption into plasma, its distribution, and its final elimination.

The neutrophil model consists of a set of six ODE, whose parameters are determined either by model fitting to clinical trial data, or leveraging literature and pre-clinical experimental information. Model identifiability analysis confirmed that parameter values are determinable given the selected model structure and the data availability.

The model was qualified for its context of use by comparing model predictions to independent clinical datasets, in order to confirm the model predictive accuracy.

To account for the variability observed in the patient population, rather than adopting a single parameterization, multiple alternative model parameterizations are determined by taking the values from distribution density functions which are determined based on clinical data. These alternative model parameterizations, which are effectively defined virtual patients, allow for capturing a likely distribution of treatment outcomes, thereby determining the fraction of patients which are expected to experience a given neutropenia grade under the tested dosing schedule regimens.

The model raw outputs consist of the longitudinal neutrophil counts in blood over the course of a 21 day treatment, these results are then processed to derive clinically relevant parameters such as the neutropenia grade, the time of toxic event, its duration, and whether neutrophil count recovery occurs.

This model based analysis can be used in conjunction with experimental evidence to reduce decision-making risks in the uncertainty of clinical development settings.

12.7 Conclusions

In the last few decades, the pharmaceutical research and development landscape has undergone profound changes. The field has progressively shifted towards more sophisticated products, driven by research advancements and by the need to meet increasingly higher standards for efficacy and safety as demanded by regulatory agencies. This shift has also paved the way for shorter cycle times for product development, a focus on personalized medicine, and a reduction in animal experiments.

This chapter has discussed the critical role of mathematical modelling and simulation in addressing these challenges. Specifically, the discipline of quantitative systems pharmacology, by integrating experimental and computational methods, provides a robust framework for analysis in the translational and clinical development stages. Many of the methodologies adopted by QSP are rooted in foundational chemical engineering principles such as mass balances, transport phenomena, and reaction kinetics. By leveraging innovative modelling approaches, the pharmaceutical industry can achieve more efficient, effective, and safer therapeutic solutions, ultimately improving patient outcomes and public health.

As the pharmaceutical industry continues to evolve, the adoption of interdisciplinary methodologies is expected to play a crucial role in driving innovation and improving therapeutic outcomes. This creates numerous opportunities for engineers to contribute to this field by leveraging the wide variety of theories and methodologies that are routinely applied in their respective fields. Engineers bring a unique perspective and skill set that can be instrumental in tackling complex biological systems, optimizing drug delivery mechanisms, and enhancing the precision of therapeutic interventions.

One of the major challenges engineers can expect when working in the pharma space is dealing with unknowns and technical limitations, which are generally not encountered to the same extent when dealing with human-made systems. In biology and pharmacology, the system under analysis is only partially understood, and valuable contributions often consist of making inferences and educated assumptions with minimal evidence and data availability. Engineers must be adept at handling uncertainty, developing robust models that can accommodate variability, and iteratively refining their approaches based on emerging data.

Moreover, the integration of machine learning and artificial intelligence with QSP models presents a promising frontier. These technologies can enhance predictive capabilities, identify novel drug targets, and streamline the drug development process.

Engineers with expertise in data science and computational modelling are well-positioned to lead these advancements, bridging the gap between experimental data and clinical application.

The future of drug development lies in the seamless integration of experimental data, computational models, and clinical insights to bring new therapeutic solutions to patients in need. By fostering collaboration between engineers, biologists, pharmacologists, and clinicians, the pharmaceutical industry can accelerate the development of innovative treatments and improve the quality of life for countless individuals. The contributions of engineers will be pivotal in this interdisciplinary effort, driving progress and ensuring that the next generation of therapies is both safe and effective.

Acknowledgments: The authors would like to thank the editors Prof. D. Bogle and Prof. T. Sosnowski for their guidance and review of this article before its publication.

References

1. Leil TA, Bertz R. Quantitative systems pharmacology can reduce attrition and improve productivity in pharmaceutical research and development. Front Pharmacol 2014;5:247.
2. Bleicher LS, van Daelen T, Honeycutt JD, Hassan M, Chandrasekhar J, Shirley W, et al. Enhanced utility of AI/ML methods during lead optimization by inclusion of 3D ligand information. Front Drug Discov 2022;2. https://doi.org/10.3389/fddsv.2022.1074797.
3. Lin X, Li X, Lin X. A review on applications of computational methods in drug screening and design. Molecules 2020;25:1375.
4. Temml V, Kutil Z. Structure-based molecular modeling in SAR analysis and lead optimization. Comput Struct Biotechnol J 2021;19:1431–44.
5. European Medicine Agency. ICH guideline M3(R2) on non-clinical safety studies for the conduct of human clinical trials and marketing authorisation for pharmaceuticals; 2009.
6. Zou P, Yu Y, Zheng N, Yang Y, Paholak HJ, Yu LX, et al. Applications of human pharmacokinetic prediction in first-in-human dose estimation. AAPS J 2012;14:262–81.
7. Kimko H, Pinheiro J. Model-based clinical drug development in the past, present and future: a commentary. Br J Clin Pharmacol 2015;79:108–16.
8. Lalonde RL, Kowalski KG, Hutmacher MM, Ewy W, Nichols DJ, Milligan PA, et al. Model-based drug development. Clin Pharmacol Ther 2007;82:21–32.
9. Milligan PA, Brown MJ, Marchant B, Martin SW, van der Graaf PH, Benson N, et al. Model-based drug development: a rational approach to efficiently accelerate drug development. Clin Pharmacol Therapeut 2013;93:502–14.
10. Azer K, Kaddi CD, Barrett JS, Bai JPF, McQuade ST, Merrill NJ, et al. History and future perspectives on the discipline of quantitative systems pharmacology modeling and its applications. Front Physiol 2021;12. https://doi.org/10.3389/fphys.2021.637999.
11. Sorger PK, Allerheiligen SRB, Abernethy DR, Altman RB, Brouwer KLR, Califano A, et al. Quantitative and systems pharmacology in the post-genomic era: new approaches to discovering drugs and understanding therapeutic mechanisms; 2011.
12. Zhang L, Sinha V, Forgue ST, Callies S, Ni L, Peck R, et al. Model-based drug development: the road to quantitative pharmacology. J Pharmacokinet Pharmacodyn 2006;33:369–93.

13. Agoram BM, Demin O. Integration not isolation: arguing the case for quantitative and systems pharmacology in drug discovery and development. Drug Discov Today 2011;16:1031–6.
14. Allerheiligen SRB. Next-generation model-based drug discovery and development: quantitative and systems pharmacology. Clin Pharmacol Ther 2010;88:135–7.
15. Manca D, editor. Quantitative systems pharmacology: models and model-based systems with applications. In: Computer aided chemical engineering. Amsterdam: Elsevier; 2018, 42.
16. Fogler HS. Elements of chemical reaction engineering, 5th ed. London, UK: Prentice Hall; 2016.
17. Aghamiri SS, Amin R, Helikar T. Recent applications of quantitative systems pharmacology and machine learning models across diseases. J Pharmacokinet Pharmacodyn 2022;49:19–37.
18. Musante C, Ramanujan S, Schmidt B, Ghobrial O, Lu J, Heatherington A. Quantitative systems pharmacology: a case for disease models. Clin Pharmacol Ther 2017;101:24–7.
19. Strimbu K, Tavel JA. What are biomarkers? Curr Opin HIV AIDS 2010;5:463–6.
20. Pletcher MJ, Pignone M. Evaluating the clinical utility of a biomarker. Circulation 2011;123:1116–24.
21. Visser Sa G, de Alwis DP, Kerbusch T, Stone JA, Allerheiligen SRB. Implementation of quantitative and systems pharmacology in large pharma. CPT Pharmacometrics Syst Pharmacol 2014;3:142.
22. Arulraj T, Wang H, Emens LA, Santa-Maria CA, Popel AS. A transcriptome-informed QSP model of metastatic triple-negative breast cancer identifies predictive biomarkers for PD-1 inhibition. Sci Adv 2023;9:eadg0289.
23. Allen RJ, Rieger TR, Musante CJ. Efficient generation and selection of virtual populations in quantitative systems pharmacology models. CPT Pharmacometrics Syst Pharmacol 2016;5:140–6.
24. Cheng Y, Straube R, Alnaif AE, Huang L, Leil TA, Schmidt BJ. Virtual populations for quantitative systems pharmacology models. In: Bai JPF, Hur J, editors. Systems medicine. New York, NY: Springer US; 2022: 129–79 pp.
25. Wang H, Arulraj T, Kimko H, Popel AS. Generating immunogenomic data-guided virtual patients using a QSP model to predict response of advanced NSCLC to PD-L1 inhibition. npj Precis Oncol 2023;7:1–14.
26. Matthews RJ, Hollinshead D, Morrison D, van der Graaf PH, Kierzek AM. QSP designer: quantitative systems pharmacology modeling with modular biological process map notation and multiple language code generation. CPT Pharmacometrics Syst Pharmacol 2023;12:889–903.
27. Gong C, Ruiz-Martinez A, Kimko H, Popel AS. A spatial quantitative systems pharmacology platform spQSP-IO for simulations of tumor-immune interactions and effects of checkpoint inhibitor immunotherapy. Cancers 2021;13:3751.
28. Ruiz-Martinez A, Gong C, Wang H, Sové RJ, Mi H, Kimko H, et al. Simulations of tumor growth and response to immunotherapy by coupling a spatial agent-based model with a whole-patient quantitative systems pharmacology model. PLoS Comput Biol 2022;18:e1010254.
29. Michaelis L, Menten ML. Die kinetik der invertinwirkung. Biochem Z 1913;49:333–69. Find this article online.
30. Hill AV. Proceedings of the physiological society: January 22, 1910. J Physiol 1910;40. https://doi.org/10.1113/jphysiol.1910.sp001386.
31. Au JL-S, Abbiati RA, Wientjes MG, Lu Z. Target site delivery and residence of nanomedicines: application of quantitative systems pharmacology. Pharmacol Rev 2019;71:157–69.
32. Flessner MF. The transport barrier in intraperitoneal therapy. Am J Physiol Ren Physiol 2005;288:F433–42.
33. Jain RK, Martin JD, Stylianopoulos T. The role of mechanical forces in tumor growth and therapy. Annu Rev Biomed Eng 2014;16:321–46.
34. Morris PD, Narracott A, von Tengg-Kobligk H, Silva Soto DA, Hsiao S, Lungu A, et al. Computational fluid dynamics modelling in cardiovascular medicine. Heart 2016;102:18–28.
35. Quarteroni A, Veneziani A, Vergara C. Geometric multiscale modeling of the cardiovascular system, between theory and practice. Comput Methods Appl Mech Eng 2016;302:193–252.
36. Zheng S, Carugo D, Mosayyebi A, Turney B, Burkhard F, Lange D, et al. Fluid mechanical modeling of the upper urinary tract. WIREs Mech Dis 2021;13:e1523.
37. Cao Y, Balthasar JP, Jusko WJ. Second-generation minimal physiologically-based pharmacokinetic model for monoclonal antibodies. J Pharmacokinet Pharmacodyn 2013;40:597–607.

38. Harms BD, Kearns JD, Su SV, Kohli N, Nielsen UB, Schoeberl B. Optimizing properties of antireceptor antibodies using kinetic computational models and experiments. Methods Enzymol 2012;502:67–87.

39. Stein A, Franklin JL, Chia VM, Arrindell D, Kormany W, Wright J, et al. Benefit–risk assessment of blinatumomab in the treatment of relapsed/refractory B-cell precursor acute lymphoblastic leukemia. Drug Saf 2019;42:587–601.

40. Wang L. Trial suggests expanded role for blinatumomab in treating ALL. Cancer Currents Blog 2023. https://www.cancer.gov/news-events/cancer-currents-blog/2023/blincyto-leukemia-minimal-residual-disease [Accessed 13 Aug 2024].

41. Betts A, van der Graaf PH. Mechanistic quantitative pharmacology strategies for the early clinical development of bispecific antibodies in oncology. Clin Pharmacol Ther 2020;108:528–41.

42. Flowers D, Bassen D, Kapitanov GI, Marcantonio D, Burke JM, Apgar JF, et al. A next generation mathematical model for the in vitro to clinical translation of T-cell engagers. J Pharmacokinet Pharmacodyn 2023;50:215–27.

43. Li R, Dere E, Kwong M, Fei M, Dave R, Masih S, et al. A bispecific modeling framework enables the prediction of efficacy, toxicity, and optimal molecular design of bispecific antibodies targeting MerTK. AAPS J 2024;26: 11.

44. Weddell J. Mechanistically modeling peripheral cytokine dynamics following bispecific dosing in solid tumors. CPT Pharmacometrics Syst Pharmacol 2023;12:1726–37.

45. Sanford M. Blinatumomab: first global approval. Drugs 2015;75:321–7.

46. Chen X, Kamperschroer C, Wong G, Xuan D. A modeling framework to characterize cytokine release upon T-cell-engaging bispecific antibody treatment: methodology and opportunities. Clin Transl Sci 2019;12: 600–8.

47. Hosseini I, Gadkar K, Stefanich E, Li C-C, Sun LL, Chu Y-W, et al. Mitigating the risk of cytokine release syndrome in a Phase I trial of CD20/CD3 bispecific antibody mosunetuzumab in NHL: impact of translational system modeling. NPJ Syst Biol Appl 2020;6:28.

48. Jiang X, Chen X, Jaiprasart P, Carpenter TJ, Zhou R, Wang W. Development of a minimal physiologically-based pharmacokinetic/pharmacodynamic model to characterize target cell depletion and cytokine release for T cell-redirecting bispecific agents in humans. Eur J Pharmaceut Sci 2020;146:105260.

49. Li R, Dere E, Kwong M, Fei M, Dave R, Masih S, et al. A bispecific modeling framework enables the prediction of efficacy, toxicity, and optimal molecular design of bispecific antibodies targeting MerTK. AAPS J 2024;26: 11.

50. Zhu M, Wu B, Brandl C, Johnson J, Wolf A, Chow A, et al. Blinatumomab, a bispecific T-cell engager (BiTE(®)) for CD-19 targeted cancer immunotherapy: clinical pharmacology and its implications. Clin Pharmacokinet 2016;55:1271–88.

51. Betts, A, Haddish-Berhane, N, Shah, DK, Van Der Graaf, PH, Barletta, F, King, L, et al., 2019. A translational quantitative systems pharmacology model for CD3 bispecific molecules: application to quantify T cell-mediated tumor cell killing by P-Cadherin LP DART®. AAPS J 21, 66.

52. Carpentier B, Pierobon P, Hivroz C, Henry N. T-cell artificial focal triggering tools: linking surface interactions with cell response. PLoS One 2009;4:e4784.

53. Nicolas L, Monneret G, Debard AL, Blesius A, Gutowski MC, Salles G, et al. Human gammadelta T cells express a higher TCR/CD3 complex density than alphabeta T cells. Clin Immunol 2001;98:358–63.

54. Ginaldi L, De Martinis M, Matutes E, Farahat N, Morilla R, Catovsky D. Levels of expression of CD19 and CD20 in chronic B cell leukaemias. J Clin Pathol 1998;51:364–9.

55. Dreier T, Lorenczewski G, Brandl C, Hoffmann P, Syring U, Hanakam F, et al. Extremely potent, rapid and costimulation-independent cytotoxic T-cell response against lymphoma cells catalyzed by a single-chain bispecific antibody. Int J Cancer 2002;100:690–7.

56. Jiang X, Chen X, Carpenter TJ, Wang J, Zhou R, Davis HM, et al. Development of a Target cell-Biologics-Effector cell (TBE) complex-based cell killing model to characterize target cell depletion by T cell redirecting bispecific agents. mAbs 2018;10:876–89.

57. Carpio C, Bouabdallah R, Ysebaert L, Sancho J-M, Salles G, Cordoba R, et al. Avadomide monotherapy in relapsed/refractory DLBCL: safety, efficacy, and a predictive gene classifier. Blood 2020;135:996–1007.
58. Abbiati RA, Pourdehnad M, Carrancio S, Pierce DW, Kasibhatla S, McConnell M, et al. Quantitative systems pharmacology modeling of avadomide-induced neutropenia enables virtual clinical dose and schedule finding studies. AAPS J 2021;23:103.
59. Wang Y, Huang SM. Commentary on fit-for-purpose models for regulatory applications. J Pharmaceut Sci 2019;108:18–20.
60. Chiu H, Trisal P, Bjorklund C, Carrancio S, Toraño EG, Guarinos C, et al. Combination lenalidomide-rituximab immunotherapy activates anti-tumour immunity and induces tumour cell death by complementary mechanisms of action in follicular lymphoma. Br J Haematol 2019;185:240–53.
61. Felmlee MA, Morris ME, Mager DE. Mechanism-based pharmacodynamic modeling. Methods Mol Biol 2012;929:583–600.
62. Goutelle S, Maurin M, Rougier F, Barbaut X, Bourguignon L, Ducher M, et al. The Hill equation: a review of its capabilities in pharmacological modelling. Fund Clin Pharmacol 2008;22:633–48.
63. Bassingthwaighte JB, Butterworth E, Jardine B, Raymond GM. Compartmental modeling in the analysis of biological systems. In: Reisfeld B, Mayeno AN, editors. Computational toxicology. Totowa, NJ: Humana Press; 2012, vol I:391–438 pp.
64. Mould D, Upton R. Basic concepts in population modeling, simulation, and model-based drug development. CPT Pharmacometrics Syst Pharmacol 2012;1:6.
65. Upton RN, Foster DJR, Abuhelwa AY. An introduction to physiologically-based pharmacokinetic models. Pediatr Anesth 2016;26:1036–46.

Ewa Dluska* and Agnieszka Markowska-Radomska*

13 A novel strategy for brain cancer treatment through a multiple emulsion system for simultaneous therapeutics delivery

Abstract: The research integrates chemical engineering principles with biological insights to overcome key barriers in glioblastoma multiforme (GBM) therapy. GBM remains one of the most aggressive and lethal brain tumours, characterised by its infiltrative growth, chemoresistance and poor prognosis. Conventional chemotherapy faces critical limitations, including restricted drug penetration across the blood–brain barrier, systemic toxicity and tumour resistance to classic treatment. Addressing these challenges, this study proposes an innovative, multiple emulsion–based drug delivery system designed to enhance the therapeutic effectiveness of GBM treatment through synergistic combinations of RNA-class molecules and chemotherapeutic agent (doxorubicin–DOX). The system utilises a pH-responsive biopolymer (carboxymethylcellulose sodium salt), facilitating controlled and selective drug release in the acidic microenvironment of tumour cells (pH 6.3), while preserving healthy tissues. The emulsion structures prepared using Couette–Taylor flow techniques, achieved high encapsulation efficiency of DOX, stability and precise control over release kinetics. The addition of siRNA targets the genetic pathways of tumour DNA repair, sensitising cancer cells to DOX and significantly reducing their viability. Experimental results demonstrated a substantial improvement in cytotoxic efficacy, with up to a 65 % reduction in cancer cell viability compared to conventional DOX solution, further amplified to about 81 % when combined with liposomal siRNA. A mathematical model of drug diffusion and chemical reaction expressing absorption by cancer cells highlights the systems' potential for personalising therapy by optimising drug dose and release profiles. This approach not only minimises systemic side effects but also provides a platform for targeted, efficient and more patient-friendly cancer treatment. This study establishes multiple emulsion as a promising carrier for dual-drug delivery system, bridging the gap between biological complexity and engineering precision. Future work will focus on *in vivo* evaluation and clinical validation to realise the potential of this approach in improving GBM patient outcomes.

Keywords: cancer treatment; multiple emulsion; delivery system; mass transfer; mathematical modelling; RNA interference

*Corresponding authors: Ewa Dluska and **Agnieszka Markowska-Radomska**, Faculty of Chemical and Process Engineering, Warsaw University of Technology, Warsaw, 00-645, Poland,
E-mail: ewa.dluska@pw.edu.pl (E. Dluska), agnieszka.markowska@pw.edu.pl (A. Markowska-Radomska).
https://orcid.org/0000-0001-8833-2744 (E. Dluska)

As per De Gruyter's policy this article has previously been published in the journal Physical Sciences Reviews. Please cite as: E. Dluska and A. Markowska-Radomska "A novel strategy for brain cancer treatment through a multiple emulsion system for simultaneous therapeutics delivery" *Physical Sciences Reviews* [Online] 2024. DOI: 10.1515/psr-2024-0064 | https://doi.org/10.1515/9783111394558-013

13.1 Introduction

In the dynamically changing field of cancer treatment, innovative strategies are continually explored to enhance therapeutic effectiveness while minimising drug doses and potential side effects from chemotherapy. One such breakthrough is gene-mediated therapy combined with chemotherapy medication delivery to act synergistically at specific sites using a single carrier or platform [1–3]. When a gene mutation causes a protein to be missing or faulty, gene therapy may be able to restore the normal function of that protein, or in contrast, via gene expression regulation, lead to cell death or slow the growth of cells with mutations. One of the processes for gene expression regulation is RNA interference by binding silencing agents such as shRNA (short hairpin RNA) and siRNA (small interfering RNA) molecules to the messenger RNAs (mRNA), forming RNA-induced silencing complexes (RISC) and cleaving targeted mRNA molecules [4–6]. For cancer therapy, siRNA functions by inhibiting target mRNA overexpression in cancer cells. Currently, several siRNA therapeutics have been approved by the US Food and Drug Administration (FDA) (e.g. patisiran, givosiran, inclisiran, lumasiran) [7, 8].

The genetic material in the naked form of RNA or DNA molecules, when inserted directly, usually does not function because of low bioavailability, resulting in rapid clearance, primarily via the kidneys. The unmodified siRNAs are rapidly degraded by nucleases in plasma, tissues and the cytoplasm [7, 9]. The chemical modifications of siRNA delay its degradation from a few minutes to hours and improve its performance *in vivo*. Thus, it is crucial to find a carrier/vector that delivers a specific gene to tumour tissue efficiently. Viral and non-viral carriers/vectors are engineered to carry and deliver the genetic material [10–13]. Certain viruses and lipid-based delivery systems are used as they can penetrate cell membranes. Significant advances have been made in the development of lipid-based delivery systems including liposomes, polymeric micelles, microemulsions and solid lipid nanoparticles [7, 14–16]. Among emulsion-based delivery systems, multiple emulsions are particularly of interest as they represent multifunctional structures.

Multiple emulsions are hierarchically organised liquid-dispersed systems having structures of 'droplets in drops' with a great potential for mass transfer processes in reactive and non-reactive multiphase systems. This includes applications in separation/extraction processes, environmental protection, the food industry, pharmaceuticals and medical and biological engineering [17–23]. Multiple emulsions can have double, triple, quadruple, quintuple or even more complex structures. Such multiphase systems create favourable conditions for surface functionalistions, co-encapsulation of the biologically and chemically active ingredients (drugs, living cells, genes, cosmetics) and their co-release in a controlled way through drop size, composition and properties of the dispersed system [19, 23–28]. Moreover, emulsion drops surfaces may be functionalised by the adsorption of specific antibodies for targeting cancerous cells. Also, an increase in the selective delivery of drugs to targeted cancer cells may be achieved by using stimuli-responsive materials as components of emulsions. This material can react in response to the presence of, or changes in external stimuli, such as pH, light, temperature, magnetic or electric fields by the changes in material properties [29, 30]. The development of a pH-responsive multiple emulsion–based delivery system, including dual drug delivery, is a significant stride forward in the quest for more effective and targeted anticancer therapeutics, as we have shown in our previous paper addressing complex medical conditions associated with brain tumours [31, 32].

Glioblastoma multiforme (GBM, Latin: glioblastoma multiforme) is a primary malignant tumour of the central nervous system (brain cancer) with one of the worst prognoses and survival rates [33]. GBM detection typically involves different imaging techniques such as computer tomography (CT) or magnetic resonance imaging (MRI) with contrast enhancement, which identifies the tumour's location, size and infiltration into surrounding brain tissues [34]. Once diagnosed, the treatment begins with maximal safe surgical resection to reduce tumour burden, followed by radiotherapy to eliminate residual cells [35] (Figure 13.1). Additionally, chemotherapy, including targeted drug therapy, is administered concurrently as maintenance therapy to enhance tumour sensitivity to treatment. Follow-up care and rehabilitation also comprise the treatment.

Despite huge progress in the field of oncology, the median survival rate for patients after diagnosis is less than 12 months [36]. One factor contributing to this low survival rate is the fact that many deep-seated and pervasive tumours are not entirely accessible or

Key Points of Classic Glioblastoma Multiforme (GBM) Therapy

I - Tumour Detection and Diagnosis

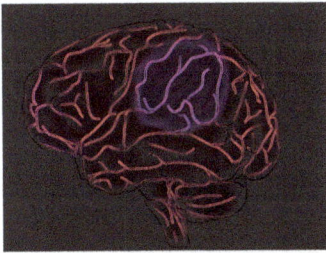

III – Radiotherapy & Chemotherapy

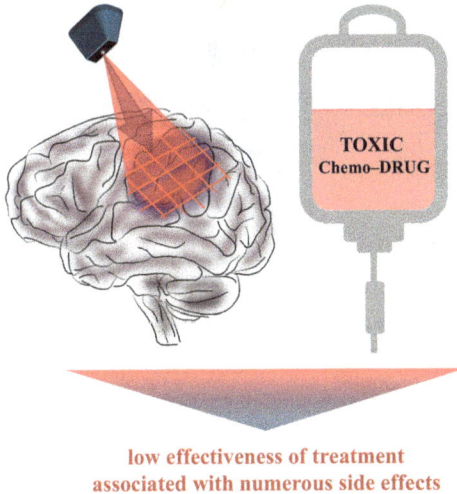

TOXIC
Chemo–DRUG

II - Surgical Resection of Tumour

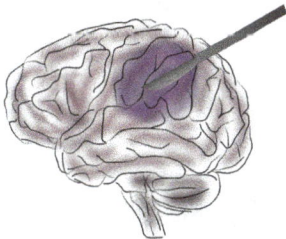

low effectiveness of treatment
associated with numerous side effects

Figure 13.1: The key points of the classic brain tumour treatment.

even visible when using current neurosurgical tools and imaging techniques. Also, the infiltrative nature of GBM leads to difficulties in its complete removal [35, 36]. In addition, the effectiveness of classic chemotherapy is usually low, which is caused by primary or early acquired chemo-resistance, significantly limited penetration of chemotherapeutics across the blood–brain barrier, and their neurotoxicity. Generally, chemotherapeutics disrupt or inhibit cell proliferation, leading to apoptosis (death) of cancer cells, but also non-cancerous cells, causing a number of side effects. The advent of both targeted and gene therapy have raised expectations for brain tumour therapy [37, 38]. However, therapeutic benefits still depend on the development of the most efficient gene vector/ carrier capable of overcoming brain tumour localisation problems. Bearing in mind the above limitations of classic GBM brain tumour therapy, we developed an injectable liquid implant/carrier in the form of multiple emulsions for delivering anticancer drugs and the RNA-class of molecules. This approach provides a real chance of increasing the effectiveness of anticancer therapy by the molecular mechanism of RNA interference and increasing the selective drug transport to cancer cells, and also reducing the toxicity of chemotherapy to healthy cells (Figure 13.2).

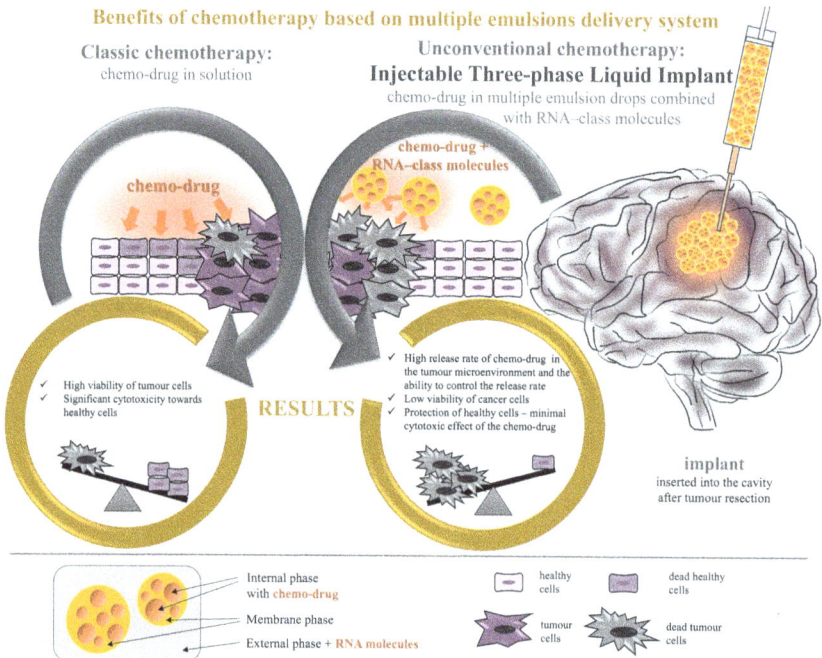

Figure 13.2: The concept of glioblastoma multiforme (GBM) therapy using emulsion-based drug delivery systems in cancer treatment supported by the RNA-class molecules and the comparison with classic therapy.

13.2 The concept of multiple emulsions as a dual drug delivery system for brain tumour treatment

In an experimental model, two therapeutic combinations were used: (i) small interfering RNA molecules (siRNAs) for silencing genes of DNA repair and (ii) chemotherapeutic drug–doxorubicin (DOX) for damaging the cancer cell's DNA. Therapeutics are delivered to cancer cells using multiple emulsions as a drug delivery system in the form of an injectable three-phase liquid implant (Figure 13.2). The proposed implant is a type of water-in-oil-in-water multiple emulsion inserted into the cavity after tumour resection, as surgery usually is the first treatment for brain tumours. The chemotherapeutic agent is encapsulated in the internal water droplets of the emulsion suspended in oil drops. The factor (stimulus) activating the process of selective DOX diffusional release from emulsion drops is a difference in pH of the tumour and healthy cells. The pH of the tumour cells' environment is acidic, whereas healthy cells have a neutral pH [38]. This fact was exploited at the stage of selecting the emulsion composition. The pH-sensitive biopolymer (sodium carboxymethylcellulose) [39, 40] was used in the external phase of the emulsion. With an acidic pH, this biopolymer, which is also adsorbing at the drop interfaces, changes the spatial arrangement of the polymer chain and decreases the viscosity of the external phase, leading to a faster release of highly toxic DOX from emulsions' drops. In addition, the selectivity of the system was also achieved by modifying the emulsion droplet surfaces. For this purpose, antibodies (N-cadherin, CD82, CD15), specific for glioblastoma cells, were attached by physical/chemical adsorption [41]. The DOX release was controlled by droplet size, emulsion structure, composition, density and viscosity of the emulsion liquid phases. During the release studies, three GBM tumour cell lines were verified, namely (U87 MG, LN229, T98G), and one non-cancerous (K21-fibroblasts). A high rate of efficiency for the emulsion was obtained considering the GBM cell's viability. After treatment with DOX, in the emulsion, results showed up to 65 % lower cancer cell viability compared to cells treated with a DOX in solution (classic chemotherapy) [31, 42]. Moreover, this efficiency was increased by another 16 % by introducing RNA molecules encapsulated in liposomes to GBM cells to induce cancer cell apoptosis (cell death) [32]. Promising results have already been obtained with one of the lowest doses of DOX tested, normally ineffective while DOX is administrated as classic chemotherapy.

13.3 Preparation of multiple emulsion–based delivery system

The multiple emulsions were prepared using a Couette–Taylor flow (CTF) apparatus, which enables intensive mixing of liquid phases through rotational and axial flows

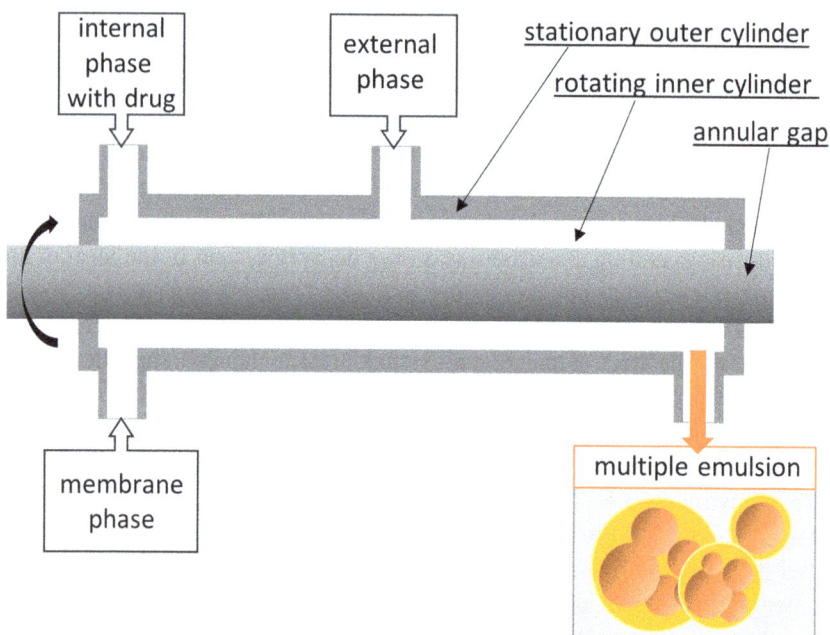

Figure 13.3: A schematic representation of a Couette–Taylor flow (CTF) contactor for preparing multiple emulsion structures with doxorubicin encapsulated in the internal droplets.

providing uniform shear flow, and high mass transfer parameters (interfacial area and mass transfer coefficient) resulting in high encapsulation efficiency and stable emulsion structures (Figure 13.3) [25, 43, 44]. The method of the preparation of different types of multiple emulsions can be found in the previous authors' works [27, 42, 43].

Initially, the internal water phase (W) containing doxorubicin hydrochloride (DOX) and the organic membrane phase (O) comprising soybean oil were mixed to form a simple W/O emulsion. Subsequently, the external water phase (W), containing pH-responsive biopolymer (sodium carboxymethylcellulose-CMC), and additionally liposomal siRNA (in the case of tests with a dual drug delivery system) were introduced to create a double W/O/W emulsion. Two types of multiple emulsions were obtained, differing in their droplet sizes and internal structures. The first emulsion (DOX-E1) featured larger membrane phase droplets encapsulating multiple smaller internal aqueous droplets. The second emulsion (DOX-E2) consisted of smaller membrane phase droplets, each containing a single internal aqueous droplet (Figure 13.4). Both emulsions achieved high encapsulation efficiencies exceeding 95 % for DOX, ensuring minimal drug loss during preparation, and were stable over a few months.

DOX-E1

$D_{32} = 28.6 \pm 0.5 \mu m$
$d_{32} = 6.8 \pm 0.5 \mu m$
$PDI_D = 1.1 \pm 0.1$
$PDI_d = 1.8 \pm 0.1$

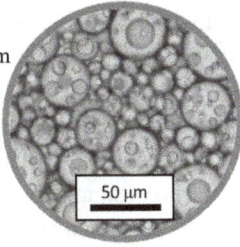

50 μm

DOX-E2

$D_{32} = 9.5 \pm 0.5 \mu m$
$d_{32} = 5.5 \pm 0.5 \mu m$
$PDI_D = 1.1 \pm 0.1$
$PDI_d = 1.8 \pm 0.1$

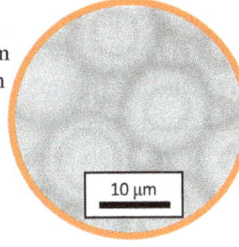

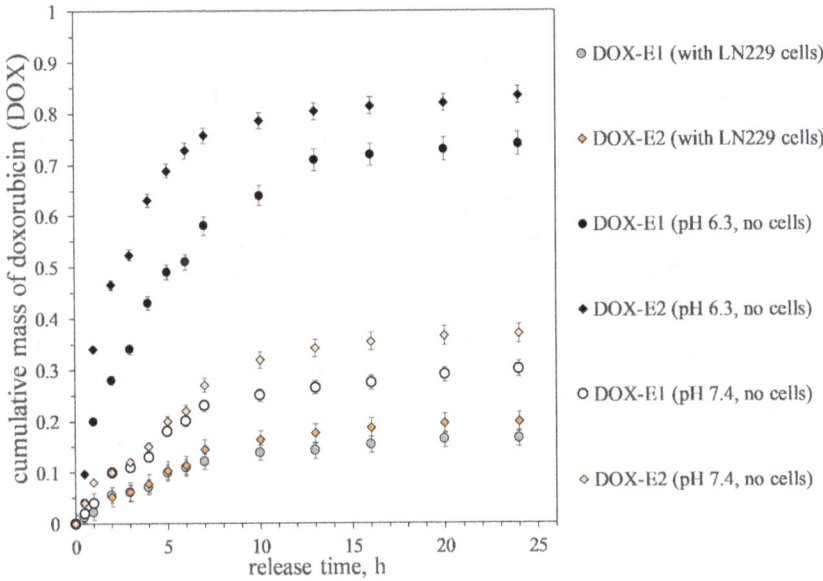

10 μm

- ◉ DOX-E1 (with LN229 cells)
- ◇ DOX-E2 (with LN229 cells)
- ● DOX-E1 (pH 6.3, no cells)
- ◆ DOX-E2 (pH 6.3, no cells)
- ○ DOX-E1 (pH 7.4, no cells)
- ◇ DOX-E2 (pH 7.4, no cells)

Figure 13.4: The structure of multiple emulsions and experimental data of the release of doxorubicin (DOX) from two emulsion formulations, DOX-E1 and DOX-E2, tested in the presence of glioblastoma multiforme cell line LN229, and in the absence of cells at pH 7.4 and pH 6.3. Data points represent mean values ± SD (error bars are not visible when errors are equal to or smaller than the symbols for individual measurements).

13.4 Drug release study in the biological system with multiple emulsion–based delivery implant and cancer cells

The studies on DOX release were focused on analysing the kinetics of drug diffusion and drug consumption by glioblastoma multiforme (GBM) cells (U87 MG, LN229). The exemplary results for LN229 cells are presented as the cumulative mass of DOX released over time for the initial concentration of doxorubicin (DOX) encapsulated in the emulsions of 0.1 μM (Figure 13.4).

The emulsions exhibited distinct structural characteristics. DOX-E1 consisted of larger membrane phase droplets encapsulating multiple smaller internal aqueous droplets, providing a more gradual drug release. In contrast, DOX-E2 had smaller, more uniformly structured membrane phase droplets with single internal droplets, which facilitated a faster release. This hierarchical structure allowed for tailored drug delivery depending on the therapeutic need. The structural differences between the emulsions directly influenced their therapeutic efficacy. The hierarchical arrangement in DOX-E1, with multiple internal droplets, allowed for controlled, sustained release, whereas the simpler structure of DOX-E2 favoured rapid release. These findings underscore the versatility of multiple emulsions for customised, local drug delivery (to a specific target site within the body) in oncological applications.

The release was further influenced by the properties of the pH-responsive biopolymer (CMC) in the external phase of the emulsions, which altered its conformation under acidic tumour microenvironment conditions, enhancing release control. In acidic conditions, the structure of CMC undergoes partial protonation, reducing its solubility and leading to conformational changes. This triggers the collapse of its polymer chains, facilitating the release of encapsulated substances. This responsiveness allows for targeted delivery, as the drug is preferentially released in the acidic microenvironment of cancer cells, which typically exhibit a pH of 6.5–6.8 while remaining stable in normal physiological conditions (pH 7.4). Experimental results confirmed that the release rates were higher in acidic pH, representative of tumour environment [31]. Cell viability studies on glioblastoma cell lines (U87MG, LN229) revealed that the multiple emulsions exhibited high toxicity towards cancerous cells. The studies confirmed the system's ability to control release rates in acidic environment. These findings highlight the potential of multiple emulsions to deliver chemotherapeutics like doxorubicin directly to tumour sites, enhancing therapeutic effectiveness while minimising off-target effects compared to conventional treatment strategies (solution of chemotherapeutic agent).

The role of multiple emulsions in controlled drug release was further explored in our research [45]. This study highlighted that carefully designing multiple emulsions composition and structure can maintain drug concentration at therapeutic levels over extended time periods. This feature is particularly beneficial for patients undergoing chemotherapy, as it may reduce the frequency of drug administration and associated side effects. Additionally, the ability of multiple emulsions to encapsulate drugs in a stable environment of the internal phase of emulsions prevents premature degradation, which is a common problem with conventional delivery systems. The structure stability of the emulsion ensured that the drugs remained effectively encapsulated until they reached the target site, making multiple emulsions an efficient carrier for long-term cancer therapies.

13.5 Evaluation of the effectiveness of a multiple emulsion–based delivery system

The cell viability results illustrate the efficacy of the proposed anticancer therapy based on synergistic delivery of siRNA and doxorubicin (DOX) via multiple emulsions. The study compared the response of glioblastoma U87 MG and LN229 cells to different treatment systems: DOX in solution (classic chemotherapy), DOX in emulsions and the combined delivery of both agents using the proposed system.

The most significant reduction in cell viability, down to about 16 % (15.84 %), was observed with the synergistic approach combining liposomal siRNA and DOX in emulsions. This effect surpassed the outcomes of single-agent therapies, such as DOX in solution or emulsions without siRNA, which achieved only partial reductions in viability. The results demonstrate the enhanced efficacy of combining targeted gene silencing with controlled drug delivery.

Our research highlights the importance of emulsion structure and release kinetics in determining therapeutic outcomes. The cytotoxicity varied between the two emulsion types. DOX-E1, with larger droplets containing multiple internal aqueous phases, showed a slower release rate, resulting in prolonged exposure and higher cytotoxicity against cancer cells. In contrast, DOX-E2, characterised by smaller droplets with single internal phases, facilitated faster release but achieved slightly lower cytotoxicity overall [31]. The emulsion system also demonstrated efficacy at lower DOX doses, which were ineffective in the classic solution form. This suggests that the emulsion-based approach could minimise drug-related side effects by reducing the required dosage while maintaining high anti-cancer efficacy.

Additionally, the inclusion of siRNA amplified the cytotoxic effect by inhibiting DNA repair mechanisms, rendering cancer cells more susceptible to DOX-induced damage. The findings suggest that the proposed emulsion-based system effectively combines chemotherapy and gene therapy, overcoming drug resistance and increasing therapeutic efficiency. This approach also demonstrates the potential to reduce systemic toxicity by maintaining effectiveness at lower drug doses.

13.6 Drug release predictions from a multiple emulsion–based delivery system: mass transfer modelling

Modern medicine responds to the needs related to treatment methods with comprehensive solutions, in which mathematical models play an increasingly important role. Mathematical models used in anti-cancer therapies can be divided into three main groups of models describing (i) tumour growth, (ii) the drug mass balance on a differential volume element in the tissue and (iii) changes at the molecular level in cancer cells exposed to drugs [46–48]. The developed model in the biological system (emulsion-based implant surrounded by cancer cells) refers to the second group. The model uses chemical engineering tools, such as the mass balance on a differential volume element in the system described by transport equations (diffusion/convection) with a chemical reaction. A mathematical model was developed for the process of diffusional transport during the release process of a drug (or drugs) from multiple emulsions and its absorption by cancer cells (drug consumption by cells as a chemical reaction). The model includes the emulsion structure and transport parameters to simulate the spatiotemporal release profiles of drug. Experimental verification of the model on GBM cells confirmed that the drug release kinetics followed the proposed model predictably across various tested doses of the drug [31]. In the considered model, the mass balance of the drug in the differential volume of the system is represented by two or three partial differential equations of mass transport, i.e. drug diffusion from the appropriate emulsion phases, i.e. from the internal emulsion droplets (step 1), through the membrane phase droplets (step 2) to the external environment (step 3), where cancer cells absorb the drug (absorption = chemical reaction). In the mathematical model, cancer tumour cells are represented by the so-called mass source terms expressed by the kinetic equation of the chemical reaction rate.

Steps 1 and 2 can be combined into a single equation, which represents the drug concentration within the implant's drops, i.e. drug concentration in the membrane phase where the drug is released from the internal droplets. In this case, two equations (presented in our paper [31]) for each dispersed phase of emulsion can be reduced to one equation (13.1). Further, equation (13.2) may be expressed as equation (13.3), when a substitute rate constant of drug consumption by cells is considered.

With fluid convection assumed to be negligible within brain tissue, the general governing equations in the considered biological system are diffusion equations coupled with a chemical reaction (equations (13.1)–(13.3)) [31]. Transport of the doxorubicin (chemo-drug) inside the implant's larger drops having radius ($0 \le r \le R$), (equation (13.1)):

$$\frac{\partial c}{\partial t} = D\nabla^2 c \tag{13.1}$$

Mass transport of the doxorubicin (chemo-drug) in the environment of cancer cells – outside the emulsion drops (r > R), (equations (13.2) and (13.3)):

$$\frac{\partial c_z}{\partial t} = D_z\nabla^2 c_z + R(c) - \frac{\partial B}{\partial t} \tag{13.2}$$

$$\frac{\partial c_z}{\partial t} = D_z\nabla^2 c_z - \Phi_R \tag{13.3}$$

Where:

c – concentration of the drug in the emulsion drop,

c_z – concentration of the drug in the external phase,

D – the effective diffusion coefficient of the drug in the dispersed phase,

D_z – the effective diffusion coefficient of the drug in the external phase,

R(c) – rate of drug consumption by cancer cells,

B – rate of drug bound or internalised per tissue volume,

Φ_R – term representing the rate of drug reaction/elimination (equation (13.4)):

$$\Phi_R = R\left(c\right) - \frac{\partial B}{\partial t} = kc_z \tag{13.4}$$

$$k = \frac{k_{app}}{1 + K_{bin}} \tag{13.5}$$

k_{app} –substitute rate constant of drug consumption by cells (equation (13.5)),

K_{bin} – the rate constant of drug binding/internalisation.

The initial conditions (equations (13.6) and (13.7)):

$$c\left(r,0\right) = mc_{s0} \tag{13.6}$$

$$c_z\left(r,0\right) = 0 \tag{13.7}$$

The boundary conditions in the centre of each domain volume of the external phase containing a single droplet of emulsion-symmetry condition:

$$\left.\frac{\partial c\left(r,t\right)}{\partial r}\right|_{r=0} = 0 \tag{13.8}$$

Boundary conditions at the interface between drop (membrane phase) and external phases $(r = R)$:

$$c\left(R,t\right) = nc_z\left(R,t\right) \tag{13.9}$$

$$\left(1 - \phi_s\right)D\left.\frac{\partial c\left(r,t\right)}{\partial r}\right|_{r=R} = D_z\left.\frac{\partial c_z\left(r,t\right)}{\partial r}\right|_{r=R} \tag{13.10}$$

$m = c/c_s$ – the partition coefficient of the drug between the membrane phase and the internal phase,

$n = c/c_z$ – the partition coefficient of the drug between the membrane phase and the external phase,

ϕ_s – volume fraction of the internal phase drops in the membrane phase drop.

The equations of the developed model contain characteristic parameters that consider the structure of the emulsion, processes occurring in the tumour environment, i.e. drug absorption by cancer cells and diffusional drug transport inside the drug carrier, i.e. emulsion, and in the tumour environment. The structure of the emulsion was evaluated through the droplet size and their volume packing parameter (fraction of the internal droplets within the larger membrane phase drops). The rates of mass transport processes are represented by appropriate parameters: (i) apparent drug diffusion coefficients inside and outside the emulsion droplets (simulation of actual transport resistances occurring in the system), (ii) mass transfer coefficients inside the emulsion membrane phase drops and the elimination (absorption) rate constants of the drug by cancer cells (reaction rate constants, e.g. first-order). The developed method of modelling drug delivery from a multiphase implant in biological systems on the background of available solutions based on the group of transport mechanism models includes some advantages. Firstly, the developed model enables planning a course of therapy and its

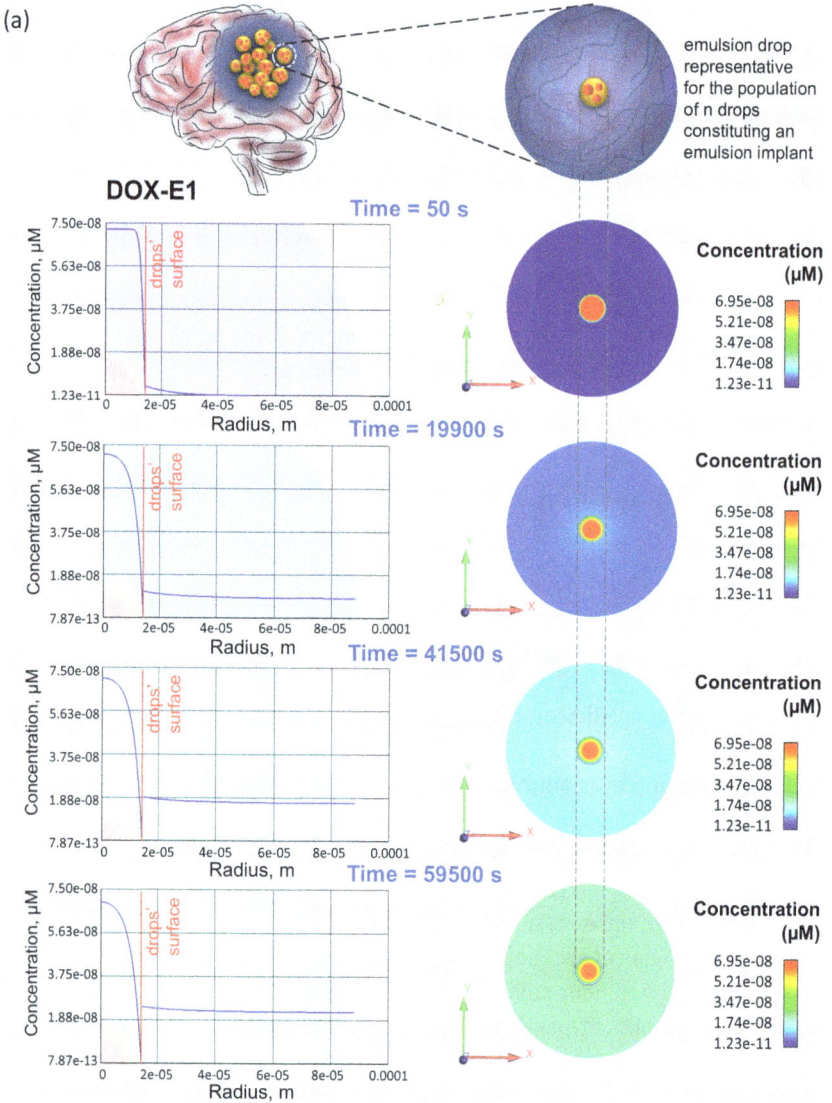

Figure 13.5: Spatial distributions of doxorubicin concentration inside and outside a representative droplet of emulsion-based implant surrounded by fluid containing LN229 cancer cells over time, for (a) DOX-E1 and (b) DOX-E2, containing doxorubicin dose of 0.1 μM. Adapted with permission from [31].

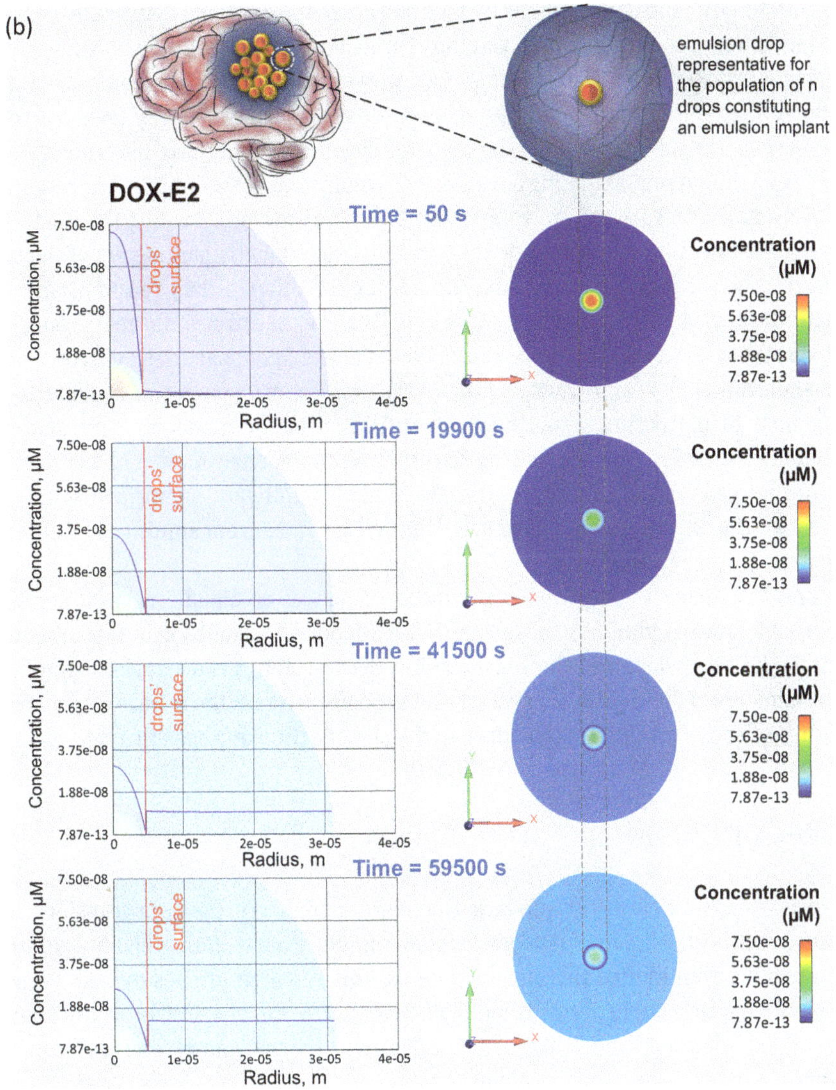

Figure 13.5: Continued.

personalisation based on the changes in the concentration of the chemotherapeutic agent in time and space in the tumour environment, and thus the selection of the drug dose and the duration of therapy depending on the type of drug and the needs of individual oncological patients. Easy selection of the drug dose is enabled by defined parameters of the emulsion carrier structure (volume fraction of drop packing and drop diameter). Secondly, the model takes into account the resistance to mass transport of the component (drug) in the tumour environment by incorporating appropriate coefficients, enabling the simulation of conditions similar to those prevailing in the natural environment of a living organism (*in vivo*). This is an important advantage of the model because most of the available solutions of mathematical models of this group consider only the mass transport resistance inside the drug carrier itself (often without analysis of its structure), and not outside the carrier, assuming a constant concentration at the interface or conditions of steady-state transport of the component or sink conditions. Finally, the model has universal features in the form of defined transport and kinetic parameters of the mass transfer process with an irreversible first-order (or other order) reaction, and also structural parameters of the carrier. Moreover, it can be used to describe mass transfer in any dispersed systems at micro and nanoscale (e.g. nanoparticles, microparticles, nanoemulsions), in which transport and formation or disappearance of mass of the component (drug) occurs. Experimental verification of the model by comparison of computational and experimental drug release rates in the environment of glioblastoma multiforme cells using CFD tools, and Mathematica software, confirmed with good agreement the experimentally observed drug release rates from emulsions of different structures (Figure 13.5) [31].

Similar good agreement with experimental data was obtained for the drug release rate in simulated conditions of acidic pH of the tumour and healthy cells (pH practically neutral) [42]. The model confirms the possibility of controlling the drug release rates with the parameters of the emulsion structure and the parameters of the release environment, and thus selectively delivering the drug to the site of action at a specific rate.

13.7 Conclusions

The proposed multiple emulsion–based delivery system represents a transformative advancement in the treatment of glioblastoma multiforme (GBM), a highly aggressive brain tumour with limited therapeutic options. This research bridges the gap between the physiological complexity of tumour environments and the precision of chemical engineering solutions, addressing key challenges such as tumour microenvironment targeting, drug resistance and systemic toxicity.

Glioblastoma's characteristic features, namely infiltrative growth, chemo-resistance and the protective blood–brain barrier, are significant obstacles to effective treatment. Traditional chemotherapeutics often lack the specificity required to differentiate between healthy and cancerous cells, resulting in substantial off-target effects. By leveraging the tumours' acidic microenvironment and incorporating pH-responsive biopolymers, the developed emulsion system ensures selective and controlled drug release. This approach not only enhances therapeutic efficacy but also minimises neurotoxicity, preserving healthy tissues.

The synergistic integration of RNA interference with chemotherapeutic agents, such as doxorubicin, further amplifies the systems' effectiveness. The RNA-based mechanism silences gene expression critical for DNA repair in cancer cells, sensitising them to chemotherapeutic damage and overcoming traditional barriers to drug effectiveness. Encapsulation within multiple emulsions provides an additional layer of protection against premature drug degradation, ensuring the stability and bioavailability of active agents until they reach the target site.

The use of Couette–Taylor flow methods to create stable, high-efficiency emulsions with tailored droplet architectures underscores the potential of engineering principles in addressing complex biological challenges. The modelling of drug transport mechanisms further enhances the system's utility, enabling the optimisation of dosing regimens and personalisation of therapy. The developed mathematical model not only predicts drug release profiles but also integrates environmental factors such as tumour pH, providing a comprehensive tool for therapy planning.

Experimental results validate the systems' capability to achieve high encapsulation efficiency and selective cytotoxicity, with significant reductions in glioblastoma cell viability even at reduced drug doses. These findings confirmed the potential of multiple emulsion as innovative and effective delivery system for cancer therapy by combining precision engineering with advanced biological insights.

Looking forward, the integration of such delivery systems with advanced imaging and diagnostic technologies could pave the way for real-time monitoring and adaptive treatment strategies. While this study demonstrates promising *in vitro* results, further research involving *in vivo* models and clinical trials will be essential to translate these findings into tangible medical applications. The potential to combine this system with additional stimuli-responsive features or multi-agent therapies also offers a rich avenue for future exploration.

The emulsion-based delivery system demonstrates significant potential for application in various other cancer types, particularly those with solid tumours and drug resistance challenges. Its versatility allows for the incorporation of different chemotherapeutic agents and RNA molecules, enabling tailored therapies for diverse malignancies. The pH-responsive characteristics of the system are especially promising for targeting tumours with acidic microenvironment, a common feature in many cancer types. This approach could thus be extended to a wide range of cancers, including breast, lung and colon cancers, offering a new avenue for more effective and targeted treatment strategies.

By merging the biological intricacies of tumour behaviour with the precision of chemical engineering methodologies, this research lays the groundwork for a new oncological treatment – one that prioritises targeted delivery, reduced toxicity and personalised patient care.

Acknowledgements: The authors would like to thank the editors David Bogle and Tomasz Sosnowski for their guidance and review of this article before its publication. The authors would like to sincerely thank AIChE Journal for granting permission to use figures from the publication: Mass transfer of anti-cancer drug delivery to brain tumours by a multiple emulsion-based implant published In: Dluska E, Markowska-Radomska A, Metera A, Rudniak L, Kosicki K. Mass transfer of anti-cancer drug delivery to brain tumours by a multiple emulsion-based implant. AICHE Journal. 2022;68:1-15. doi:10.1002/aic.17501. The study was based on published results of research funded by the National Science Centre – Poland (successfully completed grant number: 2014/13/B/ST8/04274) and by (POB Biotechnology and Biomedical Engineering) of Warsaw University of Technology within the Excellence Initiative: Research University (IDUB) programme (project BIOTECHMED-2).

References

1. Chen L, Luo J, Zhang J, Wang S, Sun Y, Liu Q, et al. Dual targeted nanoparticles for the codelivery of doxorubicin and siRNA cocktails to overcome ovarian cancer stem cells. Int J Mol Sci 2023;24:11575.
2. Chen D, Liu X, Lu X, Tian J. Nanoparticle drug delivery systems for synergistic delivery of tumor therapy. Front Pharmacol 2023;14:1111991.
3. Li X, Peng X, Zoulikha M, Boafo GF, Magar KT, Ju Y, et al. Multifunctional nanoparticle-mediated combining therapy for human diseases. Sig Transduct Target Ther 2024;9:1.
4. Chen X, Mangala LS, Rodriguez-Aguayo C, Kong X, Lopez-Berestein G, Sood AK. RNA interference-based therapy and its delivery systems. Cancer Metastasis Rev 2018;37:107–24.
5. Rao DD, Vorhies JS, Senzer N, Nemunaitis J. siRNA vs. shRNA: similarities and differences. Adv Drug Deliv Rev 2009;61:746–59.
6. Kang H, Ga YJ, Kim SH, Cho YH, Kim C, Yeh JY, et al. Small interfering RNA (siRNA)-based therapeutic applications against viruses: principles, potential, and challenges. J Biomed Sci 2023;30:88.
7. Paul A, Muralidharan A, Biswas A, Kamath BV, Joseph A, Alex AT. siRNA therapeutics and its challenges: recent advances in effective delivery for cancer therapy. OpenNano 2022;7:100063.
8. Traber GM, Yu A-M. RNAi therapeutics and novel RNA bioengineering technologies. J Pharmacol Exp Ther 2023;384:133–54.
9. Bartlett DW, Davis ME. Effect of siRNA nuclease stability on the in vitro and in vivo kinetics of siRNA-mediated gene silencing. Biotechnol Bioeng 2007;97:909–21.
10. Akhtar S, Benter IF. Nonviral delivery of synthetic siRNAs in vivo. J Clin Invest 2007;117:3623–32.
11. Gao J, Xia Z, Vohidova D, Joseph J, Luo JN, Joshi N. Progress in non-viral localized delivery of siRNA therapeutics for pulmonary diseases. Acta Pharm Sin B 2022;13:1400–28.
12. Zhang Y, Chang S, Sun J, Zhu S, Pu C, Li Y, et al. Targeted microbubbles for ultrasound mediated short hairpin RNA plasmid transfection to inhibit survivin gene expression and induce apoptosis of ovarian cancer A2780/DDP cells. Mol Pharm 2015;12:3137–45.
13. Zhao X, Yang J, Zhang J, Wang X, Chen L, Zhang C, et al. Inhibitory effect of aptamer-carbon dot nanomaterial-siRNA complex on the metastasis of hepatocellular carcinoma cells by interfering with FMRP. Eur J Pharm Biopharm 2022;174:47–55.
14. Ozpolat B, Sood AK, Lopez-Berestein G. Liposomal siRNA nanocarriers for cancer therapy. Adv Drug Deliv Rev 2014;66:110–6.
15. Sinani G, Durgun ME, Cevher E, Özsoy Y. Polymeric-micelle-based delivery systems for nucleic acids. Pharm 2023;15:2021.
16. Kalita T, Dezfouli SA, Pandey LM, Uludag H. siRNA functionalized lipid nanoparticles (LNPs) in management of diseases. Pharm 2022;14:2520.
17. Aserin A. Multiple emulsion: technology and applications. Wiley series on surface and interfacial chemistry. Hobooken, NJ: John Wiley & Sons; 2008.

18. Dluska E, Markowska-Radomska A, Metera A, Kosicki K. Hierarchically structured emulsions for brain therapy. Colloid Surf A Physicochem Eng Asp 2019;575:205–11.
19. Markowska-Radomska A, Skowronski P, Kosicki K, Dluska E. Multiple emulsions as carriers for the topical delivery of anti-inflammatory drugs. Chem Process Eng 2023;44:1–9.
20. Loya-Castro MF, Sánchez-Mejía M, Sánchez-Ramírez DR, Domínguez-Ríos R, Escareño N, Oceguera-Basurto PE, et al. Preparation of PLGA/rose Bengal colloidal particles by double emulsion and layer-by-layer for breast cancer treatment. J Colloid Interface Sci 2018;518:122–9.
21. Soriano-Ruiz JL, Suner-Carbo J, Calpena-Capmany AC, Bozal-de Febrer N, Halbaut-Bellowa L, Boix-Montañés A, et al. Clotrimazole multiple W/O/W emulsion as anticandidal agent: characterization and evaluation on skin and mucosae. Colloids Surf B Biointerfaces 2018;175:166–74.
22. Mutaliyeva B, Grigoriev D, Madybekova G, Sharipova A, Aidarova S, Saparbekova A, et al. Microencapsulation of insulin and its release using w/o/w double emulsion method. Colloids Surf A Physicochem Eng Asp 2017;521:147–52.
23. Dluska E, Metera A, Markowska-Radomska A, Tudek B. Effective cryopreservation and recovery of living cells encapsulated in multiple emulsions. Biopreserv Biobank 2019;17:468–76.
24. Luo T, Wei Z. Recent progress in food-grade double emulsions: fabrication, stability, applications, and future trends. Food Front 2023;4:1543–2096.
25. Markowska-Radomska A, Dluska E. An evaluation of a mass transfer rate at the boundary of different release mechanisms in complex liquid dispersion. Chem Eng Proc: Process Intensif 2016;101:56–71.
26. Zou Y, Wu N, Miao C, Yue H, Ma G. A novel multiple emulsion enhanced immunity via its biomimetic delivery approach. J Mater Chem B 2020;8:7365–74.
27. Dluska E, Cui Z, Markowska-Radomska A, Metera A, Kosicki K. Cryoprotection and banking of living cells in a 3D multiple emulsion-based carrier. Biotechnol J 2017;12:1–7.
28. Hema SK, Karmakar A, Das RK, Srivastava P. Simple formulation and characterization of double emulsion variant designed to carry three bioactive agents. Heliyon 2022;8:e10397.
29. Maboudi A, Lotfipour M, Rasouli M, Azhdari MH, MacLoughlin R, Bekeschus S, et al. Micelle-based nanoparticles with stimuli-responsive properties for drug delivery. Nanotechnol Rev 2024;13:20230218.
30. Chen K, Li Y, Li Y, Tan Y, Liu Y, Pan W, et al. Stimuli-responsive electrospun nanofibers for drug delivery, cancer therapy, wound dressing, and tissue engineering. J Nanobiotechnol 2023;21:237.
31. Dluska E, Markowska-Radomska A, Metera A, Rudniak L, Kosicki K. Mass transfer of anti-cancer drug delivery to brain tumours by a multiple emulsion-based implant. AIChE J 2022;68:1–15.
32. Markowska-Radomska A, Dluska E, Kosicki K. Cancer treatment based on a doxorubicin double emulsion delivery system aided by a mechanism of synthetic lethality. In: Interdisciplinary conference on drug sciences. Abstract book, Accord 2022. Warsaw, Poland: Medical University of Warsaw.
33. Mohammed S, Dinesan M, Ajayakumar T. Survival and quality of life analysis in glioblastoma multiforme with adjuvant chemoradiotherapy: a retrospective study. Rep Pract Oncol Radiother 2022;27:1026–36.
34. Thenuwara G, Curtin J, Tian F. Advances in diagnostic tools and therapeutic approaches for gliomas: a comprehensive review. Sensors 2023;23:9842.
35. Wu W, Klockow JL, Zhang M, Lafortune F, Chang E, Jin L, et al. Glioblastoma multiforme (GBM): an overview of current therapies and mechanisms of resistance. Pharmacol Res 2021;171:105780.
36. Nabian N, Ghalehtaki R, Zeinalizadeh M, Balaña C, Jablonska PA. State of the neoadjuvant therapy for glioblastoma multiforme – where do we stand? Neuro-Oncol Adv 2024;6:vdae028.
37. Malech HL, Garabedian EK, Hsieh MM. Evolution of gene therapy, historical perspective. Hematol Oncol Clin North Am 2022;36:627–45.
38. Pérez-Tomás R, Pérez-Guillén I. Lactate in the tumor microenvironment: an essential molecule in cancer progression and treatment. Cancers (Basel) 2020;12:3244.
39. Dluska E, Markowska-Radomska A, Skowronski P. A pH-responsive biopolymer-based multiple emulsion prepared in a helicoidal contactor for chemotherapeutics delivery. Polimery 2022;67:346–54.

40. Khaled B, Abdelbaki B. Rheological and electrokinetic properties of carboxymethylcellulose-water dispersions in the presence of salts. Int J Phys Sci 2012;7:1790–8.
41. Metera A, Dluska E, Markowska-Radomska A, Tudek B, Fraczyk T, Kosicki K. Functionalized multiple emulsions as platforms for targeted drug delivery. IJCEA 2017;8:305–10.
42. Dluska E, Markowska-Radomska A, Metera A, Tudek B, Kosicki K. Multiple emulsions as effective platforms for controlled anti-cancer drug delivery. Nanomed 2017;12:2183–97.
43. Dluska E, Markowska-Radomska A. Regimes of multiple emulsions of W1/O/W2 and O1/W/O2 type in the continuous Couette-Taylor flow contactor. Chem Eng Technol 2010;33:113–20.
44. Markowska-Radomska A, Dluska E. The multiple emulsion entrapping active agent produced via one-step preparation method in the liquidliquid helical flow for drug release study and modeling. Progr Colloid Polym Sci 2012;139:29–34.
45. Dluska E, Markowska-Radomska A, Metera A, Ordak M. Multiple emulsions as a biomaterial-based delivery system for the controlled release of an anti-cancer drug. J Phys Conf Ser 2020;1681:1–11.
46. Nicholson C. Diffusion and related transport mechanisms in brain tissue. Rep Prog Phys 2001;64:815–84.
47. de Montigny J, Iosif A, Breitwieser L, Manca M, Bauer R, Vavourakis V. An in silico hybrid continuum-/agent-based procedure to modelling cancer development: interrogating the interplay amongst glioma invasion, vascularity and necrosis. Methods 2021;185:94–104.
48. Preziosi L. Cancer modelling and simulation. In: Chapman & Hall/CRC mathematical biology and medicine series, v.3, 1st ed. Boca Raton, FL: CRC Press LLC; 2003.

Elnaz Jamili, Amit C. Nathwani and Vivek Dua*

14 Model-based dose selection for gene therapy for haemophilia B

Abstract: Haemophilia B, also known as the Christmas disease, named after Stephen Christmas the first patient diagnosed with this disease, is an inherited disease caused by a defect in the Factor IX Gene (*F9*). This defect manifests in insufficient production of the blood coagulation factor IX, resulting in excessive bleeding. The therapy which is mainly used involves prophylactic infusions of factor IX concentrate to improve the quality of life by minimising the episodes of bleeds. The main limitations of such a treatment plan are repeat infusions, product half-life, costs and inhibitor formation. The FIX concentration in healthy individuals is typically 90 nM and based upon the experience of the clinicians increasing FIX activity to 1–5 % of normal values has significant impact on patients' quality of life. Therefore, even a partial correction the FIX deficiency would result in improved clinical outcomes and increase the chances of patients living a near-normal life. Gene therapy has the potential to deliver this, and the fact that haemophilia B is monogenic in nature further encourages the exploration of gene delivery for this disease. In this chapter, an integrated Pharmacokinetic (PK) – Pharmacodynamic (PD) model that has been developed using the clinical data is reported. The key features of the model are that it considers the pharmacological response, i.e., plasma FIX coagulation activity level as well as the toxicological response, i.e., the level of serum alanine aminotransferase. The simulation-based PK-PD modelling approach is then used for the initial dose selection to provide clinicians with better tools to simplify the decision-making process for designing more effective treatment plans, which can be tailored to maximise efficacy while minimising toxicity for individual patients.

Keywords: gene delivery; initial dose selection; Pharmacokinetic/pharmacodynamic modelling; toxicity; efficacy

*Corresponding author: Vivek Dua, Department of Chemical Engineering, The Sargent Centre for Process Systems Engineering, University College London, Torrington Place, London WC1E 7JE, UK,
E-mail: v.dua@ucl.ac.uk. https://orcid.org/0000-0002-0165-7421
Elnaz Jamili, Department of Chemical Engineering, Centre for Process Systems Engineering, University College London, Torrington Place, London, WC1E 7JE, UK
Amit C. Nathwani, Department of Haematology, UCL Cancer Institute, University College London, London, UK

As per De Gruyter's policy this article has previously been published in the journal Physical Sciences Reviews. Please cite as: E. Jamili, A. C. Nathwani and V. Dua "Model-based dose selection for gene therapy for haemophilia B" *Physical Sciences Reviews* [Online] 2024. DOI: 10.1515/psr-2024-0057 | https://doi.org/10.1515/9783111394558-014

14.1 Introduction

14.1.1 Chemical engineering and haemophilia B

This chapter presents the collaborative work that was carried out by researchers from chemical engineering and haemophilia at University College London [1]. The problem statement and steps for developing gene therapy for haemophilia B involve statements that chemical engineers are quite familiar with. It is common for chemical engineers to collect experimental data for the process system under consideration, set up a mathematical model that captures the phenomena taking in the process system and then estimate parameters for the mathematical model that fit the data that were collected. If the data does not fit well, usually the mathematical model is revisited and/or additional experiments are carried out, in an iterative manner, until there is sufficient confidence in the model. The model is then simulated to predict system response for situations that were not necessarily covered during experimentation. This aligns with the decision that a clinician would have to take in terms of selecting dose for gene delivery for haemophilia B. While higher dose would result in higher efficacy, it would also give higher toxicity, making it a multi-objective decision-making problem. Decision making in chemical engineering also involves similar situations where, for example, one has to consider trade-offs between profit and environmental impact, yield and safety, etc. In this chapter, clinical data can be considered to be equivalent to the experimental data and integrated pharmacokinetic/pharmacodynamic model can be considered to be equivalent to the mathematical model, mentioned above.

14.1.2 Haemophilia B

Haemophilia B (HB) is a genetic bleeding disorder resulting from a deficiency or dysfunction of coagulation factor IX (FIX) caused by mutations in the gene that encodes FIX [2, 3]. Although prophylactic therapy with factor IX protein concentrates improves clinical outcomes and reduces the frequency of spontaneous bleeding, it requires frequent intravenous injections for the life-time of patients due to the short half-life of the protein, resulting in an inconvenient and expensive (£140,000 per year per patient) treatment [4]. Thus, various strategies have been investigated for the treatment of haemophilia B including the use of bioengineered coagulation factors [5] and gene-transfer therapy [6, 7]. Gene therapy is a potentially curative treatment option as it aims to restore, modify or enhance cellular functions through the introduction of a therapeutic gene into a target cell, which is demonstrated in the work by Nathwani et al. [7–13]. In the clinical trial conducted by Nathwani and colleagues, a single dose of a serotype-8-pseudotyped, self-complementary (sc) adeno-associated (AAV) vector expressing a codon-optimised version of the human factor IX (hFIXco) gene was infused in patients with severe HB whose FIX activity level is <1 % of normal values [12, 13]. hFIXco transgene was synthesised and cloned downstream of a compact synthetic liver-specific promoter (LP1) to enable packaging into scAAV vectors (scAAV2/8-LP1-hFIXco) [4]. The evaluation of safety and efficacy in HB patients, having had the peripheral-vein infusion of scAAV2/8-LP1-hFIXco, was reported in the work by Nathwani et al. [7].

Mathematical models are crucial tools for understanding the key mechanisms involved in biological systems, and for predicting the outcome of a given treatment plan. Mathematical modelling for gene delivery systems has evolved over the years, starting with the work by Ledley and Ledley [14] in which the authors developed a multi-compartment mathematical model for studying the kinetics of cellular processes. A variety of studies have illustrated how mathematical models can be applied to gene delivery systems. Most of the works have focused on the concept of mass action kinetic model to study the critical steps involved in the process [14–17]. A number of different computational methodologies have provided insights into the gene delivery process, including stochastic simulations [18], quantitative structure–activity relationship (QSAR) modelling strategy [19], mechanistic spatio-temporal and stochastic model of DNA delivery [20], semi-mechanistic model of transgene expression [21] and telecommunication model [22].

While a lot of important work has been done in the area of modelling for gene delivery systems, there are several areas that are yet to be explored adequately. We have recently developed a model-based control algorithm for both efficacy and safety to provide quantitative understanding of non-viral siRNA delivery [23]. Having explored the nature and purpose of quantitative analysis of *in vitro* experimental data in our previous work, this chapter aims to develop a novel mathematical modelling approach, based on *in vivo* clinical data, for gene transfer of adeno-associated viral vectors in patients with haemophilia B. In this work, an integrated pharmacokinetic/pharmacodynamic model is developed using compartment modelling to describe the behaviour of scAAV2/8-LP1-hFIXco vectors in patients, which is then used in a simulation-based modelling platform for the initial dose selection with the goal of predicting the pharmacokinetics and pharmacodynamics of the vector during the therapy. A promising platform for gene delivery systems is provided by using modelling techniques to determine the initial dose selection that can be used in clinical trial simulations to determine optimal dosing recommendations.

14.2 Methods

14.2.1 Clinical data

Nathwani et al. [7] aimed to assess the efficacy and safety of factor IX gene therapy in patients with severe HB by evaluating the stability of transgene expression and monitoring the hepatocellular toxicity. The authors also reported the vector genomes in plasma, urine, stool, semen and saliva, which were collected from patients at regular intervals in order to assess vector shedding following systemic administration of scAAV2/

8-LP1-hFIXco. The clinical data are used to build an integrated PK/PD model so as to be capable of providing a platform to guide initial dose selection.

14.2.2 Pharmacokinetic modelling

Physiologically based pharmacokinetic (PBPK) models, while being able to offer a more realistic picture of vector kinetics by modelling the real physiological space in the human body, are very complex and typically require more clinical data in more compartments for the validation of the models, which is not readily available in clinical trials [24]. Therefore, a mechanistically lumped PK model was developed based on the available clinical data. The PK model comprised of two compartments, plasma (P) and body fluids (BFs), to illustrate the simultaneous kinetics of both plasma and metabolites (Figures 14.1 and 14.2). The body fluids, which encompass data from urinary, stool, semen and saliva, were lumped into a single compartment to represent the elimination process. This approach was adopted because the parallel effluxes can be merged and represented within a unified compartment [24, 25]. Mathematically,

$$\frac{dC_P}{dt} = -\theta_d\, C_P - \theta_{el.0}\, C_P \tag{14.1}$$

$$C_P\,(t = 0) = C_{P0}$$

$$\frac{dC_{BF}}{dt} = \theta_{el.0}\, C_P - \theta_{el.1}\, C_{BF} \tag{14.2}$$

$$C_{BF}\,(t = 0) = C_{BF0}$$

where C_P (vector genome/mL) and C_{BF} (vector genome/mL) are the vector concentrations in patient plasma and body fluids, respectively. θ_d (day^{-1}) represents the distribution rate constant while $\theta_{el.0}$ (day^{-1}) and $\theta_{el.1}$ (day^{-1}) are the elimination rate constants.

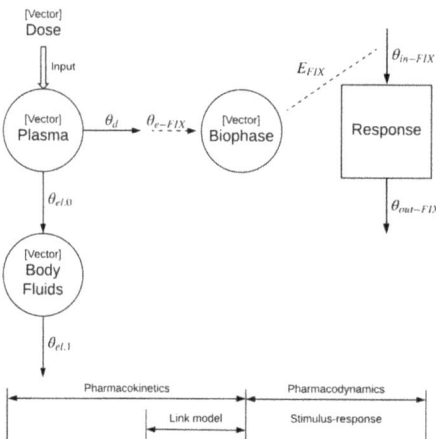

Figure 14.1: Schematic representation illustrating the relationship between kinetics and dynamics of the vector when considering the pharmacological response (plasma FIX coagulation activity level).

The developed pharmacokinetic model serves as a platform for a quantitative evaluation of gene delivery. Equation (14.1) captures the rate of change of the vector concentration in patient plasma after a single intravenous infusion of vector.

14.2.3 Pharmacodynamic modelling

Human factor IX (hFIX) is a coagulation protein, which is synthesised in the liver and encoded in a gene located on the X chromosome [26, 27]. Hepatocytes, which are the most common cells type in the liver, directly secrete factor IX into the bloodstream, where it circulates in an inactive form until needed in a response to an injury that damages the blood vessel wall [28]. Since FIX is naturally synthesised in the liver, the site of action for scAAV2/8-LP1-hFIXco vectors is located in the liver compartment.

In order to develop a mathematical model, the plasma FIX activity has been considered as the pharmacological effect (response), which can be treated as an objective function to be maximised in a gene delivery optimal control problem. A physiological indirect response model with stimulation of factors controlling the response was thought to be appropriate to describe the vector pharmacodynamics. This is because of the time delay between the observed pharmacological effects and vector concentration in plasma as the pharmacological responses take time to be developed. The temporal displacement could be due to the vector tissue distribution phenomena to reach the site of action, liver. To this purpose, a dynamic model must be developed to link the vector concentration in the biophase or effect compartment to a response compartment. The effect compartment model, which is also known as the link model, can be considered as a first-order distribution model relating the vector concentration in plasma and the biophase using a first-order constant. Once the vector is transferred to the liver, a cascade of biological events may take place resulting in a functional response, which can be viewed as a link model. Schematic illustration of the integrated PK/PD model is shown in Figure 14.1.

While a more detailed representation of an integrated PK/PD approach can be developed by incorporating the liver compartment into the PK model, the model structure, which was developed and used in this work, had been simplified to only include the plasma and other body fluids compartments. This is due to a lack of available data as liver biopsies are required.

Considering the pharmacological analysis, the rate of change of the vector concentration in the effect (biophase) compartment, C_{e_FIX} (vector genome/mL), can be modelled as:

$$\frac{dC_{e\_FIX}}{dt} = \theta_{e\_FIX} C_P - \theta_{in\_FIX} C_{e\_FIX} \tag{14.3}$$

where C_P (vector genome/ml) is the concentration of vector in the plasma compartment of the pharmacokinetic model, linked to the effect compartment, with the first-order rate constant $\theta_{e\_FIX} \left(day^{-1} \right)$.

The plasma FIX coagulation activity level, R_{FIX} (% of the normal value – IU/deciliter), which is of interest in our case, is formulated as a function of the concentration in the effect compartment with the use of an effect-concentration model. The differential equation for the observed pharmacological effect, factor IX activity level, can be expressed as:

$$\frac{dR_{FIX}}{dt} = \theta_{in\_FIX}\, E_{FIX} - \theta_{out\_FIX}\, R_{FIX} \tag{14.4}$$

where the *rate in* and *rate out* of the response compartment are governed by $\theta_{in\_FIX}\left(\text{day}^{-1}\right)$ and $\theta_{out\_FIX}\left(\text{day}^{-1}\right)$.

Note that the effect compartment model should be selected with an appropriate effect equation. In this study, the response is modelled by means of a linear transduction function in which the vector concentration is proportionally related to a pharmacological response [29]. Therefore,

$$E_{FIX} = k\, C_{e\_FIX} \tag{14.5}$$

where k is the slope parameter, which is assumed to be $k = 1$ in order to simplify the model to help to mitigate the numerical difficulties.

14.2.4 Incorporating the toxicological model

The PD model may be extended to incorporate the toxicological responses that capture the liver toxicity, which was observed in the clinical study by Nathwani and colleagues as the primary endpoint of their study was the safety evaluation of the vector infusion at different doses. The reported level of serum alanine aminotransferase (ALT) over time demonstrates the hepatocellular toxicity. ALT is an enzyme which is found in serum and organ tissues such as liver. The ALT level is the most widely used clinical biomarker of liver function, which may be elevated as a result of the leakage from the damaged hepatocytes into the plasma following hepatocellular injury [30].

In this section, the structure of the PD model has been kept the same as in Section 14.2.3. Assuming an indirect response model with stimulation of factors controlling the toxicological response (Figure 14.2), the rate of change of the vector concentration in the effect (biophase) compartment, C_{e_ALT} (vector genome/mL), can be modelled as:

$$\frac{dC_{e\_ALT}}{dt} = \theta_{e\_ALT}\, C_P - \theta_{in\_ALT}\, C_{e\_ALT} \tag{14.6}$$

where C_P (vector genome/mL) is the concentration of vector in the plasma compartment of the pharmacokinetic model, linked to the effect compartment, with the first-order rate constant $\theta_{e\_ALT}\left(\text{day}^{-1}\right)$.

The ALT level, R_{ALT} (IU/L), is formulated as a function of the concentration in the effect compartment with the use of an effect-concentration model:

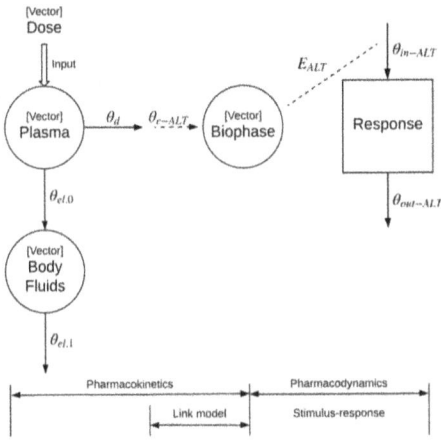

Figure 14.2: Schematic representation illustrating the relationship between kinetics and dynamics of the vector when considering the toxicological response (ALT level).

$$\frac{dR_{ALT}}{dt} = \theta_{in\_ALT}\, E_{ALT} - \theta_{out\_ALT}\, R_{ALT} \tag{14.7}$$

$$E_{ALT} = k\, C_{e\_ALT} \tag{14.8}$$

where the *rate in* and *rate out* of the response compartment are governed by $\theta_{in\_ALT}\,(\mathrm{day}^{-1})$ and $\theta_{out\_ALT}\,(\mathrm{day}^{-1})$, and $k = 1$.

14.3 Results and discussion

The proposed modelling framework will be evaluated for three patients with severe HB who had received intermediate dose of vector, 6×10^{11} vector genomes (vg) per kilogram (kg) of body weight, (patient 4), and high dose of vector, 2×10^{12} vg per kg, (patients 6 and 9). The mean weight was 80.7 kg. Table 14.1 summarises the key characteristics of the patients.

Table 14.1: Key characteristics of the patients at baseline, according to vector dose. Adapted from Nathwani et al. [7].

Characteristic	Vector dose, 6×10^{11} vg/kg	Vector dose, 2×10^{12} vg/kg	
	Patient 4	Patient 6	Patient 9
Sex	Male	Male	Male
Age (yr)	29	27	44
Factor IX prophylaxis	Once weekly	Three times weekly	On demand
HIV status	Negative	Negative	Negative
Hepatitis C status	Negative	Negative	Positive

The results obtained from this study will be presented in two parts. First, the results of the parameter estimation problem will be discussed in Section 14.3.1. Then, a number of dynamic simulations will be presented in Section 14.3.2 for initial dose selection.

14.3.1 Parameter estimation

Having the clinical data and the PK/PD model, given by Equations (14.1)–(14.8), the parameter estimation problem was formulated as an optimisation problem and solved using the analytical solutions of the PK and PD models, which were obtained by using Mathematica. Since the spread of values in the PK clinical data set is large, the PK parameter estimation problem was performed using both absolute and scaled objective functions. The full set of model parameters and state variables are listed in Table 14.2.

The generic mathematical formulation of the parameter estimation problem is as follows:

Table 14.2: Model parameters and state variables of the PK/PD model.

Symbol	Description	Units
Ψ_k	The vector of the state variables in compartment k	
C_P	Vector concentration in the plasma compartment	vg/mL
C_{BF}	Vector concentration in the body fluids compartment	vg/mL
C_{e_FIX}	Vector concentration in the biophase (effect) compartment when considering the pharmacological response (FIX coagulation activity level)	vg/mL
C_{e_ALT}	Vector concentration in the biophase (effect) compartment when considering the toxicological response (ALT level)	vg/mL
R_{FIX}	Plasma factor IX coagulation activity level	IU/dL
R_{ALT}	ALT level	IU/L
θ	The vector of the model parameters	
θ_d	Distribution rate constant	day^{-1}
$\theta_{el.0}$	Elimination rate constant	day^{-1}
$\theta_{el.1}$	Elimination rate constant	day^{-1}
θ_{e_FIX}	Rate constant linking a kinetic model and a dynamic model when considering the pharmacological response (FIX coagulation activity level)	day^{-1}
θ_{e_ALT}	Rate constant linking a kinetic model and a dynamic model when considering the toxicological response (ALT level)	day^{-1}
θ_{in_FIX}	The *rate in* of the pharmacological response compartment (R_{FIX})	day^{-1}
θ_{out_FIX}	The *rate out* of the pharmacological response compartment (R_{FIX})	day^{-1}
θ_{in_ALT}	The *rate in* of the toxicological response compartment (R_{ALT})	day^{-1}
θ_{out_ALT}	The *rate out* of the toxicological response compartment (R_{ALT})	day^{-1}
Err$_{absolute}$	Absolute objective function	
Err$_{scaled}$	Scaled objective function	
$\widehat{\Psi}_k$	The vector of the observed clinical data in compartment k	

$$\text{Err}_{\text{absolute}} = \min_{\theta, \Psi(t)} \sum_{p \in P} \sum_{k \in K} \left\{ \Psi_k(t_p) - \widehat{\Psi}_k(t_p) \right\}^2 \tag{14.9}$$

or

$$\text{Err}_{\text{scaled}} = \min_{\theta, \Psi(t)} \sum_{p \in P} \sum_{k \in K} \left\{ \frac{\Psi_k(t_p) - \widehat{\Psi}_k(t_p)}{\widehat{\Psi}_k(t_p)} \right\}^2 \tag{14.10}$$

subject to the analytical solutions of the PK/PD model. For more details, please see Equations (14.1)–(14.6) in the Supplementary Appendix.

To carry out parameter estimation for the system, first, PK/PD parameters were estimated individually for each patient, which could be useful for the development of personalised gene therapy. Then, PK and PD parameters were estimated for all patients simultaneously, which were used for the initial dose selection, aiming at predicting the physiological response of a patient to a dose of vector. For individually estimated PK/PD parameters, the analysis was dependent on the initial vector concentration, whereas the simultaneous parameter estimation was dose-dependent. Tables 14.3 and 14.4 summarise the parameter estimation results for individually and simultaneously estimated parameters. The estimated parameter values were then used for dynamic simulations using Orthogonal Collocation on Finite Elements (OCFE), which were carried out for the validation of the model, with a view to pave the way for control of gene delivery in future work. Note that the model parameters are specific to a patient and may vary between patients (inter-patient) and also within individual patients (intra-patient). There are different factors that affect inter- and intra-patient variability, such as age, sex, body weight, health condition and activity levels.

In order to visualise the variance between the estimated PK/PD parameters across different patients, the results are also graphically shown in Figure 14.3. Note that in the following figure, P.4, P.6 and P.9 refer to Patient 4, Patient 6 and Patient 9, respectively, where the PK and PD parameters were estimated individually for each patient. However, P.4-6-9 refers to the population modelling approach in which each PK and PD parameters were estimated for all patients simultaneously.

In Figure 14.3, the variability of the estimated model parameters across different patients could be associated with the inter-patient variability, suggesting that the personalised gene therapy using an individual modelling approach would make more sense because the pharmacokinetics and pharmacodynamics of the vector can vary between patients. However, to gain more insights into the process, both the individual modelling approach (solving the parameter estimation problem for each patient individually) and the population modelling approach (solving the parameter estimation problem for all patients simultaneously) were considered in the present work.

It is important to note here that the estimated model parameters could vary for different initial guesses used for the parameter estimation problem. Difficulties arise from both the existence of local minima and non-identifiability [31]. The solver may find different local minima when started from different starting points due to the non-

Table 14.3: Estimated PK/PD model parameters, individually for each patient.

		Patient 4 (P.4)		
		Estimated parameters (day^{-1})		
PK model	Absolute OBJ[a]	θ_d = 1.5710559	$\theta_{el.0}$ = 1.0506840	$\theta_{el.1}$ = 2.1366106
	Scaled OBJ[b]	θ_d = 2.5971076	$\theta_{el.0}$ = 0.0247028	$\theta_{el.1}$ = 0.4823376
PD model	FIX	θ_{e_FIX} = 9.7701316	θ_{in_FIX} = 0.0016288	θ_{out_FIX} = 0.0631596
	ALT	θ_{e_ALT} = 18.4752261	θ_{in_ALT} = 0.0005428	θ_{out_ALT} = 0.0074621
		Patient 6 (P.6)		
		Estimated parameters (day^{-1})		
PK model	Absolute OBJ[a]	θ_d = 2.1140705	$\theta_{el.0}$ = 0.0073093	$\theta_{el.1}$ = 0.5635716
	Scaled OBJ[b]	θ_d = 2.0194024	$\theta_{el.0}$ = 0.0910754	$\theta_{el.1}$ = 1.7344535
PD model	FIX	θ_{e_FIX} = 21.1668725	θ_{in_FIX} = 0.0003748	θ_{out_FIX} = 0.0158966
	ALT	θ_{e_ALT} = 0.3656878	θ_{in_ALT} = 0.0028681	θ_{out_ALT} = 0.0005408
		Patient 9 (P.9)		
		Estimated parameters (day^{-1})		
PK model	Absolute OBJ[a]	θ_d = 0.1593991	$\theta_{el.0}$ = 1.1246204	$\theta_{el.1}$ = 0.6580731
	Scaled OBJ[b]	θ_d = 0.9911402	$\theta_{el.0}$ = 0.3439847	$\theta_{el.1}$ = 0.4674078
PD model	FIX	θ_{e_FIX} = 2.0086934	θ_{in_FIX} = 0.0012088	θ_{out_FIX} = 0.0038267
	ALT	θ_{e_ALT} = 6.4510203	θ_{in_ALT} = 0.0010856	θ_{out_ALT} = 0.0033077

[a]Solved the parameter estimation problem using an absolute objective function (Equation (14.9)). [b]Solved the parameter estimation problem using a scaled objective function (Equation (14.10)).

Table 14.4: Estimated PK/PD model parameters, for all patients simultaneously.

		Patients 4, 6 and 9 (P.4-6-9)		
		Estimated parameters (day^{-1})		
PK model	Absolute OBJ[a]	θ_d = 1.5511141	$\theta_{el.0}$ = 0.4723049	$\theta_{el.1}$ = 0.7640243
	Scaled OBJ[b]	θ_d = 7.1957447	$\theta_{el.0}$ = 2.0910047	$\theta_{el.1}$ = 1.7113180
PD model	FIX	θ_{e_FIX} = 11.2140501	θ_{in_FIX} = 0.0005731	θ_{out_FIX} = 0.0737731
	ALT	θ_{e_ALT} = 0.6582939	θ_{in_ALT} = 0.0007284	θ_{out_ALT} = 0.0014742

[a]Solved the parameter estimation problem using an absolute objective function (Equation (14.9)). [b]Solved the parameter estimation problem using a scaled objective function (Equation (14.10)).

convexity of the objective function. Global optimisation-based algorithms were applied; however, the model was unable to converge to find a global optimal solution. Furthermore, the identifiability issue is concerned with the theoretical existence of unique solutions to the parameter estimation problem. Hence, there are various sets of parameter values that fit the clinical data equally well. Different strategies, such as model

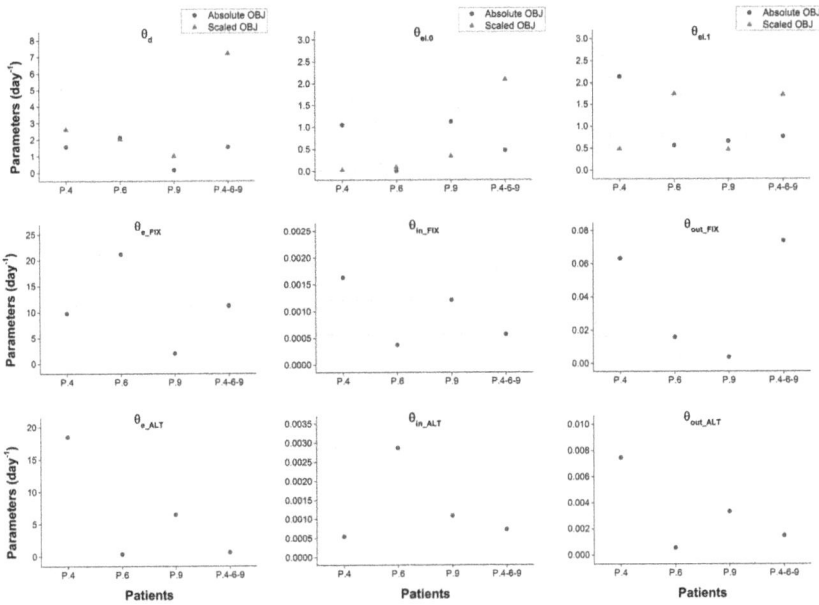

Figure 14.3: Estimated PK/PD parameters across different patients.

reformulation, model reduction, or generating additional clinical data can be used to overcome the identifiability problem [31]. Sensitivity analysis was performed to investigate the sensitivities of state variables relative to small changes in model parameters at the steady state (Tables 14.5 and 14.6). All relative sensitivities of model variables to changes in parameters are smaller than one in absolute value, meaning that perturbations in value of the parameters are attenuated.

The results obtained from the PK/PD analysis using an individual modelling are shown in Figures 14.4–14.6, while the results illustrated in Figures 14.7–14.9 present the PK/PD analysis using a population modelling. The parameter estimation and the simulation results obtained from the work have been qualitatively verified by using the compartmental modelling approach. As can be seen from the following figures, the dynamic simulations agree closely with the parameter estimation results, and the model predictions are in good accordance with the clinical data. However, depending on the type of the objective function and the choice of individual modelling approach or population modelling approach, various results of the study highlighted several feasible configurations of the system. Such considerations were taken into account to aid decision making for further research. The values of the objective function obtained for each case study are reported in Tables 14.7 and 14.8, which give an indication of the solution accuracy. According to the results, the objective function values observed for the PD parameter estimation are much higher than those obtained for the PK parameter estimation. This is because of the extensive PD data set and the widespread existence of

Table 14.5: Model sensitivity matrix for the individual modelling approach.

Parameters	Individual modelling approach											
	Patient 4				Patient 6				Patient 9			
	C_P	C_{BF}	R_{FIX}	R_{ALT}	C_P	C_{BF}	R_{FIX}	R_{ALT}	C_P	C_{BF}	R_{FIX}	R_{ALT}
$\theta_{d\_absolute}$	-0.000001	-0.000001	–	–	-0.000002	-0.000001	-0.2	-0.14	-0.000001	-0.000001	-0.03	-0.08
$\theta_{el,0\_absolute}$	-0.000001	-0.000001	–	–	-0.000001	0.000001	-0.01	-0.01	-0.000002	-0.000001	-0.18	-0.57
$\theta_{el,1\_absolute}$	–	-0.000002	–	–	–	-0.000003	–	–	–	-0.000002	–	–
θ_{d_scaled}	-0.000002	-0.000003	-0.04	-0.6	-0.000002	-0.000001	–	–	-0.000002	-0.000001	–	–
$\theta_{el,0\_scaled}$	-0.000001	0.000002	-0.01	-0.01	-0.000001	0.000001	–	–	-0.000001	0.000001	–	–
$\theta_{el,1\_scaled}$	–	-0.000025	–	–	–	-0.000002	–	–	–	-0.000002	–	–
θ_{e_FIX}	–	–	0.03	–	–	–	0.18	–	–	–	0.18	–
θ_{in_FIX}	–	–	-0.03	–	–	–	0.11	–	–	–	0.17	–
θ_{out_FIX}	–	–	-0.04	–	–	–	-0.21	–	–	–	-0.27	–
θ_{e_ALT}	–	–	–	0.57	–	–	–	0.12	–	–	–	0.62
θ_{in_ALT}	–	–	–	0.3	–	–	–	-0.02	–	–	–	0.48
θ_{out_ALT}	–	–	–	-0.68	–	–	–	-0.44	–	–	–	-0.81

Table 14.6: Model sensitivity matrix for the population modelling approach.

Parameters	Population modelling approach											
	Patient 4				Patient 6				Patient 9			
	C_P	C_{BF}	R_{FIX}	R_{ALT}	C_P	C_{BF}	R_{FIX}	R_{ALT}	C_P	C_{BF}	R_{FIX}	R_{ALT}
$\theta_{d\_absolute}$	-0.000002	-0.000001	-0.03	-0.1	-0.000002	-0.000001	-0.15	-0.53	-0.000002	-0.000001	-0.22	-0.49
$\theta_{el.0\_absolute}$	-0.000001	0.000001	-0.01	-0.03	-0.000001	0.000001	-0.05	-0.16	-0.000001	0.000001	-0.07	-0.15
$\theta_{el.1\_absolute}$	—	-0.000002	—	—	—	-0.000004	—	—	—	-0.000002	—	—
θ_{d_scaled}	-0.000001	-0.000001	—	—	-0.000001	-0.000001	—	—	-0.000001	-0.000001	—	—
$\theta_{el.0\_scaled}$	-0.000001	0.000001	—	—	-0.000001	0.000001	—	—	-0.000001	0.000001	—	—
$\theta_{el.1\_scaled}$	—	-0.000002	—	—	—	-0.000002	—	—	—	-0.000002	—	—
θ_{e_FIX}	—	—	0.03	—	—	—	0.17	—	—	—	0.27	—
θ_{in_FIX}	—	—	0.01	—	—	—	0.05	—	—	—	0.19	—
θ_{out_FIX}	—	—	-0.04	—	—	—	-0.19	—	—	—	-0.3	—
θ_{e_ALT}	—	—	—	0.12	—	—	—	0.66	—	—	—	0.6
θ_{in_ALT}	—	—	—	0.07	—	—	—	0.31	—	—	—	0.48
θ_{out_ALT}	—	—	—	-0.56	—	—	—	-0.74	—	—	—	-0.55

Patient 4

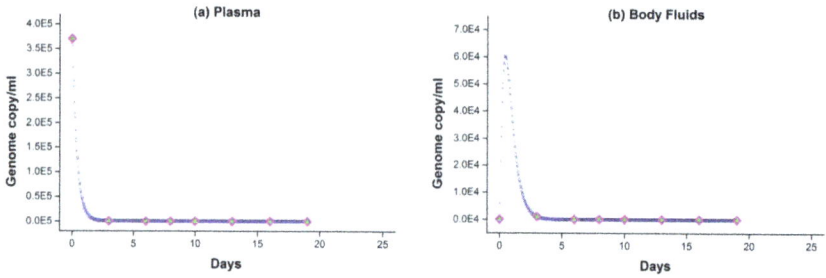

Patient 6

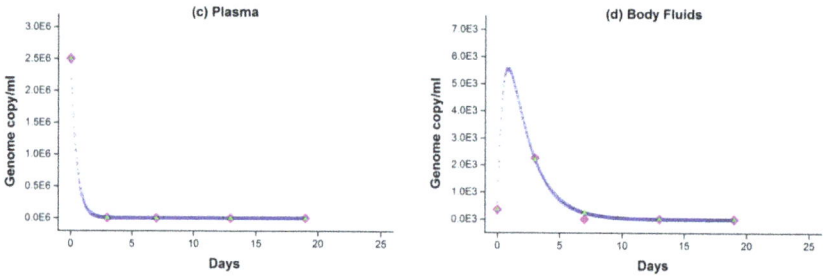

Patient 9

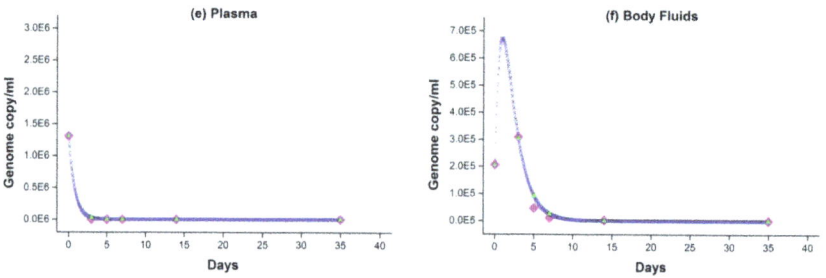

◆ Clinical data
· Parameter estimation using analytical solution
· Model simulation for estimated parameters using OCFE

Figure 14.4: Pharmacokinetic analysis, individually for each patient – comparison of the PK model predictions (using an absolute objective function) with the clinical data.

Patient 4

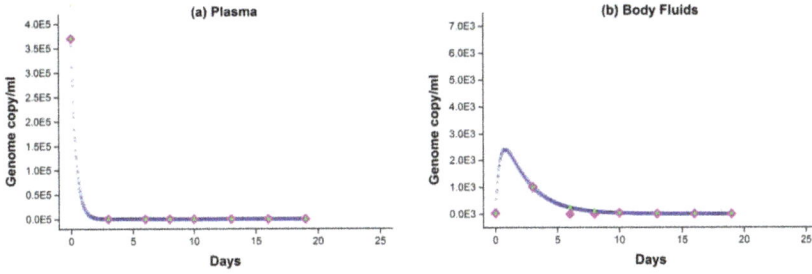

Patient 6

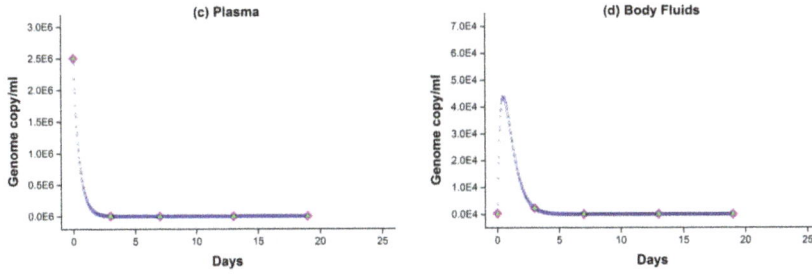

Patient 9

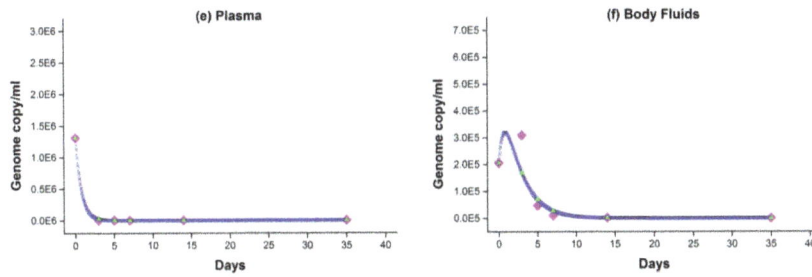

◆ Clinical data
· Parameter estimation using analytical solution
  Model simulation for estimated parameters using OCFE

Figure 14.5: Pharmacokinetic analysis, individually for each patient – comparison of the PK model predictions (using a scaled objective function) with the clinical data.

Patient 4

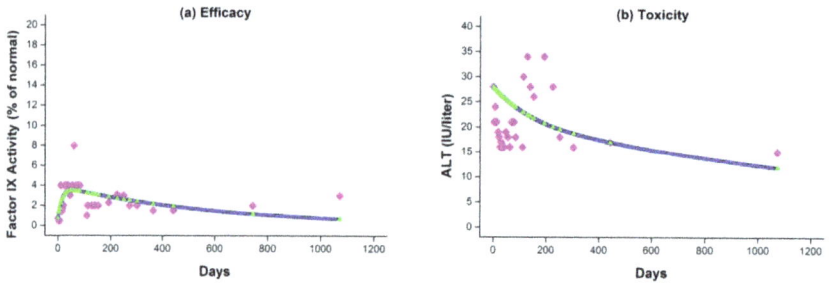

(a) Efficacy

(b) Toxicity

Patient 6

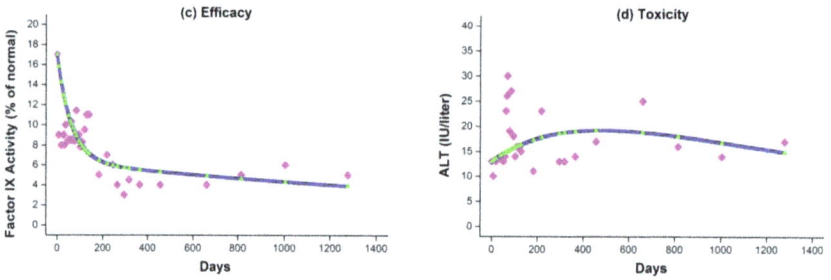

(c) Efficacy

(d) Toxicity

Patient 9

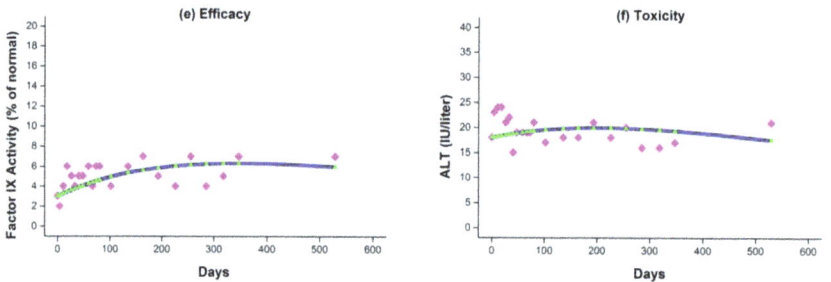

(e) Efficacy

(f) Toxicity

- Clinical data
- Parameter estimation using analytical solution
- Model simulation for estimated parameters using OCFE

Figure 14.6: Pharmacodynamic analysis, individually for each patient – comparison of the PD model predictions (using an absolute objective function) with the clinical data.

Patient 4

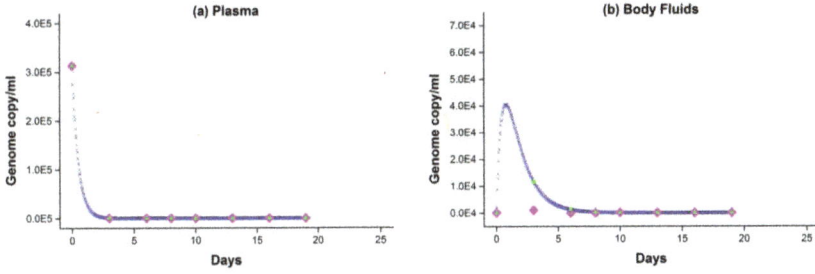

Patient 6

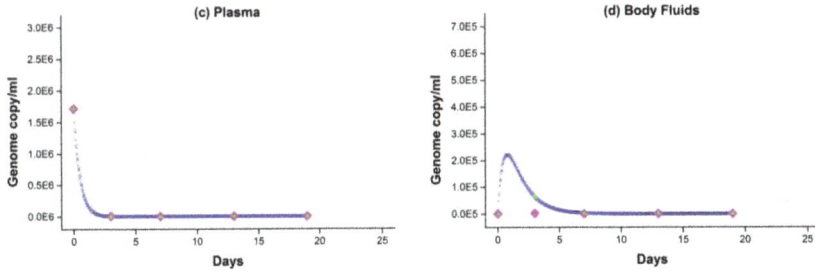

Patient 9

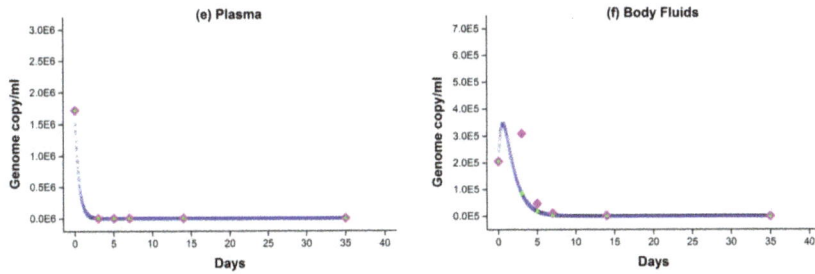

- ◆ Clinical data
- Parameter estimation using analytical solution
- Model simulation for estimated parameters using OCFE

Figure 14.7: Pharmacokinetic analysis, for all patients simultaneously – comparison of the PK model predictions (using an absolute objective function) with the clinical data.

Patient 4

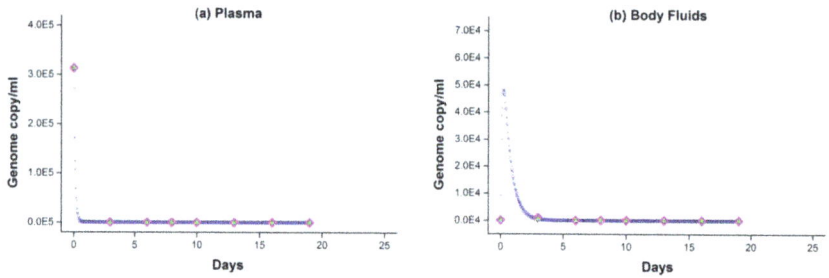

(a) Plasma

(b) Body Fluids

Patient 6

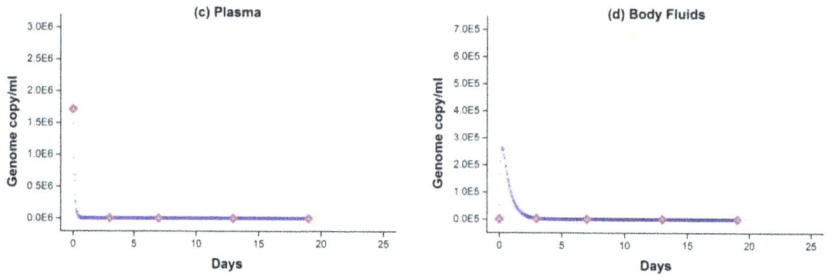

(c) Plasma

(d) Body Fluids

Patient 9

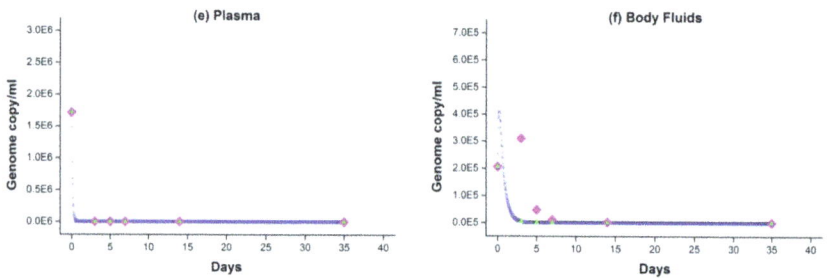

(e) Plasma

(f) Body Fluids

◆ Clinical data
Parameter estimation using analytical solution
Model simulation for estimated parameters using OCFE

Figure 14.8: Pharmacokinetic analysis, for all patients simultaneously – comparison of the PK model predictions (using a scaled objective function) with the clinical data.

Patient 4

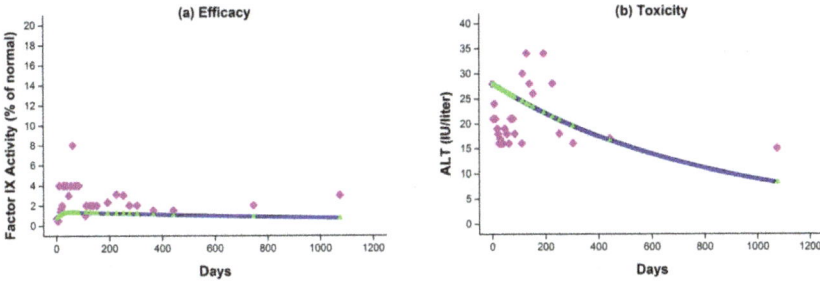

Patient 6

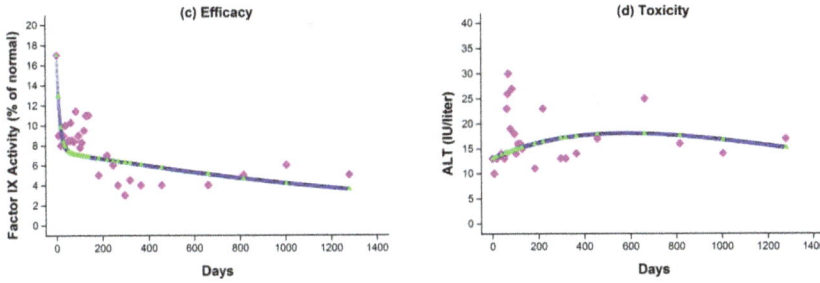

Patient 9

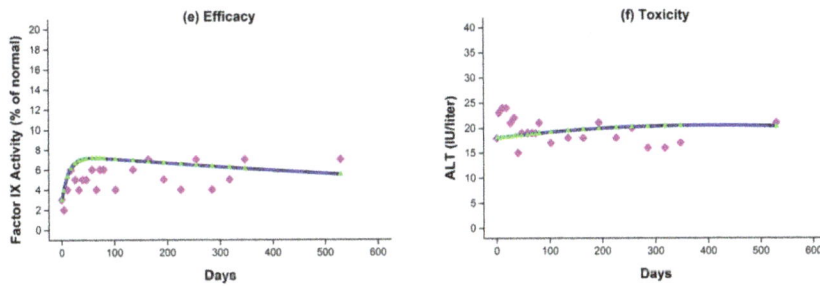

- ◆ Clinical data
- ◆ Parameter estimation using analytical solution
- · Model simulation for estimated parameters using OCFE

Figure 14.9: Pharmacodynamic analysis, for all patients simultaneously – comparison of the PD model predictions (using an absolute objective function) with the clinical data.

Table 14.7: Computational results for the individual modelling approach.

Patient 4		
	Objective function values	**Corresponding figures**
PK model	$Err_{absolute} = 1.2013 \times 10^{-5}$	Figure 14.4(a) and (b)
	$Err_{scaled} = 1.667 \times 10^{-16}$	Figure 14.5(a) and (b)
PD model – FIX	$Err_{absolute} = 52.140$	Figure 14.6(a)
PD model – ALT	$Err_{absolute} = 1,399.890$	Figure 14.6(b)

Patient 6		
	Objective function values	**Corresponding figures**
PK model	$Err_{absolute} = 1.0396 \times 10^{-5}$	Figure 14.4(c) and (d)
	$Err_{scaled} = 2.990$	Figure 14.5(c) and (d)
PD model – FIX	$Err_{absolute} = 200.021$	Figure 14.6(c)
PD model – ALT	$Err_{absolute} = 799.967$	Figure 14.6(d)

Patient 9		
	Objective function values	**Corresponding figures**
PK model	$Err_{absolute} = 3 \times 10^{-1}$	Figure 14.4(e) and (f)
	$Err_{scaled} = 2.997$	Figure 14.5(e) and (f)
PD model – FIX	$Err_{absolute} = 37.134$	Figure 14.6(e)
PD model – ALT	$Err_{absolute} = 187.068$	Figure 14.6(f)

Table 14.8: Computational results for the population modelling approach.

Patients 4, 6, and 9		
	Objective function values	**Corresponding figures**
PK model	$Err_{absolute} = 1,481.198$	Figure 14.7
	$Err_{scaled} = 10.270$	Figure 14.8
PD model – FIX	$Err_{absolute} = 1,011.102$	Figure 14.9(a), (c), and (e)
PD model – ALT	$Err_{absolute} = 4,167.984$	Figure 14.9(b), (d), and (f)

fluctuations in the PD clinical data. Another potential contributor is the existence of hypothetical effect compartment that acts as a link between the PK and PD models. However, the analysis shows that a good match is obtained between the clinical data and the model predictions. The pharmacokinetic analysis in this work demonstrates how the overall performance of the PK parameter estimation problem depends on the optimisation algorithms and the objective functions. Making such comparisons between an absolute objective function and a scaled objective function leads to the fact that using a scaling factor may cause an algorithm to determine a different optimal solution. The absolute and scaled objective function values vary with no observable trend. Hence, based on a trade-off between the objective function values and the simulation results, a decision is made to use a set of parameters for subsequent computational studies.

14.3.2 Initial dose selection

This section aims to explore how the simulation-based modelling approach can assist in the initial dose selection. In this work, the initial doses used for the simulations are calculated based on the following assumptions: (i) the average plasma volume is 50 mL/kg [32] and (ii) there is a linear relationship between the dose administered (after conversion from vg/kg to vg/mL) and the initial vector concentration in plasma.

Linear regression is one of the most commonly used techniques to investigate the relationship between two quantitative variables [33]. Therefore, a linear regression analysis was carried out to determine the equation of the regression line, which is as follows and shown in Figure 14.10: Initial vector concentration in plasma = $5 \times 10^{-5} \times$ Dose − 287,000.

For comparison purposes, the dynamic simulations were carried out for different time periods and for various initial bolus doses. The PK/PD profiles are shown in Figures 14.11–14.14.

As can be seen in Figures 14.11b, 14.12b, 14.13b, and 14.14b, the vector is expected to be eliminated from the body within 10 days after administration. The simulation results (Figures 14.11–14.14) demonstrated that the increase in both factor IX activity and ALT level is dose-dependent, which is one of the key findings that is consistent with the work by Nathwani et al. [7]. In a recent study by Nathwani and Tuddenham [34], the authors reported that the highest level of transgene expression of between 8 % and 12 % of normal

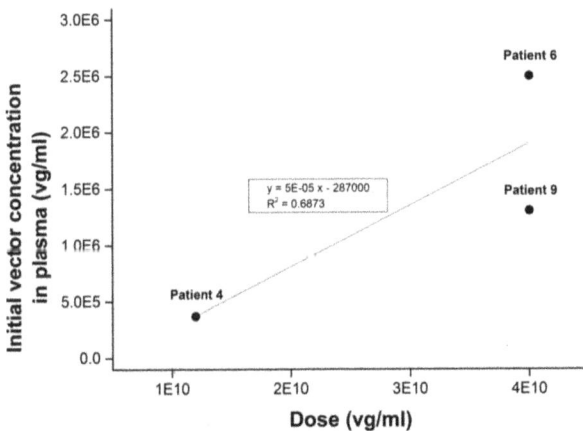

Figure 14.10: Linear regression curve between the dose administered and the initial vector concentration in plasma.

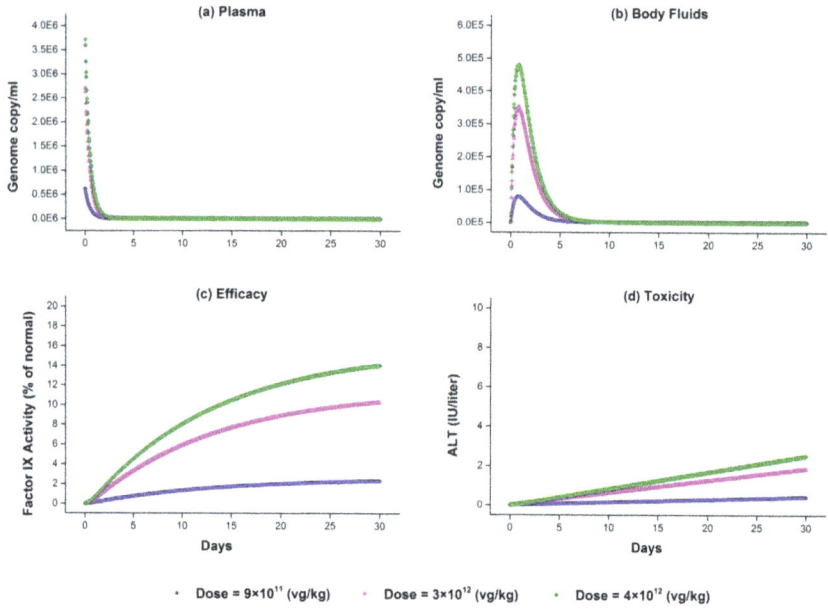

Figure 14.11: Population pharmacokinetic and pharmacodynamic results over a period of 30 days for different initial bolus doses.

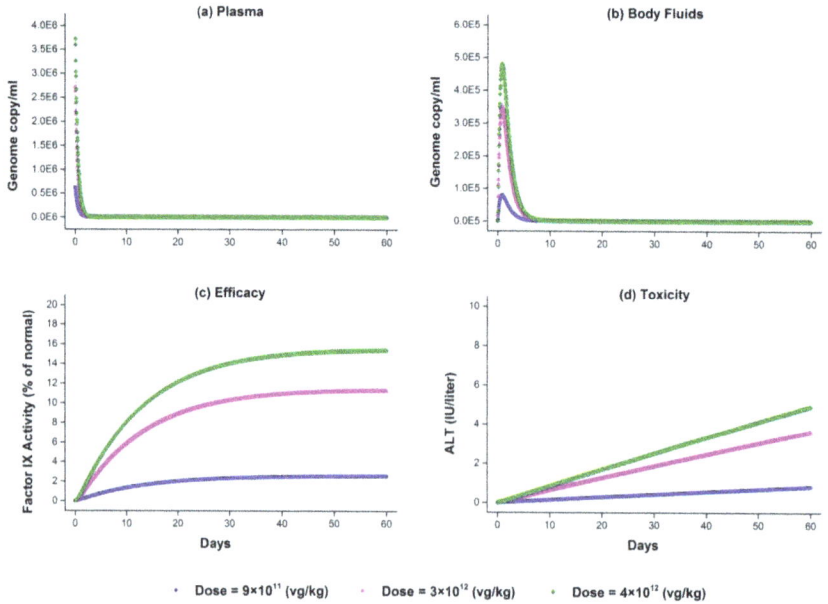

Figure 14.12: Population pharmacokinetic and pharmacodynamic results over a period of 60 days for different initial bolus doses.

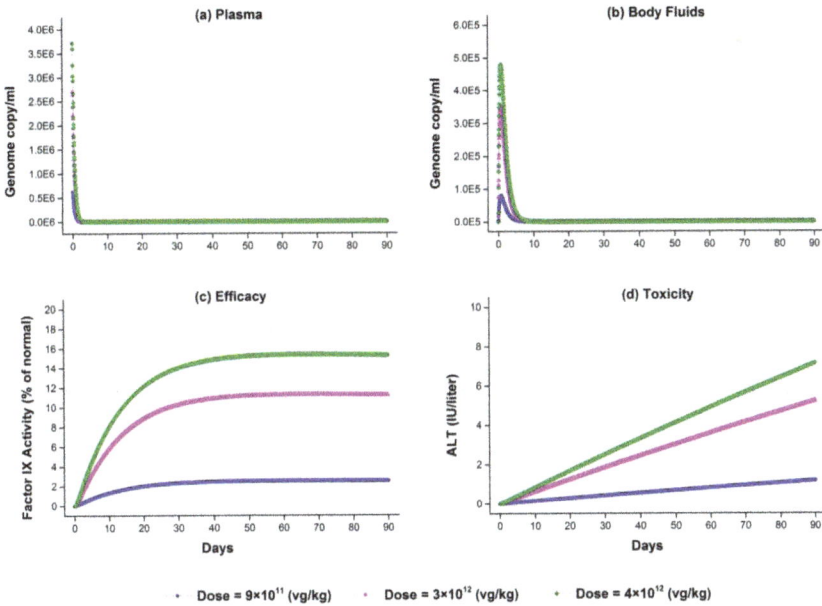

Figure 14.13: Population pharmacokinetic and pharmacodynamic results over a period of 90 days for different initial bolus doses.

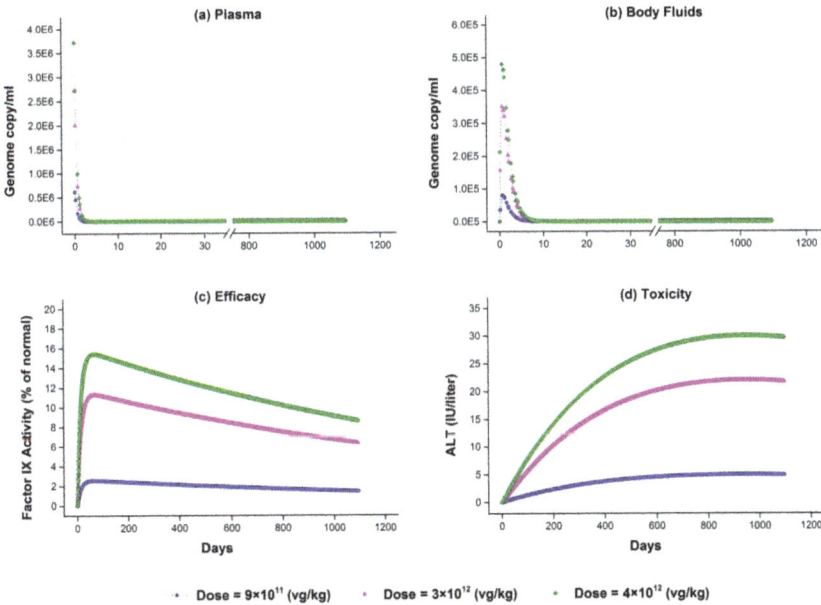

Figure 14.14: Population pharmacokinetic and pharmacodynamic results over a period of 3 years for different initial bolus doses.

was observed in the patients treated at the dose level of 2×10^{12} vg/kg, which remained stable up to 6 weeks after gene transfer. The simulation results in this chapter (Figures 14.12c, 14.13c, and 14.14c) lead to similar conclusion where FIX activity levels between 11 % and 15 % of normal can be observed for the high-dose subjects (dose level of 3×10^{12} vg/kg and 4×10^{12} vg/kg), which remained stable within 3 months after infusion. However, the ALT levels are increased consistently, especially in higher dose cohorts, which subsequently leads to a relative reduction in factor IX levels (about 55 % reduction). According to Nathwani et al. [7], the increase in the ALT level is associated with a decline in factor IX activity levels, suggesting a loss of transduced hepatocytes. Despite the drop in the level of expression, the simulation analysis found evidence for long-term efficacy as the FIX expression levels are maintained in the 6–10 % range in the high-dose patients within a period of 3 years (Figure 14.14c), suggesting a reduction in FIX concentrate usage. This is in line with the findings reported by Nathwani and Tuddenham [34], demonstrating that the transgenic FIX activity levels have remained stable over a period of 10 years follow-up and reduced the need for treatments with FIX concentrates.

14.4 Conclusions

In this chapter, a mathematical modelling approach was developed for gene transfer of adeno-associated viral vectors in patients with haemophilia B. The model-based platform discussed in this chapter incorporates the pharmacokinetics and pharmacodynamics of the scAAV2/8-LP1-hFIXco vectors. The PK/PD model parameters were estimated using the analytical solution of the model, individually for each patient in a dose-independent manner and for all patients simultaneously in a dose-dependent manner. A number of dynamic simulations were also carried out using OCFE for the validation of the model, demonstrating the simulation results are comparable to that obtained from parameter estimation. The simulation-based PK/PD modelling approach was then used for the initial dose selection to provide clinicians with better tools to make the decision-making process simpler for designing more effective treatment plans, which can be tailored to maximise efficacy while minimising toxicity for individual patients.

Acknowledgements: The authors would like to thank the editors David Bogle and Tomasz Sosnowski for their guidance and review of this article before its publication.

References

1. Jamili E, Nathwani AC, Dua V. Mathematical modelling of gene delivery in patients with haemophilia B. Chem Eng Sci 2023;281:119073.
2. George LA, Sullivan SK, Giermasz A, Rasko JEJ, Samelson-Jones BJ, Ducore J, et al. Hemophilia B gene therapy with a high-specific-activity factor IX variant. N Engl J Med 2017;377:2215–27.

3. Ramaswamy S, Tonnu N, Tachikawa K, Limphong P, Vega JB, Karmali PP, et al. Systemic delivery of factor IX messenger RNA for protein replacement therapy. Proc Natl Acad Sci USA 2017;114:E1941–E19.

4. Patel N, Reiss U, Davidoff AM, Nathwani AC. Progress towards gene therapy for haemophilia B. Int J Hematol 2014;99:372–6.

5. Powell JS, Pasi KJ, Ragni MV, Ozelo MC, Valentino LA, Mahlangu JN, et al. Phase 3 study of recombinant factor IX Fc fusion protein in hemophilia B. N Engl J Med 2013;369:2313–23.

6. Manno CS, Arruda VR, Pierce GF, Glader B, Ragni M, Rasko J, et al. Successful transduction of liver in hemophilia by AAV-Factor IX and limitations imposed by the host immune response. Nat Med 2006;12: 342–7.

7. Nathwani AC, Reiss UM, Tuddenham EGD, Rosales C, Chowdary P, McIntosh J, et al. Long-term safety and efficacy of factor IX gene therapy in hemophilia B. N Engl J Med 2014;371:1994–2004.

8. Nathwani AC, Davidoff A, Hanawa H, Zhou JF, Vanin EF, Nienhuis AW. Factors influencing in vivo transduction by recombinant adeno-associated viral vectors expressing the human factor IX cDNA. Blood 2001;97:1258–65.

9. Nathwani AC, Davidoff AM, Tuddenham EGD. Gene therapy for hemophilia. Hematol Oncol Clin N Am 2017; 31:853–68.

10. Nathwani AC, Gray JT, McIntosh J, Ng CYC, Zhou JF, Spence Y, et al. Safe and efficient transduction of the liver after peripheral vein infusion of self- complementary AAV vector results in stable therapeutic expression of human FIX in nonhuman primates. Blood 2007;109:1414–21.

11. Nathwani AC, Gray JT, Ng CYC, Zhou JF, Spence Y, Waddington SN, et al. Self-complementary adeno-associated virus vectors containing a novel liver-specific human factor IX expression cassette enable highly efficient transduction of murine and nonhuman primate liver. Blood 2006;107:2653–61.

12. Nathwani AC, Rosales C, McIntosh J, Rastegarlari G, Nathwani D, Raj D, et al. Long-term safety and efficacy following systemic administration of a self- complementary AAV vector encoding human FIX pseudotyped with serotype 5 and 8 capsid proteins. Mol Ther 2011;19:876–85.

13. Nathwani AC, Tuddenham EGD, Rangarajan S, Rosales C, McIntosh J, Linch DC, et al. Adenovirus-associated virus vector-mediated gene transfer in hemophilia B. N Engl J Med 2011;365:2357–65.

14. Ledley TS, Ledley FD. Multicompartment, numerical-model of cellular events in the pharmacokinetics of gene therapies. Hum Gene Ther 1994;5:679–91.

15. Banks GA, Roselli RJ, Chen R, Giorgio TD. A model for the analysis of nonviral gene therapy. Gene Ther 2003; 10:1766–75.

16. Varga CM, Hong K, Lauffenburger DA. Quantitative analysis of synthetic gene delivery vector design properties. Mol Ther 2001;4:438–46.

17. Varga CM, Tedford NC, Thomas M, Klibanov AM, Griffith LG, Lauffenburger DA. Quantitative comparison of polyethylenimine formulations and adenoviral vectors in terms of intracellular gene delivery processes. Gene Ther 2005;12:1023–32.

18. Dinh AT, Pangarkar C, Theofanous T, Mitragotri S. Understanding intracellular transport processes pertinent to synthetic gene delivery via stochastic simulations and sensitivity analyses. Biophys J 2007;92: 831–46.

19. Horobin RW, Weissig V. A QSAR-modeling perspective on cationic transfection lipids. 1. predicting efficiency and understanding mechanisms. J Gene Med 2005;7:1023–34.

20. Jandt U, Shao S, Wirth M, Zeng AP. Spatiotemporal modeling and analysis of transient gene delivery. Biotechnol Bioeng 2011;108:2205–17.

21. Berraondo P, Gonzalez-Aseguinolaza G, Troconiz IF. Semi-mechanistic pharmacodynamic modelling of gene expression and silencing processes. Eur J Pharmaceut Sci 2009;37:418–26.

22. Martin TM, Wysocki BJ, Wysocki TA, Pannier AK. Identifying intracellular pDNA losses from a model of nonviral gene delivery. IEEE Trans NanoBiosci 2015;14:455–64.

23. Jamili E, Dua V. Optimal model-based control of non-viral siRNA delivery. Biotechnol Bioeng 2018;115: 1866–77.

24. Holz M, Fahr A. Compartment modeling. Adv Drug Deliv Rev 2001;48:249–64.
25. Nestorov I. Whole body pharmacokinetic models. Clin Pharmacokinet 2003;42:883–908.
26. Howard EL, Becker KCD, Rusconi CP, Becker RC. Factor IXa inhibitors as novel anticoagulants. Arterioscler Thromb Vasc Biol 2007;27:722–7.
27. Tsang TC, Bentley DR, Mibashan RS, Giannelli F. A factor-IX mutation, verified by direct genomic sequencing, causes haemophilia-B by a novel mechanism. EMBO J 1988;7:3009–15.
28. Franchini M, Frattini F, Crestani S, Bonfanti C. Haemophilia B: current pharmacotherapy and future directions. Expet Opin Pharmacother 2012;13:2053–63.
29. Gabrielsson J, Weiner D. Pharmacokinetic and pharmacodynamic data analysis: concepts and applications, 4th ed. Sweden: Swedish Pharmaceutical Press; 2010.
30. Washington IM, Van Hoosier G. Clinical biochemistry and hematology. In: Suckow MA, Stevens KA, Wilson RP, editors. The laboratory rabbit, guinea pig, hamster, and other rodents. American college of laboratory animal medicine series. San Diego: Elsevier Academic Press Inc; 2012:57–116 pp.
31. Degasperi A, Fey D, Kholodenko BN. Performance of objective functions and optimisation procedures for parameter estimation in system biology models. NPJ Syst Biol Appl 2017;3:20.
32. Yiengst MJ, Shock NW. Blood and plasma volume in adult males. J Appl Physiol 1962;17:195.
33. Bewick V, Cheek L, Ball J. Statistics review 7: correlation and regression. Crit Care 2003;7:451–9.
34. Nathwani AC, Tuddenham EGD. Haemophilia, the journey in search of a cure. 1960-2020. Br J Haematol 2020;191:573–8.

Supplementary Material: This article contains supplementary material (https://doi.org/10.1515/psr-2024-0057).

Sonia Sarnelli, Manuel Cardamone, Ernesto Reverchon and
Lucia Baldino*

15 Lipid-based nanoparticles for nucleic acids delivery

Abstract: This chapter highlights challenges and advancements in the production of lipid-based nanoparticles (LNPs) and their application in nucleic acid-based therapies. Recently, mRNA-based vaccines for COVID-19 immunization revealed that the use of nucleic acids is a promising strategy to develop treatments at high therapeutic efficiency and reduced side effects. In this context, LNPs emerged as favourable vehicles for nucleic acids delivery (like mRNA and DNA), due to their biocompatibility, bioavailability, and versatility. The four main components employed to produce LNPs loaded with mRNA are: cationic or ionizable lipids, helper lipids, cholesterol, and PEGylated lipids. Several conventional techniques have been proposed over the years to produce this kind of nanoparticles. However, they show many drawbacks that hinder the direct production of vesicles characterized by a nanometric size, high encapsulation efficiency of the active pharmaceutical ingredient, and prolonged stability. Processes assisted by supercritical fluids (in particular, supercritical CO_2) can represent a sustainable and interesting alternative to produce LNPs without using post-processing steps for solvent removal and size reduction that are time-consuming procedures, lead to a large loss of nucleic acids, and negatively influence the general productivity of the process.

Keywords: nucleic acid; lipid-based nanoparticles; cationic and ionizable lipids; PEG-lipids; cholesterol; conventional and innovative

15.1 Historical background of nucleic acids

The history of nucleic acids started in 1869, when Friedrich Miescher isolated a new substance within the cell nucleus, that he called "nuclein" [1]. This molecule, characterized by a high concentration of phosphorus, showed high resistance to enzymes involved in the degradation of proteins and lipids. In 1944, Oswald Avery and co-workers identified DNA as the molecule of heredity [2]. This discovery indicated that DNA is the carrier of the genetic information [3]. However, understanding the structure of this molecule did not

*Corresponding author: Lucia Baldino, Department of Industrial Engineering, University of Salerno, Via Giovanni Paolo II, 132, 84084, Fisciano, SA, Italy, E-mail: lbaldino@unisa.it. https://orcid.org/0000-0001-7015-0803
Sonia Sarnelli, Manuel Cardamone and Ernesto Reverchon, Department of Industrial Engineering, University of Salerno, Via Giovanni Paolo II, 132, 84084, Fisciano, SA, Italy

As per De Gruyter's policy this article has previously been published in the journal Physical Sciences Reviews. Please cite as: S. Sarnelli, M. Cardamone, E. Reverchon and L. Baldino "Lipid-based nanoparticles for nucleic acids delivery" *Physical Sciences Reviews* [Online] 2025. DOI: 10.1515/psr-2025-0001 | https://doi.org/10.1515/9783111394558-015

occur until 1953, when James Watson and Francis Crick foresaw the existence of a double helix structure and published the article "Molecular Structure of Nucleic Acids: A Structure for Deoxyribose Nucleic Acid" [4]. Five years later, Crick defined the central dogma of molecular biology in an article titled "On protein synthesis", stating that the flow of genetic information is unidirectional, from DNA to messenger RNA (mRNA) up to protein synthesis [5].

15.1.1 The evolution of medicine: from conventional drugs to nucleic acid-based therapies

The pharmaceutical industry has relied on low molecular weight drugs for a long time; but the introduction of nucleic acid-based therapies is revolutionizing modern medicine [6]. This innovative field exploits the unique properties of nucleic acids, such as plasmid deoxyribonucleic acid (pDNA), messenger ribonucleic acid (mRNA), small interfering ribonucleic acid (siRNA), micro ribonucleic acid (miRNA) and antisense oligonucleotides, to address a large variety of medical diseases, including rare genetic illnesses, complex disorders (e.g., cancer, diabetes, and cardiovascular disease) and viral infections, such as human immunodeficiency virus (HIV) [7]. More specifically, nucleic acid-based therapies operate at the genetic level, allowing precision interventions that are often unachievable by using traditional drugs [8]. For example, mRNA-based vaccines emerged as promising candidates for preventing infectious diseases during COVID-19 pandemic. These vaccines act transmitting instructions to cells, inducing them to produce a specific protein able to activate an immune response [9].

Unlike conventional drugs, nucleic acid-based therapies could offer highly customized treatments to target cells. In this way, it is possible to operate on biological processes at their origin, correcting defective genes, blocking disease progression or producing specific therapeutic proteins [10]. This approach not only increases the range of treatable diseases; but, it also reduces the risk of side effects commonly associated with less specific treatments [11]. Therefore, the development of nucleic acid-based therapies represents a main goal for many pharmaceutical industries, and can be considered as the beginning of a new era of medical breakthroughs, providing hope for the treatment of challenging diseases [12].

15.1.2 Analogies and differences between DNA and RNA

DNA and RNA are biological macromolecules composed of nucleotide subunits. Each nucleotide includes a phosphate group, a pentose sugar and a nitrogen base [13]. The main differences between these two types of nucleic acids are related to composition, structure, and function. In particular, the composition of DNA differs from that of RNA for the presence of deoxyribose that replaces ribose in RNA. Furthermore, nitrogen bases of

DNA include adenine (A), thymine (T), cytosine (C), and guanine (G); whereas uracil (U) substitutes thymine in RNA [14].

In terms of structure, DNA is a double-stranded helical molecule stabilised by hydrogen bonds between complementary bases (A bonds with T, and C bonds with G). RNA instead is a single-stranded molecule that exhibits greater structural flexibility and could assume different functional forms [15]. However, the hydrophilic character, the high molecular weight and the presence of negatively charged phosphate groups hinder the cellular transport of DNA and RNA [16]. Because of the structural and functional differences between these nucleic acids, their functions in cellular processes and the strategies required for their therapeutic delivery are different [17].

15.1.3 mRNA-based therapies

Historically, DNA was the most widely used molecule in gene therapy, as its structure and function were well known. Recently, mRNA-based approaches have gained a significant attention, since they show higher therapeutic efficiency [18]. Therefore, researchers expressed great interest in the development of mRNA-based therapies, with the aim of moving from experimental phases to practical clinical applications [19]. Messenger RNA is a large molecule, typically up to 10^6 Da that transports the genetic information necessary for cells to synthesise specific proteins from DNA to ribosomes within the cytoplasm [20]. mRNA is composed of five key regions; among these, the most important one is the open reading frame (ORF) or "coding sequence", since it represents the part of the molecule that is read and translated ribosomes to produce the desired protein [21]. All the other regions are located at the end of the molecule and contribute to the stability and translation efficiency of mRNA [21].

mRNA shows great potential in several therapeutic applications, including protein replacement therapy. The cells of the patient are induced to produce specific (missing or defective) proteins, offering a potential treatment for genetic diseases such as cystic fibrosis, haemophilia and other rare diseases [22]. mRNA-based therapies directly address the root cause at the cellular level, avoiding genetic integration [23]. The development of tailored-made vaccines for cancer fight is another important area where mRNA-based therapies are emerging. In this case, mRNA could identify tumour-specific neoantigens; i.e., mutated proteins expressed by cancer cells [24]. mRNA-based therapies can also be exploited for the treatment of infectious diseases. mRNA-based vaccine represents an innovative approach to immunization, as demonstrated by the anti-COVID-19 vaccines, developed by Pfizer-BioNTech and Moderna, during the pandemic caused by SARS-CoV-2 virus [25]. The success of mRNA-based vaccines in the fight against COVID-19 has paved the way for the development of new mRNA-based vaccines to treat other infectious diseases, including seasonal flu and malaria [26].

15.1.3.1 Challenges for mRNA delivery

One of the main challenges regarding mRNA as a therapeutic agent is related to its high instability. Indeed, without an appropriate protection, mRNA could be rapidly degraded by nucleases (i.e., specific enzymes located in the intracellular and/or extracellular environment) before reaching the target site [27]. Endocytosis and endosomal escape represent an additional obstacle for mRNA intracellular delivery [28].

Generally, the term "endocytosis" refers to the process by which cells internalise molecules that are present in the extracellular environment, modifying the shape of the plasmatic membrane (Figure 15.1a). In this way, the material could be introduced into the cell forming a vesicle called "endosome" (Figure 15.1b) [29]. This mechanism is essential for the absorption of mRNA encapsulated within endosomes, that act as a sort of temporary storage compartment [30]. However, to ensure that mRNA could perform its therapeutic effect, it should escape from the endosome, since the translation mechanism (Figure 15.1d) that leads to protein expression takes place in the cytoplasm. This critical process, known as "endosomal escape" (Figure 15.1c), is essential to prevent the degradation of mRNA within the acid environment of the endosome [31–33].

Endosomal escape could be favoured using specific carriers for mRNA delivery, constituted of cationic lipids (i.e., positively charged lipids) [34]. They should interact with the negatively charged endosomal membrane, allowing the release of mRNA inside the cytoplasm and avoiding its degradation within the endosomal environment [35]. mRNA delivery vectors should be properly designed to ensure effective transfection and correct expression of the protein. In addition, they should protect mRNA from enzymatic

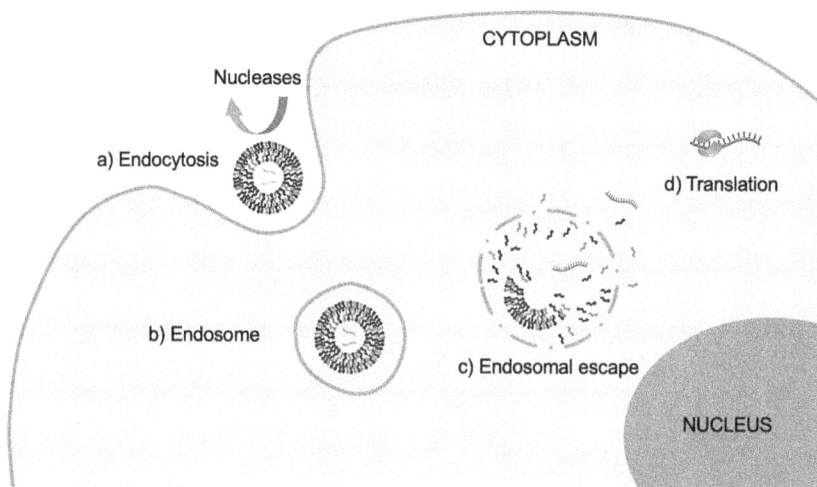

Figure 15.1: Endocytosis and endosomal escape of mRNA-loaded nanoparticle.

degradation by nucleases, ensure the integrity and functionality of mRNA and allow high transfection efficiency [36].

15.2 RNA delivery systems

Vectors designed to overcome the challenges associated with an efficient and specific delivery of different types of RNA into cells are divided in two main categories: viral and non-viral vectors [37].

15.2.1 Viral vectors

Viral vectors are obtained from genetically modified viruses (such as adenoviruses, retroviruses, lentiviruses, and adeno-associated viruses) and take advantage from the capacity of a virus to infect the host cell and duplicate the genetic material inside it [38, 39]. They allow high transfection efficiency both *in vivo* and *in vitro* and can provide a long-term expression of nucleic acids [40]. The main drawbacks associated with viral vectors are related to the occurrence of immune reactions, the risk of insertional mutagenesis and the possibility of producing new pathogenic viruses by recombination with viruses available in the host cell [41]. In addition, viral vectors show a limited nucleic acid cargo capacity, usually between 5 and 10 kilobase pairs. Therefore, only molecules with limited sizes can be transported [42]. Viral vectors are also highly complex, show limited potential for targeted delivery and have high production costs [42]. For these reasons, in recent years, there has been a growing interest in non-viral vectors, as an alternative and promising method to safely deliver RNA.

15.2.2 Non-viral vectors

Non-viral vectors, like lipid-based nanocarriers, polymer-based nanoparticles, and inorganic nanoparticles are proposed as an alternative method to obtain a safe and targeted delivery of genetic material [43]. Unlike viral vectors, they are cheap, easy to prepare, stable and applicable to all cells and tissues [44, 45]. Non-viral vectors also show low toxicity and can deliver large amounts of genetic material, without inducing undesirable inflammatory or immune responses [46, 47]. Among non-viral vectors, lipid-based nanoparticles are considered the "gold standard" for nucleic acid delivery, since they show a structure that resembles the one of natural cell membranes. They have also been clinically approved by the Food and Drug Administration (FDA) in the development of mRNA-based vaccines for COVID-19 and are characterized by high biocompatibility [48–50].

15.2.2.1 Lipid-based systems

Lipid-based nanoparticles are engineered to deliver RNA into target cells, protecting it from enzymatic degradation and enhancing cellular uptake [51]. Lipid-based nanoparticles also allow the sustained release of nucleic acids, opening new paths in the treatment of genetic disorders, cancers, infectious diseases (e.g., HIV, hepatitis C, etc.) and neurological disorders (such as Parkinson and Alzheimer) [52]. Lipid-based systems can be classified according to their composition and physical properties in liposomes, niosomes, lipid nanoparticles (including solid-lipid nanoparticles and nanostructured lipid carriers) and lipid nanoemulsions [53]. Their structure is shown in Figure 15.2.

15.2.2.1.1 Liposomes
Liposomes are spherical vesicles (usually 50–500 nm in diameter) widely used to encapsulate both hydrophilic and hydrophobic drugs, since they are composed of an internal aqueous core surrounded by one (or more) phospholipid bilayers [54]. Liposomes can be formed by both natural and synthetic phospholipids, with different amounts of cholesterol to improve the bilayer properties [55]. However, the main challenge for the encapsulation of hydrophilic RNA into conventional liposomes is the low encapsulation efficiency achieved when the lipid bilayer is composed of only phosphatidylcholine [56]. To overcome this limitation, cationic liposomes have been developed, adding cationic or ionizable lipids to the formulation that promote electrostatic interaction with the negative charge of nucleic acids [57, 58]. For example, Dhaliwal et al. [59] developed cationic liposomes encapsulating mRNA for its delivery to the brain by the

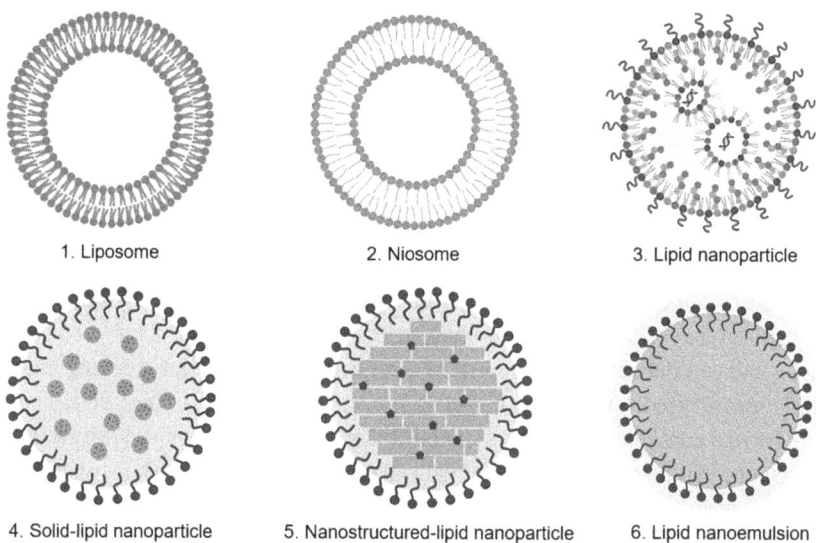

| 1. Liposome | 2. Niosome | 3. Lipid nanoparticle |
| 4. Solid-lipid nanoparticle | 5. Nanostructured-lipid nanoparticle | 6. Lipid nanoemulsion |

Figure 15.2: Schematic representation of lipid-based systems. Imagine 2 and 3 are created by bioRender. com.

intranasal route. Cationic liposomes were prepared by lipid film hydration, using 1,2-dipalmitoyl-sn-glycero-3-phosphocholine (DPPC), cholesterol, and 1,2-dioleoyl-3-trimethylammonium-propanechloride salt (DOTAP) as lipids. DOTAP was used as a cationic lipid to increase the encapsulation efficiency of mRNA, improve cellular uptake and lead to the formation of a more stable structure.

15.2.2.1.2 Niosomes

Niosomes are non-ionic surfactant-based vesicles with a structure similar the one of liposomes. However, compared to liposomes, niosomes are more stable and cheaper, since they are composed of surfactants such as polysorbate (Tween®), sorbitan mono-oleate (Span®) and polyoxyethylene stearyl ether (Brij®) [60]. The two main parameters that affect the choice of surfactants and the geometry of vesicles are the hydrophilic-lipophilic balance (HLB) and the critical packing parameter (CPP) [61]. HLB is a dimensionless parameter defined as the ratio between the hydrophilic and the hydrophobic groups of the surfactant; HLB values between 4 and 8 are suitable for the formation of niosomes [62]. CPP, instead, can be calculated from the volume of the non-polar hydrophobic group, the area of the polar hydrophilic head group and the critical length of the non-polar group of the surfactant. Surfactants with a CPP value between 1/2 and 1 produce bilayer vesicles [63]. Niosomes are considered a novel and promising system for the encapsulation of nucleic acids. For example, Hemati et al. [64] prepared cationic PEGylated niosomes to encapsulate anti-cancer drugs and siRNA for the treatment of a cancer by recombination therapy. DOTAP was used as a cationic lipid to encapsulate siRNA in niosomes; distearoyl phosphoethanolamine-polyethylene glycol (DSPE-PEG2000), instead, was added to improve the bioavailability of the drug and increase the blood circulation time.

15.2.2.1.3 Lipid nanoparticles (LNPs)

Lipid nanoparticles (LNPs) are widely used to encapsulate and deliver different types of nucleic acids and can be divided in two main categories: solid-lipid nanoparticles (SLNs) and nanostructured lipid carriers (NLCs) [65]. Unlike conventional liposomes, that are composed of liquid-crystalline lipid bilayers, SLNs are made of solid lipids; NLCs, instead, are obtained by using a mixture of solid and liquid-crystalline lipids [53]. The versatility of LNPs and their bioavailability make them promising vectors for the treatment of genetic or infectious diseases and cancer [66]. Research is focusing on the development of ionizable lipids that play a key role in LNP-based formulations by promoting the endosomal escape and minimizing toxicity issues related to the use of large amounts of cationic lipids [67].

15.2.2.1.4 Solid lipid nanoparticles (SLNs)

Solid lipid nanoparticles are colloidal carriers with a solid lipidic core containing the drug, surrounded by a surfactant layer to stabilize the structure in an aqueous environment. SLNs exhibit higher encapsulation efficiency for hydrophobic drugs and differ from the other lipid-based systems not only for the preparation method, but also for the use of organic solvents [68]. SLNs containing DOTAP and 1,2-dioleoyl-3-dimethylammonium propane (DODAP) as cationic lipids have been studied for DNA and RNA delivery. However, the application of these carriers is limited since the effective encapsulation of negatively charged hydrophilic RNA within the hydrophobic core remains a challenge [69].

15.2.2.1.5 Nanostructured lipid carriers (NLCs)

Nanostructured lipid carriers (NLCs) can be considered an advanced form of SLNs, developed to reduce issues related to drug loading efficiency and drug solubility [53]. They are composed of a mixture of solid and liquid lipids, in contrast to SLNs. This combination leads to structural defects within the lipid matrix, creating additional space that improves drug solubility and loading capacity [70]. NLCs are also studied to deliver hydrophilic nucleic acids. For example, Şenel et al. [71] developed NLCs to co-deliver siRNA and a small chemotherapeutic drug to cancer cells. DOTAP was used as a cationic lipid to promote the encapsulation of siRNA.

15.2.2.1.6 Lipid nanoemulsions

Nanoemulsions are oil-in-water (o/w) or water-in-oil (w/o) dispersions, with droplet sizes typically ranging from 20 to 200 nm. Cationic nanoemulsions have been developed to transport nucleic acids, using the same lipids to obtain cationic liposomes. For example, Borrajo et al. [72] developed ionizable nanoemulsions for mRNA delivery in the central nervous system. However, the main advantage of lipid nanoemulsions, related to the possibility of solubilizing both hydrophilic and hydrophobic drugs, is counterbalanced by challenges related to their stability and particle size control [73].

15.2.3 Composition of lipid-based nanocarriers for RNA delivery

Lipid-based nanocarriers designed for the encapsulation of genetic material typically consist of four main components: a cationic or ionizable lipids, a helper lipid, cholesterol, and a PEGylated lipid [53]. Each component plays a key role, contributing to stability, bioavailability, protection of the encapsulated material, cellular uptake, and endosomal escape. Several studies have been carried out to enhance the efficiency of these nanocarriers [74, 75]. However, further research is required to improve their potential. The optimization of the molar ratio between lipid components and the molar ratio between lipids and nucleic acids is essential for the development of a nucleic acid delivery system [76].

15.2.3.1 Cationic or ionizable lipids

The poly-anionic structure, high molecular weight and hydrophilicity nature of nucleic acids hinder their diffusion across cell membranes. Therefore, positively charged

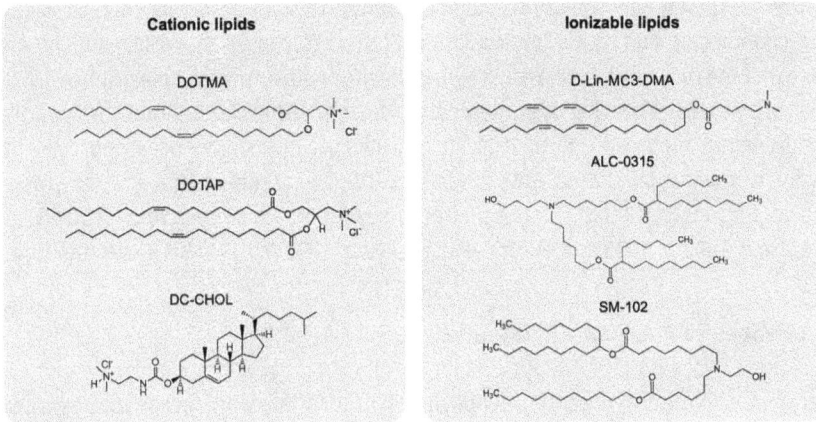

Figure 15.3: Cationic and ionizable lipids generally adopted for nucleic acids delivery.

ionizable or cationic lipids are necessary for the formulation of nanocarriers for RNA delivery (Figure 15.3).

Briefly, cationic/ionizable lipids ensure high encapsulation efficiencies due to the interactions with the negatively charged phosphate backbone of nucleic acids and promote the destabilization of endosomal membrane to release nucleic acids into the cytoplasm [53]. Cationic lipids are permanently charged molecules, in which the charge of lipid remains the same at different pH [77]. One of the earliest cationic lipids developed for nucleic acids delivery is N-[1-(2,3-dioleoyloxy)propyl]-N,N,N-trimethylammonium chloride (DOTMA), characterized by a quaternary ammonium head group bonded to hydrocarbon tails [78]. Other cationic lipids frequently used are DOTAP, dimethyldioctadecylammonium bromide (DDAB) or cholesterol derivatives such as 3β[N-(N',N'-dimethylaminoethane)-carbamoyl] cholesterol (DC-Chol) [79, 80]. However, the presence of permanent charges on the lipid structure could lead to cytotoxicity issues and rapid clearance of the circulating drug due to phagocytosis, hindering its ability to reach the target site [81, 82].

To overcome these limitations, researchers and pharmaceutical companies developed a new class of pH-sensitive amphiphilic molecules, called ionizable lipids, where the charge of the head group depends on pH [83, 84]. Most of the ionizable lipids is designed to be neutral under physiological conditions (pH ~ 7.4); but, they can become positively charged when in an acidic environment (pH < 6.0). This characteristic reduces the occurrence of side effects, offering advantages for RNA delivery. More specifically, during the production of nanoparticles, low pH conditions ensure electrostatic interactions between lipids and nucleic acids, maximizing the encapsulation efficiency. After the production, pH is regulated to physiological values, to ensure that the formulation is suitable for injection. When the lipid nanoparticle reaches the cytoplasm, ionizable lipids also contribute to endosomal escape, since the pH value inside this compartment drops to about 5–6 [83, 84]. The endosomal pH makes the ionizable lipid positively charged again, attracting counterions and water molecules. This process causes the disruption of the membrane and the release of the cargo, in a phenomenon called "proton sponge effect" [81].

There are several libraries of cationic and ionizable lipids that allow the identification of the better molecules. Until 2024, three ionizable lipids have been approved by the FDA for human applications: MC3 (DLin-MC3-DMA), contained in *Onpattro®* (patisiran, siRNA therapy); ALC-0315, contained in Pfizer-BioNTech's *Comirnaty®* (COVID-19 mRNA vaccine) and SM-102 used in Moderna *Spikevax®* (COVID-19 mRNA vaccine) [85].

15.2.3.2 Nitrogen to Phosphate (N/P) ratio

A key parameter that influences the encapsulation of RNA into lipid nanoparticles is the Nitrogen to Phosphate (N/P) ratio, defined as the molar ratio between positively charged lipids and negatively charged nucleic acid [86]. An optimal N/P value ensures an efficient electrostatic complexation and good cellular uptake, avoiding cytotoxicity issues. A low N/P ratio could result in low RNA encapsulation efficiencies, leading to weak therapeutic results. The optimal N/P ratio is usually in the range of 3–6; but, it could be also higher [86, 87]. For example, Carrasco et al. [88] prepared mRNA lipid nanoparticles changing the N/P ratio from 2 to 16. They found that mRNA encapsulation efficiency decreased for low values of N/P ratio. The selection of the optimal value of N/P ratio depends on several parameters: nature and length of the nucleic acid (e.g., mRNA, siRNA, microRNA, etc.), properties of cationic or ionizable lipids, and desired characteristics of lipid nanoparticles, expressed in terms of size, Zeta-potential and encapsulation efficiency [53]. This highlights the importance of a tailored optimization for a therapeutic success.

15.2.3.3 Helper lipids

Other components of nucleic acid delivery systems are "helper lipids" that are usually phospholipids. They show the ability of spontaneously organizing themselves in a lipid layer, contributing to endosomal escape and providing high stability to the nanoparticle structure [89, 90]. The helper lipids commonly used for nucleic acid delivery are DSPC (distearoylphosphatidylcholine), DPPC (dipalmitoylphosphatidylcholine) and DOPE (dioleoylphosphatidylethanolamine) (Figure 15.4) [91]. For example, DSPC is one of the components of currently FDA-approved LNPs for nucleic acid delivery. This phospholipid confers rigidity to the lipid bilayer, due to the fully saturated acyl chains, forming a rigid structure that prolongs the stability and the circulation of the drug [91]. DOPE, instead, is a non-saturated phospholipid with double bonds in its acyl chains. This structure confers more flexibility to the lipidic membrane, compared with DSPC [92]. DOPE is known for the ability to adopt an inverted hexagonal shape under low pH: this phase transition could facilitate the endosomal escape [93]. Therefore, the optimization of this lipid component is required for the development of new drugs that are more effective and safe.

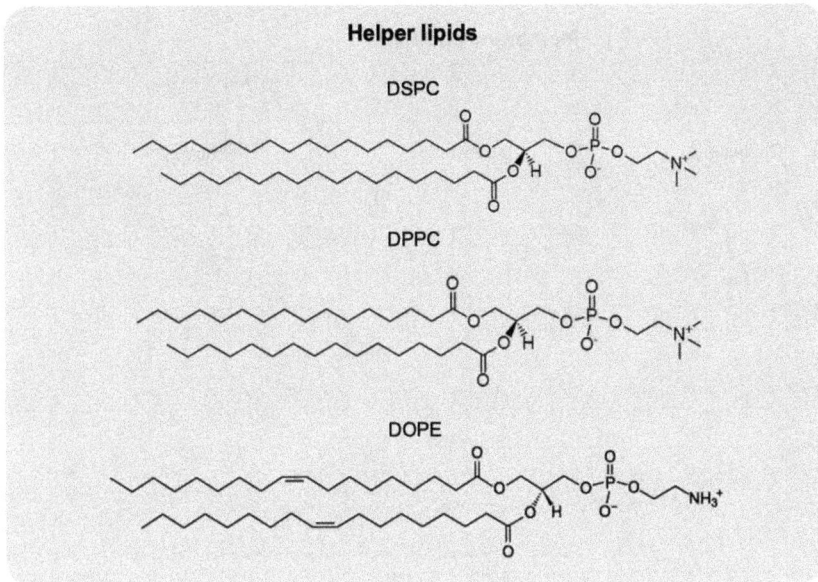

Figure 15.4: Helper lipids commonly used to produce lipid-based nanoparticles loaded with nucleic acids.

15.2.3.4 Cholesterol

Cholesterol is the most commonly lipid used to produce RNA-loaded lipid nanoparticles. It provides high rigidity and stability to the bilayer, reducing the leakage of the encapsulated material through the lipid membrane and prolonging the release of nucleic acid. The presence of cholesterol also facilitates the cellular uptake of LNPs by endocytosis, since it enhances the interaction between the nanoparticle and the cell membrane [94]. The amount of cholesterol added to the lipid-based formulation could vary between 10 and 50 % of the total molar lipid composition. However, an insufficient quantity of cholesterol could negatively affect the stability of nanoparticles; on the contrary, an excess of cholesterol will result in the formation of insoluble crystallites, providing an excessive rigidity to vesicles membrane. Therefore, optimizing this parameter is fundamental to obtain the best formulation for producing lipid nanoparticles, in terms of stability and entrapment efficiency of nucleic acid. Research is presently focused on the study of alternative membrane additives to cholesterol with similar properties, such as beta-sitosterol, squalene, fucosterol or other cholesterol derivatives, as shown in Figure 15.5 [53].

15.2.3.5 PEGylated lipids

PEGylated lipids are a class of polyethylene glycol (PEG) derivates, composed of a hydrophobic portion of alkyl chains and a hydrophilic part containing PEG. The coverage of

Membrane additives

Cholesterol   β-sitosterol   Fucosterol

Squalene

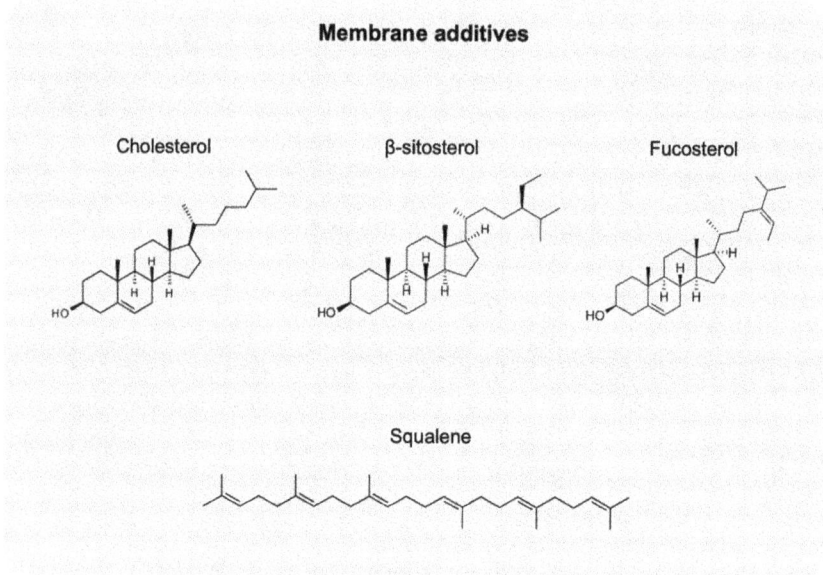

Figure 15.5: Cholesterol and membrane additives with similar properties.

lipid nanoparticles using PEGylation results in "stealth" nanocarriers with a prolonged circulation time [95]. In detail, the presence of PEG-lipids can minimize the adsorption of opsonin on the external surface of nanoparticles, avoiding the rapid clearance of nanovesicles by the immune system [96, 97]. The length of PEG chains also affects the behaviour of lipid nanoparticles: PEG-lipids at low molecular weight are unable to protect lipid nanoparticles from protein adsorption; whereas PEG-lipids with too high molecular weight hinder endosomal escape. Therefore, the optimal value is around 2 kDa [98]. Distearoylphosphatidylethanolamine-PEG2000 (DSPE-PEG2000) and dimyristoylglycerol-PEG2000 (DMG-PEG2000), shown in Figure 15.6, are frequently used to produce stealth

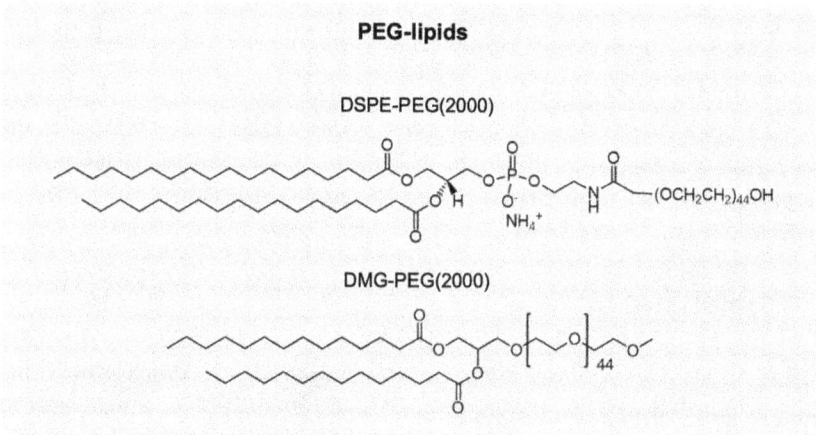

PEG-lipids

DSPE-PEG(2000)

$-(OCH_2CH_2)_{44}OH$

NH_4^+

DMG-PEG(2000)

44

Figure 15.6: PEG-lipids frequently used to produce stealth nanocarriers.

nanocarriers loaded with RNA [99, 100]. The amount of PEG-lipids added to the formulation is the lowest compared with the other lipid components, ranging from 0.5 to 2.5 %
of the total molar concentration. However, the optimization of this parameter is essential,
since a large amount of PEG-lipids could result in the production of anti-PEG antibodies
that are divided in two main categories: immunoglobulin M (IgM) and immunoglobulin G
(IgG) [101].

15.3 Conventional and innovative methods to produce lipid-based systems

Many techniques have been developed to produce lipid-based nanocarriers. They influence relevant properties of lipid vesicles, such as mean size, drug encapsulation efficiency, stability over time, and solvent residue. The most important methods proposed in
the scientific literature can be divided in two different categories: conventional and
innovative techniques.

15.3.1 Conventional techniques

15.3.1.1 Thin-film hydration

The thin film hydration (TFH), also known as Bangham method, is widely used to produce
lipid vesicles. Lipids or surfactants are dissolved in an organic solvent (e.g., ethanol,
methanol, chloroform), that is evaporated forming a thin lipid layer on the flask wall.
Then, the film is hydrated using an aqueous solution containing the hydrophilic drug and
agitated to form lipid nanovesicles [102]. Although this method is simple to carry out, it
shows several drawbacks mainly related to low drug encapsulation efficiency, difficulty
in controlling particle size, use of a large amount of organic solvent and difficulty to scale-
up. Additional steps, such as sonication and extrusion, are required to obtain nanovesicles instead of microvesicles [103].

15.3.1.2 Ethanol injection

In ethanol injection, lipids or surfactants are solubilized in ethanol; then, this solution is
rapidly injected through a needle into a stirred aqueous solution containing the hydrophilic principle [104]. After the diffusion of ethanol in the aqueous solution, the dissolved
lipids precipitate into bilayer lipid fragments, forming lipid vesicles like liposomes. A
vaporization step is required to remove the high residual of ethanol in the final suspension. Therefore, the structure of vesicles could be damaged and their size changed,
resulting in lipid particles with a diameter up to 900 nm [105]. In addition, this process can

lead to low encapsulation efficiencies: less than 20 % for the encapsulation of hydrophilic compounds, whereas it is more appropriate for the encapsulation of hydrophobic compounds [106].

15.3.1.3 Reverse-phase evaporation

Reverse-phase evaporation is a variation of thin-film hydration, and it is based on the formation of inverted micelles or water-in-oil emulsion. The organic phase is formed of lipids dissolved in an organic solvent (like ethanol, diethyl ether, or isopropyl ether); the aqueous phase contains, instead, the hydrophilic drug. A lipid film is formed after the evaporation of the organic solvent under reduced pressure. The lipids are, then, redissolved in an organic phase and the aqueous phase is added forming a water-in-oil-emulsion. Under reduced pressure, the organic solvent is removed, forming a viscous gel and finally an aqueous suspension containing nanovesicles [107]. Lipid vesicles produced using this method are characterized by high encapsulation efficiency compared with Bangham method. However, also in this case, multiple extrusion steps are necessary to obtain vesicles characterized by a nanometric size [108].

15.3.1.4 Spray-drying

Spray-drying is a method suitable for lipids that have a melting point above 70 °C [109]. The organic solution is prepared dissolving lipids or surfactants in an organic solvent, such as chloroform or methanol and, then, the encapsulated material is added. The obtained solution is spray-dried at different temperature conditions, even up to 120 °C. The spray-dried material is hydrated with water, and lipid-based microparticles are spontaneously formed. Particles size and size distribution obtained using this method are very large. Therefore, also this method is generally combined with extrusion steps to obtain nanometric lipid vesicles [110].

15.3.2 Innovative techniques

Conventional techniques are simple to perform and do not require expensive and sophisticated equipments. However, they are batch and time-consuming processes that show some limitations, especially related to an insufficient control of particle size. Therefore, innovative techniques, such as microfluidic or supercritical carbon dioxide assisted processes, have been proposed.

15.3.2.1 Microfluidic

Microfluidic devices are widely used to produce different types of nanoparticles, including lipid-based ones. The process involves the rapid mixing of an organic phase containing lipids with a water phase in which the active principle is solubilized (e.g., DNA or RNA) using micrometric channels [111]. T-junction is among the easiest kinds of microchannel, consisting of two inlets that collide at an angle, forming a junction. The aqueous solution dissolves in the organic medium, causing a decrease of lipids solubility: this phenomenon is referred as "supersaturation" and leads to the precipitation of lipid nanoparticles [112]. This method is highly versatile and cost-effective and can allow a continuous production with a good control of particle size. However, the main drawback is related to its low productivity, that limits its industrial applicability.

15.3.2.2 Supercritical CO$_2$-based processes

Processes based on supercritical carbon dioxide (SC-CO$_2$) take advantage from the unique properties of CO$_2$ when it is above its critical condition (T_c = 31.1 °C and P_c = 73.8 bar). Indeed, in supercritical conditions, CO$_2$ shows a viscosity closer to the one of a gas and a density closer to the one of a liquid, with high permeability and high solvent power [113]. Supercritical CO$_2$-based processes are classified as green production techniques since SC-CO$_2$ is non-toxic, non-flammable and inexpensive, and can work in continuous-mode. Moreover, supercritical processes can also allow the production of nanometer-sized lipid vesicles in one-step (i.e., without using post-treatments like extrusion or sonication) and working under mild operating conditions [114].

Supercritical antisolvent process (SAS) uses SC-CO$_2$ as an antisolvent to obtain powder samples, called proliposomes [115]. Liposomes can be obtained after the hydration of proliposomes with an aqueous solution containing the hydrophilic active compound. In detail, an organic solution containing lipids is sprayed into a high-pressure vessel. SC-CO$_2$ acts as an antisolvent, removing the organic solvent (like ethanol) and causing the precipitation of proliposomes with micrometric size (ranging from 0.1 µm to 100 µm) [114, 116]. However, this process demonstrated to be more suitable for the encapsulation of hydrophobic compounds, since they are solubilized in the organic phase; the encapsulation of hydrophilic compounds, instead, is generally low because they are added after the formation of the lipid bilayer [117, 118].

Supercritical reverse phase evaporation (SCRPE) involves the use of SC-CO$_2$ as a cosolvent, to obtain large lipid vesicles, between 200 and 1,200 nm [119]. The operating conditions are pressure in the range of 12–25 MPa and temperature typically around to 60 °C. For this process, an organic solution of lipids or surfactants and SC-CO$_2$ are fed into a high-pressure vessel. Then, an aqueous solution containing the drug is introduced into the same vessel. The formation of liposomes or other lipid-nanoparticles occurs when the system is depressurized [120]. Therefore, this process is discontinuous and would not be suitable for a large-scale production [121].

A promising and continuous process for producing lipid nanovesicles is called SuperSomes [122]. In this case, lipids dissolved in ethanol are continuously fed into a saturator that works at 100 bar and 40 °C. SC-CO$_2$ is introduced in the same vessel, filled with stainless steel packings. The contact between these two phases induces the formation of a gas expanded liquid, that goes to the formation chamber at the same conditions of the saturator. The hydrophilic active compound solubilized in water is sprayed through an injector in the formation chamber, allowing the formation of inverse-micelles. The double layer is formed when micelles fall into an aqueous bulk located at the bottom of the formation chamber. During the process, ethanol is separated from CO_2 and recovered in a separator; the aqueous suspension of nanovesicles, instead, is discharged at fixed time intervals [123]. This process allows the production of large volumes of nanometric lipid-vesicles (typically around 200 nm in size), with high encapsulation efficiencies (larger than 80 %) and without using further additional steps [124]. Moreover, solvent residues are very low, making this process safe for pharmaceutical applications.

15.4 Discussion, conclusions and future perspectives

Nucleic acid-based therapies have shown great potential in the last few years. Indeed, several nucleic acid-based drugs are undergoing clinical trials with promising results. There is also a growing interest in the development of advanced treatments for diseases like cancer, diabetes, genetic disorders and viral infections, predicting a bright future for DNA- or RNA-based therapeutic drug. The development of lipid-based carriers able to deliver nucleic acids into the cytoplasm or nucleus of the cell is fundamental for the clinical transposition of these innovative treatments. Therefore, new approaches are emerging, based on the modification of the composition or surface properties of lipid-based nanoparticles, to selectively target nucleic acids toward specific tissues. This strategy is called "Selective ORgan Targeting" (SORT) and, although it is still in an early stage of development, it could open new possibilities to make treatments more safe and effective [125, 126].

Another important issue is related to production methods, since a reliable and scalable process is needed to make these innovative treatments available. The encapsulation of nucleic acids in LNPs though traditional processes is not sustainable, due to poor reproducibility and productivity. New production methods are being optimized, to produce homogenous nanoparticles, with high encapsulation efficiencies and in agreement with the current good manufacturing practices (cGMPs) [127]. Frequently adopted LNPs production methods belong to the "bottom-up" category: in this case, individual molecules are assembled into the final nanoparticle. These techniques are usually based on the use of large amount of solvent that must be removed at the end of the process to satisfy the limitations imposed by pharmaceutical companies. To minimize the needs of solvents and post-production treatments, innovative processes are being developed. Although not yet commercially available, supercritical CO_2-assisted processes, like SuperSomes, have a great potential in advancing the production of nucleic acid delivery systems. Indeed, they could play a key role in reducing the environmental impact, by minimizing the use of organic solvents, and can largely improve the encapsulation efficiency of this valuable and expensive biomolecules.

Acknowledgments: The authors would like to thank the editors David Bogle and Tomasz Sosnowski for their guidance and review of this article before its publication.

References

1. Dahm R. Discovering DNA: Friedrich Miescher and the early years of nucleic acid research. Hum Genet 2008;122:565–81.
2. Mahadevan S. Oswald Avery and the identification of DNA as the genetic material. Resonance 2007;12: 4–11.
3. Laurentin Táriba HE. DNA as hereditary material. In: Agricultural genetics: from the DNA molecule to population management. Switzerland: Springer Nature; 2023:9–17 pp.
4. Watson JD, Crick FH. Molecular structure of nucleic acids: a structure for deoxyribose nucleic acid. Nature 1953;171:737–8.
5. Crick FH. On protein synthesis. Symp Soc Exp Biol 1958;12:138–63, 8.
6. Zogg H, Singh R, Ro S. Current advances in RNA therapeutics for human diseases. Int J Mol Sci 2022;23: 2736.
7. Yamada Y. Nucleic acid drugs – current status, issues, and expectations for exosomes. Cancers 2021;13: 5002.
8. Landmesser U, Poller W, Tsimikas S, Most P, Paneni F, Lüscher TF. From traditional pharmacological towards nucleic acid-based therapies for cardiovascular diseases. Eur Heart J 2020;41:3884–99.
9. Rzymski P, Szuster-Ciesielska A, Dzieciątkowski T, Gwenzi W, Fal A. mRNA vaccines: the future of prevention of viral infections? J Med Virol 2023;95:e28572.
10. Kulkarni JA, Witzigmann D, Thomson SB, Chen S, Leavitt BR, Cullis PR, et al. The current landscape of nucleic acid therapeutics. Nat Nanotechnol 2021;16:630–43.
11. Liu L, Gao H, Guo C, Liu T, Li N, Qian Q. Therapeutic mechanism of nucleic acid drugs. ChemistrySelect 2021;6:903–16.
12. Belgrad J, Fakih HH, Khvorova A. Nucleic acid therapeutics: successes, milestones, and upcoming innovation. Nucl Acid Ther 2024;34:52–72.
13. Lefferts, C.L., Lefferts, J.A. (2017). Essential concepts and techniques in molecular biology. In: Coleman W., Tsongalis G., editors. The molecular basis of human cancer. New York, NY: Humana Press. https://doi.org/ 10.1007/978-1-59745-458-2_2.
14. Rahman AU. Nucleic acid structure. In: Fundamentals of cellular and molecular biology. Bentham Science Publishers; 2024:15–35 pp. https://doi.org/10.2174/9789815238037124010004.
15. Kato D. Exploring the dynamic world of DNA and RNA: from structure to function and beyond. INOSR Appl Sci 2024;12:57–62.
16. Jiang Z, Thayumanavan S. Non-cationic material design for nucleic acid delivery. Adv Ther 2020;3:1900206.
17. Wang C, Yuan F. A comprehensive comparison of DNA and RNA vaccines. Adv Drug Deliv Rev 2024:115340. https://doi.org/10.1016/j.addr.2024.115340.
18. Qin S, Tang X, Chen Y, Chen K, Fan N, Xiao W, et al. mRNA-based therapeutics: powerful and versatile tools to combat diseases. Signal Transduct Target Ther 2022;7:166.
19. Shi Y, Shi M, Wang Y, You J. Progress and prospects of mRNA-based drugs in pre-clinical and clinical applications. Signal Transduct Target Ther 2024;9:322.
20. Clancy S, Brown W. Translation: DNA to mRNA to protein. Nat Educ 2008;1:101.
21. Kim SC, Sekhon SS, Shin WR, Ahn G, Cho BK, Ahn JY, et al. Modifications of mRNA vaccine structural elements for improving mRNA stability and translation efficiency. Mol Cell Toxicol 2022:1–8. https://doi. org/10.1007/s13273-021-00171-4.

22. Shen G, Liu J, Yang H, Xie N, Yang Y. mRNA therapies: pioneering a new era in rare genetic disease treatment. J Contr Release 2024;369:696–721.
23. Tavernier G, Andries O, Demeester J, Sanders NN, De Smedt SC, Rejman J. mRNA as gene therapeutic: how to control protein expression. J Contr Release 2011;150:238–47.
24. Trivedi V, Yang C, Klippel K, Yegorov O, von Roemeling C, Hoang-Minh L, et al. mRNA-based precision targeting of neoantigens and tumor-associated antigens in malignant brain tumors. Genome Med 2024; 16:17.
25. Pardi N, Krammer F. mRNA vaccines for infectious diseases—advances, challenges and opportunities. Nat Rev Drug Discov 2024:1–24. https://doi.org/10.1038/s41573-024-01042-y.
26. Russell CA, Fouchier RA, Ghaswalla P, Park Y, Vicic N, Ananworanich J, et al. Seasonal influenza vaccine performance and the potential benefits of mRNA vaccines. Hum Vaccin Immunother 2024;20:2336357.
27. Kiaie SH, Majidi Zolbanin N, Ahmadi A, Bagherifar R, Valizadeh H, Kashanchi F, et al. Recent advances in mRNA-LNP therapeutics: immunological and pharmacological aspects. J Nanobiotechnol 2022;20:276.
28. Chatterjee S, Kon E, Sharma P, Peer D. Endosomal escape: a bottleneck for LNP-mediated therapeutics. Proc Natl Acad Sci 2024;121. https://doi.org/10.1073/pnas.2307800120.
29. de Almeida MS, Susnik E, Drasler B, Taladriz-Blanco P, Petri-Fink A, Rothen-Rutishauser B. Understanding nanoparticle endocytosis to improve targeting strategies in nanomedicine. Chem Soc Rev 2021;50: 5397–434.
30. Grau M, Wagner E. Strategies and mechanisms for endosomal escape of therapeutic nucleic acids. Curr Opin Chem Biol 2024;81:102506.
31. Liu H, Chen MZ, Payne T, Porter CJ, Pouton CW, Johnston AP. Beyond the endosomal bottleneck: understanding the efficiency of mRNA/LNP delivery. Adv Funct Mater 2024;34:2404510.
32. Mehta MJ, Kim HJ, Lim SB, Naito M, Miyata K. Recent progress in the endosomal escape mechanism and chemical structures of polycations for nucleic acid delivery. Macromol Biosci 2024;24:2300366.
33. Barbier AJ, Jiang AY, Zhang P, Wooster R, Anderson DG. The clinical progress of mRNA vaccines and immunotherapies. Nat Biotechnol 2022;40:840–54.
34. Debisschop A, Bogaert B, Muntean C, De Smedt SC, Raemdonck K. Beyond chloroquine: cationic amphiphilic drugs as endosomal escape enhancers for nucleic acid therapeutics. Curr Opin Chem Biol 2022;83:102531.
35. Eygeris Y, Gupta M, Kim J, Sahay G. Chemistry of lipid nanoparticles for RNA delivery. Acc Chem Res 2021; 55:2–12.
36. Li X, Qi J, Wang J, Hu W, Zhou W, Wang Y, et al. Nanoparticle technology for mRNA: delivery strategy, clinical application and developmental landscape. Theranostics 2024;14:738.
37. Yildiz SN, Entezari M, Paskeh MDA, Mirzaei S, Kalbasi A, Zabolian A, et al. Nanoliposomes as nonviral vectors in cancer gene therapy. Media Commun 2024;5:e583.
38. Zhao Z, Anselmo AC, Mitragotri S. Viral vector-based gene therapies in the clinic. Bioeng Transl Med 2022; 7:10258.
39. Sung YK, Kim SW. Recent advances in the development of gene delivery systems. Biomater Res 2019;23:8.
40. Lundstrom K. Viral vectors in gene therapy: where do we stand in 2023? Viruses 2023;15:698.
41. Butt MH, Zaman M, Ahmad A, Khan R, Mallhi TH, Hasan MM, et al. Appraisal for the potential of viral and nonviral vectors in gene therapy: a review. Genes 2022;13:1370.
42. Siebart JC, Chan CS, Yao X, Su FY, Kwong GA. In vivo gene delivery to immune cells. Curr Opin Biotechnol 2024;88:103169.
43. Yan Y, Liu XY, Lu A, Wang XY, Jiang LX, Wang JC. Non-viral vectors for RNA delivery. J Contr Release 2022; 342:241–79.
44. Jain M, Yu X, Schneck JP, Green JJ. Nanoparticle targeting strategies for lipid and polymer-based gene delivery to immune cells in vivo. Small Sci 2024;4:2400248.
45. Liu L, Yang J, Men K, He Z, Luo M, Qian Z, et al. Current status of nonviral vectors for gene therapy in China. Hum Gene Ther 2018;29:110–20.

46. Panchal SS, Vasava DV. Synthetic biodegradable polymeric materials in non-viral gene delivery. Int J Polym Mater Polym Biomater 2024;73:478–89.

47. Rao D, Ganguli M. Non-viral delivery of nucleic acid for treatment of rare diseases of the muscle. J Biosci 2024;49:27.

48. Malabadi RB, Meti NT, Chalannavar RK. Applications of nanotechnology in vaccine development for coronavirus (SARS-CoV-2) disease (Covid-19). Int J Res Sci Innov 2021;8:191–8.

49. Baden LR, El Sahly HM, Essink B, Kotloff K, Frey S, Novak R, et al. Efficacy and safety of the mRNA-1273 SARS-CoV-2 vaccine. N Engl J Med 2021;384:403–16.

50. Jacob EM, Huang J, Chen M. Lipid nanoparticle-based mRNA vaccines: a new Frontier in precision oncology. Precis Clin Med 2024;7. https://doi.org/10.1093/pcmedi/pbae017.

51. Shin MD, Shukla S, Chung YH, Beiss V, Chan SK, Ortega-Rivera OA, et al. COVID-19 vaccine development and a potential nanomaterial path forward. Nat Nanotechnol 2020;15:646–55.

52. Amer MH. Gene therapy for cancer: present status and future perspective. Mol Cell Ther 2014;2:1–19.

53. Haque MA, Shrestha A, Mikelis CM, Mattheolabakis G. Comprehensive analysis of lipid nanoparticle formulation and preparation for RNA delivery. Int J Pharm X 2024:100283. https://doi.org/10.1016/j.ijpx.2024.100283.

54. Senjab R, Alsawaftah NM, AbuWatfa W, Husseini G. Advances in liposomal nanotechnology: from concept to clinics. RSC Pharm 2024;1:928–48.

55. Liu C, Zhang L, Zhu W, Guo R, Sun H, Chen X, et al. Barriers and strategies of cationic liposomes for cancer gene therapy. Mol Ther Methods Clin Dev 2020;18:751–64.

56. Berger M, Lechanteur A, Evrard B, Piel G. Innovative lipoplexes formulations with enhanced siRNA efficacy for cancer treatment: where are we now? Int J Pharm 2021;605:120851.

57. Hattori Y, Tang M. Effect of cationic and neutral lipids in cationic liposomes on antibody production induced by systemic administration of mRNA lipoplexes into mice. J Drug Deliv Sci Technol 2024;100: 106034.

58. Guéguen C, Chimol TB, Briand M, Renaud K, Seiler M, Ziesel M, et al. Evaluating how cationic lipid affects mRNA-LNP physical properties and biodistribution. Eur J Pharm Biopharm 2024;195:114077.

59. Dhaliwal HK, Fan Y, Kim J, Amiji MM. Intranasal delivery and transfection of mRNA therapeutics in the brain using cationic liposomes. Mol Pharm 2020;17:1996–2005.

60. Riccardi D, Baldino L, Reverchon E. Liposomes, transfersomes and niosomes: production methods and their applications in the vaccinal field. J Transl Med 2024;22:339.

61. Thabet Y, Elsabahy M, Eissa NG. Methods for preparation of niosomes: a focus on thin-film hydration method. Methods 2022;199:9–15.

62. Kazi KM, Mandal AS, Biswas N, Guha A, Chatterjee S, Behera M, et al. Niosome: a future of targeted drug delivery systems. J Adv Pharm Technol Res 2010;1:374–80.

63. Yasamineh S, Yasamineh P, Kalajahi HG, Gholizadeh O, Yekanipour Z, Afkhami H, et al. A state-of-the-art review on the recent advances of niosomes as a targeted drug delivery system. Int J Pharm 2022;624: 121878.

64. Hemati M, Haghiralsadat F, Yazdian F, Jafari F, Moradi A, Malekpour-Dehkordi Z. Development and characterization of a novel cationic PEGylated niosome-encapsulated forms of doxorubicin, quercetin and siRNA for the treatment of cancer by using combination therapy. Artif Cells Nanomed Biotechnol 2019;47: 1295–311.

65. Liu GW, Guzman EB, Menon N, Langer RS. Lipid nanoparticles for nucleic acid delivery to endothelial cells. Pharm Res 2023;40:3–25.

66. Jung HN, Lee SY, Lee S, Youn H, Im HJ. Lipid nanoparticles for delivery of RNA therapeutics: current status and the role of in vivo imaging. Theranostics 2022;12:7509.

67. Swetha K, Kotla NG, Tunki L, Jayaraj A, Bhargava SK, Hu H, et al. Recent advances in the lipid nanoparticle-mediated delivery of mRNA vaccines. Vaccines 2023;11:658.

68. Xu L, Wang X, Liu Y, Yang G, Falconer RJ, Zhao CX. Lipid nanoparticles for drug delivery. Adv NanoBiomed Res 2022;2:2100109.
69. Tsakiri M, Zivko C, Demetzos C, Mahairaki V. Lipid-based nanoparticles and RNA as innovative neuro-therapeutics. Front Pharmacol 2022;13:900610.
70. Khan S, Sharma A, Jain V. An overview of nanostructured lipid carriers and its application in drug delivery through different routes. Adv Pharmaceut Bull 2022;13:446.
71. Şenel B, Basaran E, Akyıl E, Güven UM, Büyükköroğlu G. Co-delivery of siRNA and docetaxel to cancer cells by NLC for therapy. ACS Omega 2024;9:11671–85.
72. Borrajo ML, Quijano A, Lapuhs P, Rodriguez-Perez AI, Anthiya S, Labandeira-Garcia JL, et al. Ionizable nanoemulsions for RNA delivery into the central nervous system – importance of diffusivity. J Contr Release 2024;372:295–303.
73. Yi XH, Guo P, Wen WC, Lun Wong H. Lipid-based nanocarriers for RNA delivery. Curr Pharm Des 2015;21:3140–7.
74. Sun M, Dang UJ, Yuan Y, Psaras AM, Osipitan O, Brooks TA, et al. Optimization of DOTAP/chol cationic lipid nanoparticles for mRNA, pDNA, and oligonucleotide delivery. AAPS PharmSciTech 2022;23:135.
75. Li W, Chen L, Gu Z, Chen Z, Li H, Cheng Z, et al. Co-delivery of microRNA-150 and quercetin by lipid nanoparticles (LNPs) for the targeted treatment of age-related macular degeneration (AMD). J Contr Release 2023;355:358–70.
76. Mendes BB, Conniot J, Avital A, Yao D, Jiang X, Zhou X, et al. Nanodelivery of nucleic acids. Nat Rev 2022;24. https://doi.org/10.1038/s43586-022-00104-y.
77. Ponti F, Campolungo M, Melchiori C, Bono N, Candiani G. Cationic lipids for gene delivery: many players, one goal. Chem Phys Lipids 2021;235. https://doi.org/10.1016/j.chemphyslip.2020.105032.
78. Balazs DA, Godbey WT. Liposomes for use in gene delivery. J Drug Deliv 2011;1.
79. Zhu Z, Zhang L, Sheng R, Chen J. Microfluidic-based cationic cholesterol lipid siRNA delivery nanosystem: highly efficient in vitro gene silencing and the intracellular behavior. Int J Mol Sci 2022;7:23.
80. Yan D, Lu H, Kaur A, Fu R, Wang N, The JH, et al. Development and optimisation of cationic lipid nanoparticles for mRNA delivery. BioRixiv 2023.
81. Mrksich K, Padilla MS, Mitchell MJ. Breaking the final barrier: evolution of cationic and ionizable lipid structure in lipid nanoparticles to escape the endosome. Adv Drug Deliv Rev 2024;214:115446.
82. Lee Y, Jeong M, Park J, Jung H, Lee H. Immunogenicity of lipid nanoparticles and its impact on the efficacy of mRNA vaccines and therapeutics. EMM 2023;55:2085–96.
83. Schlich M, Palomba R, Costabile G, Mizrahy S, Pannuzzo M, Peer D, et al. Cytosolic delivery of nucleic acids: the case of ionizable lipid nanoparticles. Bioeng Transl Med 2021;6:e10213.
84. Patel P, Ibrahim NM, Cheng K. The importance of apparent pKa in the development of nanoparticles encapsulating siRNA and mRNA. Trends Pharmacol Sci 2021;42:448–60.
85. Chaudhary N, Weissman D, Whitehead KA. mRNA vaccines for infectious diseases: principles, delivery and clinical translation. Nat Rev Drug Discov 2021;20:817–38.
86. Catenacci L, Rossi R, Sechi F, Buonocore D, Sorrenti M, Perteghella S, et al. Effect of lipid nanoparticle physico-chemical properties and composition on their interaction with the immune system. Pharmaceutics 2024;22:1521.
87. Okuda K, Sato Y, Iwakawa K, Sasaki K, Okabe N, Maeki M, et al. On the size-regulation of RNA-loaded lipid nanoparticles synthesized by microfluidic device. J Contr Release 2022;348:648–59.
88. Carrasco MJ, Alishetty S, Alameh MG, Said H, Wright L, Paige M, et al. Ionization and structural properties of mRNA lipid nanoparticles influence expression in intramuscular and intravascular administration. Commun Biol 2021;4:956.
89. Cheng X, Lee RJ. The role of helper lipids in lipid nanoparticles (LNPs) designed for oligonucleotide delivery. Adv Drug Deliv Rev 2016;99:129–37.
90. Zong Y, Lin Y, Wei T, Cheng Q. Lipid nanoparticle (LNP) enables mRNA delivery for cancer therapy. Adv Mater 2023;35:51.

91. Albertsen CH, Kulkarni JA, Witzigmann D, Lind M, Petersson K, Simonsen JB. The role of lipid components in lipid nanoparticles for vaccines and gene therapy. Adv Drug Deliv Rev 2022;188. https://doi.org/10.1016/j.addr.2022.114416.

92. Oguma T, Kanazawa T, Kaneko YK, Sato R, Serizawa M, Ooka A, et al. Effects of phospholipid type and particle size on lipid nanoparticle distribution in vivo and in pancreatic islets. J Contr Release 2024;373: 917–28.

93. Ahmad A, Khan JM, Haque S. Strategies in the design of endosomolytic agents for facilitating endosomal escape in nanoparticles. Biochimie 2019;160:61–75.

94. Pozzi D, Marchini C, Cardarelli F, Amenitsch H, Garulli C, Bifone A, et al. Transfection efficiency boost of cholesterol-containing lipoplexes. Biochim Biophys Acta 2012;1818:9.

95. Chen D, Ganesh S, Wang W, Amiji M. Plasma protein adsorption and biological identity of systemically administered nanoparticles. Nanomed 2017:2113–35. https://doi.org/10.2217/nnm-2017-0178.

96. Gao P. Exploring the latest breakthroughs in lipid nanoparticle-mediated delivery: a deep dive into lipid innovation and intracellular discovery. Bull Biomed Sci 2023;1:21–46.

97. Jeong M, Lee Y, Park J, Jung H, Lee H. Lipid nanoparticles (LNPs) for in vivo RNA delivery and their breakthrough technology for future applications. Adv Drug Deliv Rev 2023;200. https://doi.org/10.1016/j.addr.2023.114990.

98. Pozzi D, Colapicchioni V, Caracciolo G, Piovesana S, Capriotti AL, Palchetti S, et al. Effect of polyethyleneglycol (PEG) chain length on the bio–nano-interactions between PEGylated lipid nanoparticles and biological fluids: from nanostructure to uptake in cancer cells†. Nanoscale 2014;5.

99. Fedorovskiy AG, Antropov DN, Dome AS, Puchkov PA, Makarova DM, Konopleva MV, et al. Novel efficient lipid-based delivery systems enable a delayed uptake and sustained expression of mRNA in human cells and mouse tissues. MDPI Pharm 2024;16:5.

100. Huang C, Zhang Y, Su J, Guan X, Chen S, Xu X, et al. Liver-specific ionizable lipid nanoparticles mediated efficient RNA interference to clear "Bad cholesterol". Int J Nanomed 2023;18. https://doi.org/10.2147/ijn.s434908.

101. Li Z, Ma A, Miller I, Starnes R, Talkington A, Stone CA, et al. Development of anti-PEG IgG/IgM/IgE ELISA assays for profiling anti-PEG immunoglobulin response in PEG-sensitized individuals and patients with alpha-gal allergy. J Contr Release 2024;366:342–8.

102. Azmin MN, Florence AT, Handjani-Vila RM, Stuart JFB, Vanlerberghe G, Whittaker JS. The effect of non-ionic surfactant vesicle (niosome) entrapment on the absorption and distribution of methotrexate in mice. J Pharm Pharmacol 1985;37:237–42.

103. Wang J, He W, Cheng L, Zhang H, Wang Y, Liu C, et al. A modified thin film method for large scale production of dimeric artesunate phospholipid liposomes and comparison with conventional approaches. Int J Pharm 2022;619:121714.

104. Fang JY, Hong CT, Chiu WT, Wang YY. Effect of liposomes and niosomes on skin permeation of enoxacin. Int J Pharm 2001;219:61–72.

105. Charcosset C, Juban A, Valour JP, Urbaniak S, Fessi H. Preparation of liposomes at large scale using the ethanol injection method: effect of scale-up and injection devices. Chem Eng Res Des 2015;94:508–15.

106. Trucillo P, Campardelli R, Reverchon E. Liposomes: from bangham to supercritical fluids. Processes 2020; 8:1022.

107. Guinedi AS, Mortada ND, Mansour S, Hathout RM. Preparation and evaluation of reverse-phase evaporation and multilamellar niosomes as ophthalmic carriers of acetazolamide. Int J Pharm 2005;306: 71–82.

108. Arora RK, Kumar V, Pal R, Ruhil P. Liposomes: a novel approach as a carrier. World J Pharm Res 2018;7: 323–42.

109. Samimi S, Maghsoudnia N, Eftekhari RB, Dorkoosh F. Lipid-based nanoparticles for drug delivery systems. In: Characterization and biology of nanomaterials for drug delivery. Amsterdam: Elsevier; 2019:47–76 pp.

110. Kukuchi K, Yamauchi H, Hirota S. A spray-drying method for mass production of liposomes. Chem Pharm Bull 1991;39:1522–7.
111. Zhang G, Sun J. Lipid in chips: a brief review of liposomes formation by microfluidics. Int J Nanomed 2021; 16:7391–416.
112. Lopes C, Cristóvão J, Silvério V, Lino PR, Fonte P. Microfluidic production of mRNA-loaded lipid nanoparticles for vaccine applications. Expert Opin Drug Deliv 2022;19:1381–95.
113. Kankala RK, Zhang YS, Wang SB, Lee CH, Chen AZ. Supercritical fluid technology: an emphasis on drug delivery and related biomedical applications. Adv Healthcare Mater 2017;6:1700433.
114. William B, Noémie P, Brigitte E, Géraldine P. Supercritical fluid methods: an alternative to conventional methods to prepare liposomes. Chem Eng J 2020;383. https://doi.org/10.1016/j.cej.2019.123106.
115. Khan I, Edes K, Alsaadi I, Al-Khaial MQ, Bnyan R, Khan SA, et al. Investigation of spray drying parameters to formulate novel spray-dried proliposome powder formulations followed by their aerosolization performance. Pharmaceutics 2024;16:1541.
116. Lesoin L, Crampon C, Boutin O, Badens E. Preparation of liposomes using the supercritical anti-solvent (SAS) process and comparison with a conventional method. J Supercrit Fluids 2011;57:162–74.
117. Maja L, Željko K, Mateja P. Sustainable technologies for liposome preparation. J Supercrit Fluids 2020;165. https://doi.org/10.1016/j.supflu.2020.104984.
118. William B, Noémie P, Brigitte E, Géraldine P. Supercritical fluid methods: an alternative to conventional methods to prepare liposomes. Chem Eng J 2020;383. https://doi.org/10.1016/j.cej.2019.123106.
119. Imura T, Otake K, Hashimoto S, Gotoh T, Yuasa M, Yokoyama S, et al. Preparation and physicochemical properties of various soybean lecithin liposomes using supercritical reverse phase evaporation method. Colloids Surf B Biointerfaces 2003;27:133–40.
120. Chai C, Park J. Food liposomes: structures, components, preparations, and applications. Food Chem 2024; 432:137228.
121. Lesoin L, Boutin O, Crampon C, Badens E. CO_2/water/surfactant ternary systems and liposome formation using supercritical CO_2: a review. Colloids Surf A Physicochem Eng Asp 2011;377:1–14.
122. Baldino L, Reverchon E. Niosomes formation using a continuous supercritical CO_2 assisted process. J CO2 Util 2021;52:101669.
123. Baldino L, Riccardi D, Reverchon E. Production of PEGylated vancomycin-loaded niosomes by a continuous supercritical CO_2 assisted process. Nanomaterials 2024;14:846.
124. Baldino L, Riccardi D, Reverchon E. Liposomes and niosomes production by a supercritical CO2 assisted process for topical applications: a comparative study. J Supercrit Fluids 2024;212:106342.
125. Cheng Q, Wei T, Farbiak L, Johnson LT, Dilliard SA, Siegwart DJ. Selective organ targeting (SORT) nanoparticles for tissue-specific mRNA delivery and CRISPR–Cas gene editing. Nat Nanotechnol 2020;15: 313–20.
126. Dilliard SA, Cheng Q, Siegwart DJ. On the mechanism of tissue-specific mRNA delivery by selective organ targeting nanoparticles. Proc Natl Acad Sci 2021;118. https://doi.org/10.1073/pnas.2109256118.
127. Shegokar R, Nakach M. Large-scale manufacturing of nanoparticles – an industrial outlook. Drug Deliv Aspects 2020;4:57–77.

Index

www.ingramcontent.com/pod-product-compliance
Lightning Source LLC
Chambersburg PA
CBHW080657220326
41598CB00033B/5234